Medical Microbiology for
Health Professionals

JUDY GNARPE

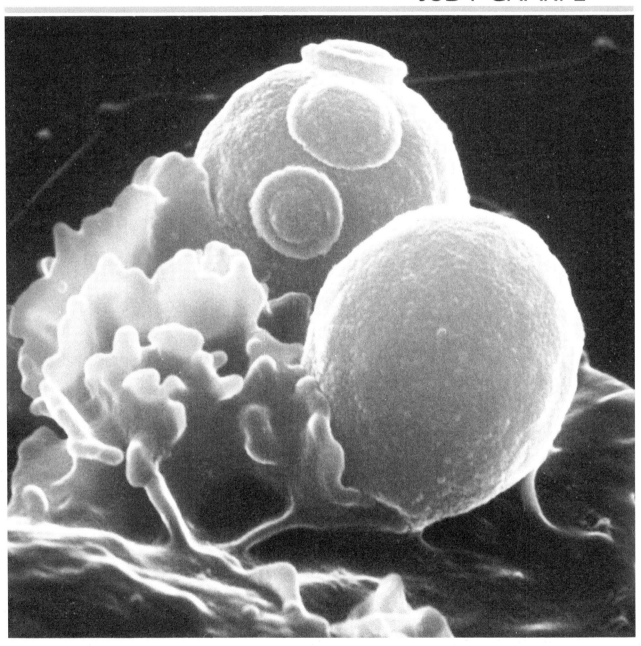

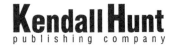

Kendall Hunt
publishing company

Cover image provided by the author.

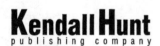

www.kendallhunt.com
Send all inquiries to:
4050 Westmark Drive
Dubuque, IA 52004-1840

Printed in the United States of America
10 9 8 7 6 5 4 3 2 1

Contents

Preface

Medical microbiology and immunology are key elements required by all who engage in a health-related career. I have been frustrated by the lack of clinical relevance in most of the textbooks that are available and, in addition, do not like having to assign a new version of the text every other year.

The result is my attempt to make things easier for you, and I hope that I have succeeded. This workbook is really my notes for the course and the bare bones of what you will need in terms of course content. Websites and recommended resources are listed at the end of every chapter if you need or want to learn more. There are many excellent resources on the Internet, and we have an excellent online library at the University of Alberta.

Judy Gnarpe, DrMedSci, RM(CCM), PG DipMedEd

Course coordinator, MMI 133

Learning Objectives by Chapter:

CHAPTER 1

1. Describe the theory of spontaneous generation and germ theory of disease.

2. Recognize key players in the development of microbiology as a science, and know the key discoveries made by important researchers (Koch, Pasteur, Lister, Gram, Jenner, Fleming, Reed, Salk).

3. Recognize Koch's postulates.

4. Order microorganisms according to size.

5. Describe the naming conventions of microorganisms at the genus and species level (bacteria, parasites, and fungi); understand how viruses are named.

6. List differences between prokaryotes and eukaryotes.

CHAPTER 2

1. Describe Gram staining: the procedure and the reactions, and give an example of bacteria that stain Gram positive, bacteria that stain Gram negative, and bacteria that must be visualized with other stains (i.e., acid-fast).

2. Differentiate between different bacterial morphologies.

3. Describe the major components of the prokaryote and its functions.

4. Understand how bacteria metabolize nutrients and the types of respiration involved.

5. Categorize organisms according to their growth characteristics; understand how different media can support growth and identification of organisms, and define plasmolysis.

6. Identify how common biofilms are formed, and describe their roles in disease.

CHAPTER 3

1. Differentiate among bacteria, virus, and prions.

2. Describe the general structure of an enveloped and nonenveloped virus.

3. Understand how a virus replicates using a host cell.

4. Explain how a virus can be a causative agent for cancer.

5. Discriminate between active, latent, and chronic infections with virus.

6. Understand the pathogenic mechanism for prions, and give examples of prion diseases.

CHAPTER 4

1. Differentiate fungi from bacteria; identify fungi as eukaryotes.
2. Identify fungal components that can be used as a target for antifungal therapy.
3. Describe the characteristics of dimorphic fungi.
4. Define three types of fungal infections (superficial, cutaneous, systemic).
5. Define opportunistic, and give examples of opportunistic infections.

CHAPTER 5

1. Differentiate between protozoa and metazoa.
2. Describe how different parasitic organisms cause disease in humans, and list the organisms causing specific diseases.
3. Identify some commonly occurring ectoparasitic infections and their causes.
4. Describe the epidemiology of parasitic infections.

CHAPTER 6

1. Define common terms used to describe disinfection, sterilization, and nosocomial infection, and identify a few major causes of nosocomial infections.
2. Explain how we can control the environment in a hospital or a laboratory.
3. Define and describe the process of sterilization.
4. Identify the spore test as a method of quality control for autoclaving processes.
5. Identify chemicals that can be used to sterilize objects and surfaces.
6. Explain why alcohol-based hand sanitizers are not as effective against endospores and naked virus as hand washing.

CHAPTER 7

1. List some problems associated with chemotherapy for bacteria, viruses, fungi, and parasites.
2. Define mechanisms of antibiotic resistance.
3. Define spectrum of activity, broad-spectrum drugs, MIC, SIR, drug of choice, bactericidal, and bacteriostatic.
4. List five modes of activity for antimicrobials, and learn the examples given.

5. Explain why monitoring antibiotic levels should be done in some patients for some antimicrobials.

6. List the common superbugs, and identify the reason they are classed as superbugs.

CHAPTER 8

1. List the major components of the innate first line of defense.

2. List and define the cell types involved in the second line of defense.

3. Describe the mechanisms in diapedesis, chemotaxis, and phagocytosis.

4. Explain how opsonization increases the efficiency of the immune system.

5. Differentiate between MHC I and MHC II.

CHAPTER 9

1. Describe the components of the adaptive immune system and their functions.

2. List the five types of antibody and their functions in health and disease.

3. Differentiate between the functions of MHC I and MHC II.

4. Differentiate between necrosis and apoptosis.

5. Explain how a defect in T-helper cells can cause immunodeficiency.

CHAPTER 10

1. Describe the four types of hypersensitivity, and give an example of each.

2. Describe the different types of vaccine formulations, and give an example of each.

3. Differentiate among the four types of immune responses.

4. Identify reasons for the use of passive administration of immunoglobulins in protective passive immunity.

CHAPTER 11

1. Define primary and opportunistic pathogen.

2. Describe superantigens and the mechanism of action.

3. Identify the portal of entry for common organisms.

4. Define virulence factors, and explain how tropism determines whether an infection will occur.

5. List some of the effects that viruses exert on host cells to cause disease.

CHAPTER 12

1. Differentiate between normal flora (normal microbiota) and transient flora.
2. Define terms used to describe disease and the course of disease.
3. Identify the mechanisms by which diseases are transmitted.
4. Define the common epidemiological terms relating to burden of disease.
5. Differentiate between acute and chronic disease.

CHAPTER 13

1. Explain why the skin is a good barrier to infection.
2. Identify the normal flora of skin.
3. Describe common causes of bacterial, viral, fungal, and parasitic skin infections.
4. Identify commonly occurring infections when skin is breached.
5. Describe problems arising from the use of artificial devices.
6. Define the different levels of infection affecting the skin (cellulitis, gangrene, etc.).

CHAPTER 14

1. Describe how infections can disrupt the normal functioning of the eye.
2. Define the different types of infections according to the site of infection (conjunctivitis, keratitis, etc.).
3. List the immune defense mechanisms in the eye.
4. Describe risk factors for eye infections.
5. Identify commonly encountered eye infections, their causative agents, and their clinical appearances.

CHAPTER 15

1. Describe the defense mechanisms against infection in the upper respiratory tract.
2. List some common causes of pharyngitis, including the common cold.
3. Describe the cause and pathogenicity of EBV causing infectious mononucleosis .
4. Discuss the pathogenicity of S. pyogenes.
5. Discuss the pathogenicity of C. diphtheriae.
6. List causes of otitis media and epiglottis.
7. Discuss the cause and pathogenicity of whooping cough.

CHAPTER 16

1. Discuss *Mycobacterium tuberculosis* pathogenicity, latent infection, and active disease.

2. Describe pneumonia caused by *S. pneumoniae* and its pathogenicity.

3. Identify and discuss characteristics of some viral causes of LRTI: RSV, parainfluenza, and influenza A.

4. Define antigenic shift and antigenic drift in influenza A.

CHAPTER 17

1. Identify the major defenses to infection in the mouth.

2. Describe the major bacterial species in the mouth contributing to dental caries and periodontal disease and the pathogenesis (e.g., biofilm formation).

3. Describe the pathogenesis of *Actinomyces* species causing "lumpy jaw."

4. Describe the clinical syndrome caused by the mumps virus.

5. Discuss the pathogenicity of *Helicobacter pylori* as a cause of peptic and duodenal ulcers.

CHAPTER 18

1. Differentiate between intoxications and infections with emphasis on individual organisms.

2. Define dysentery and gastroenteritis.

3. Describe the major causes of intoxications and gastroenteritis.

4. Identify some clinical features of viral intestinal infections with norovirus, rotavirus, hepatitis A, and hepatitis E.

CHAPTER 19

1. Describe the components of the urinary tract.

2. Identify the levels of urinary tract infection according to the organ affected.

3. Explain how asymptomatic urinary tract infections can cause disease.

4. Identify the main causes of urinary tract infections in different populations.

5. List parameters used in the urine sediment test for demonstrating kidney damage.

6. Determine important considerations for collecting representative specimens.

CHAPTER 20

1. List some characteristics bacteria and viruses causing STI have in common.
2. Describe how STI are transmitted, and how they can be prevented.
3. Rank the STI according to their severity regarding location and effect on reproductive health.
4. List major complications from STI.
5. Identify the major causes of STI and characteristics of infection.
6. Discern the effects of asymptomatic infection on reproductive health.

CHAPTER 21

1. Explain why the newborn and young infant are very susceptible to infection.
2. List common causes of congenital infections.
3. Identify the effects of common infectious diseases in the neonate.
4. Describe preventative measures for congenital infection.

CHAPTER 22

1. Identify the major route by which CNS infections occur.
2. List the most common causes of acute and chronic meningitis.
3. Differentiate meningitis from encephalitis.
4. Describe tetanus and botulism and the mechanisms of pathogenicity.
5. Discuss the diseases caused by poliovirus, leprosy, rabies, and West Nile fever.
6. Identify BSE as a TSE, and discuss how the agent can cause irreversible brain damage.

CHAPTER 23

1. Describe the role of the cardiovascular and lymphatic systems in spreading disease.
2. Identify endotoxin as a major cause of a systemic inflammatory response, and describe the three major activating events.
3. Define lymphangitis, septicemia, and septic shock.
4. Discuss the causative agents and clinical events in anthrax, Lyme disease, plague, and tularemia.
5. Describe the syndromes and causative agents of hepatitis B, hepatitis C, and hepatitis D.

6. Review the cause and clinical symptoms of malaria.

7. Identify yellow fever as the prototype for flaviviruses, and discuss the disease in relation to dengue fever and West Nile fever.

CHAPTER 24

1. Describe HIV as the cause of AIDS.

2. Explain how the HIV virus integrates into the human genome.

3. Identify how the immune system of patients with HIV is compromised.

4. Define opportunistic infections, and describe some of the common indicator infections.

5. Identify elements of HAARTS.

6. List major health risks to healthcare workers.

CHAPTER 25

1. Describe the most commonly used routine culture media for human pathogens.

2. Differentiate between aerobic and anaerobic cultures.

3. List the methods used routinely to identify bacteria.

4. Explain how hemolytic reactions, the coagulase test, and the catalase test can help to differentiate Gram-positive organisms from one another.

5. Familiarize yourself with the techniques that can be used for identification.

Chapter 1

Introduction to Medical Microbiology and Immunology

Learning Objectives

1. Describe the theory of spontaneous generation and germ theory of disease.

2. Recognize key players in the development of microbiology as a science, and know the key discoveries made by important researchers (Koch, Pasteur, Lister, Gram, Jenner, Fleming, Reed, Salk).

3. Recognize Koch's postulates.

4. Order microorganisms according to size.

5. Describe the naming conventions of microorganisms at the genus and species level (bacteria, parasites, and fungi); understand how viruses are named.

6. List differences between prokaryotes and eukaryotes.

Historical Perspective

You are not expected to know all of the dates and names, but you should have an idea of how the science developed and what famous scientists, such as Koch, Pasteur, Semmelweis, and Salk, were responsible for.

-Although microorganisms were known to exist until the discovery of the microscope, the idea that disease/decay could be caused by some entity was not foreign.

-Ancient Egyptians developed the practice of embalming to prevent the decay of their dead, not knowing that the embalming fluid was actually killing the bacteria causing the putrefaction of flesh

-For smallpox prevention, the practice of variolation was used, where material from the scab of a smallpox victim was administered to a healthy individual. No one really knows how old this practice is; there are reports from India as early as 1500 BC, and the Chinese people were masters of variolation at an early stage.

-The first "vaccines" were likely ground up scab material from smallpox victims, which were then administered nasally, stimulating a respiratory infection. Later material was introduced through a local skin scratch, and this method proved to be safer, caused a milder disease while still providing protection.

1590–1595: Zacharias Janssen, a Dutch eyeglass maker, invented the simple microscope and then followed this invention up with a compound microscope using several lenses. The attainable magnification at this time was about 9X.

1665: Robert Hooke used the compound microscope and, by studying a cork, discovered the cell as the smallest building block of tissues.

1668: Francesco Redi tried to disprove the theory of spontaneous generation with an experiment: six jars of decaying meat, three with lids to keep flies out, and three without lids. Maggots grew in the jars without lids. He concluded that maggots developed from flies. It was the first blow to the theory of **spontaneous generation** (a belief that living matter could arise from nonliving matter).

1673: Anton van Leeuwenhoek improved the microscope lenses to magnify up to about 200X; he was the first to report live microorganisms through magnifying lenses—"animalcules"—from his own dental plaque.

1767: Lazzaro Spallanzani experimented with boiled and unboiled gravy, observing that the boiled gravy did not spoil, whereas the unboiled gravy did spoil. He decided that "spontaneous generation" must be false.

1798: Robert Jenner created the first vaccination (smallpox). He postulated that exposure to a poxvirus would confer some immunity to the serious disease caused by smallpox. It was well known that milkmaids who had contracted vaccinia (cowpox) did not develop smallpox. He took scrapings from cowpox blisters and inoculated an 8-year-old boy, then challenged him with a smallpox infection. Thankfully, it worked! Vacca = cow (Lat.).

1840: Ignatius Semmelweis demonstrated that childbirth fever was caused by the hospital staff infecting patients. Women who delivered babies in the hospital often died of septic complications after delivery, but those who delivered at home did not. Semmelweis discovered that his medical students and colleagues were coming directly from work in the autopsy room to examine newly delivered mothers. Hand washing becomes important!

1854: John Snow found contaminated water from a well to be the cause of a cholera epidemic. He is dubbed the "father of epidemiology."

1858: Rudolf Virchow developed the theory that living cells could only come from other living cells, known as biogenesis.

1861-1885: Louis Pasteur disproved the theory of spontaneous generation once and for all. He designed a series of experiments that conclusively proved that living matter could only arise from living matter. He also demonstrated that microbial life could be destroyed by heat—the basis for "aseptic technique" process of pasteurization. Also while studying yeast, he adopts the terminology "aerobic" and "anaerobic."

Germ theory of disease: Pasteur thought that just as microorganisms could spoil beverages such as beer and milk, microorganisms could also cause disease in animals and man.

Pasteur was responsible for the **first artificially attenuated vaccine** to chicken cholera and later, anthrax and rabies.

1867: Joseph Lister applied the germ theory to surgical-medical procedures. He used phenol (carbolic acid) to wash surgical wounds to prevent infection. He is credited for discovering that microorganisms cause wound infections.

1876: Robert Koch validated the **germ theory of disease**: he found the cause of anthrax, cultured it on artificial media, then infected animals and produced the disease.

1882: Koch isolated and identified *Mycobacterium tuberculosis* as the causative agent of tuberculosis.

1883: Koch isolated and identified *Vibrio cholerae* as the causative agent for cholera.

1884: **"Koch's postulates"** were formulated. These were guidelines to be followed to determine whether the cause of a disease was a microorganism.

1. The same organism must be present in every case of the disease.

2. The organism must be grown in pure culture from a diseased human or animal.

3. The organism must then cause the same disease if inoculated into a healthy human or animal.

4. The same organism must be found from samples of the inoculated population.

1884: *Escherichia coli* was described by Theodor Escherich.

1884: Elie Metchnikoff described **phagocytosis**: the first description of an immune mechanism!

1884: Hans Christian Gram developed and described **Gram's stain.**

1887: Julius Richard Petri developed the petri plate for cultivation of bacteria on solid media.

1890: Emil von Behring and collaborators developed the process for producing **diphtheria antitoxin**. It was the first directed therapy to a specific infectious disease.

1891: Paul Ehrlich proposed **antibodies** for immunity.

1892: William Welch identified *Clostridium perfringens* as cause of gas gangrene.

1892: Dmitri Iwanowski gave the first demonstration of a **filterable infectious agent (virus)** smaller than bacteria.

1899: Ronald Ross published the life cycle of the **malarial parasite**.

1900: Walter Reed showed that **Yellow Fever** is caused by a virus transmitted by a mosquito. It is the first human disease where virus is implicated.

1905: *Treponema pallidum* was identified as cause of syphilis.

1909: Ricketts proved that **Rocky Mountain Spotted Fever** is caused by Rickettsia.

1910: **Chemotherapy**. Ehrlich found salvarsan (arsenic) to be effective against syphilis: the first synthetic antimicrobial and first specific chemotherapeutic agent.

1910: **Typhus** was found to pass from human to human via body lice.

1911: Peyton Rous discovered that a virus causes cancer in a chicken: the **first demonstration that a virus can cause cancer**.

1918: Worldwide **Influenza A (H1N1) pandemic** killed more people than the war.

1928: Frederick Griffith discovered **transformation** in bacteria. This led to the understanding about DNA.

1928: Alexander Fleming **discovered penicillin** (chemicals produced naturally by bacteria and fungi to act against other organisms are called **antibiotics**).

1934: **Electron microscope** was invented.

1938: Successful vaccine against **Yellow Fever** was derived.

1940: Ernst Boris Chain and Howard Florey made the first observation that bacteria can produce an enzyme that inactivates penicillin (**beta-lactamase** or penicillinase).

1953: Jonas Salk developed the **polio vaccine** (inactivated).

1983: **Human Immunodeficiency Virus** was proved to be the cause of HIV/AIDS.

1984: Barry Marshall, Stuart Goodwin, and Robin Warren proved **stomach ulcers** were caused by *Helicobacter pylori*.

1995: First **bacterial DNA sequence was mapped** (*H. influenzae*).

2003: **Human genome was mapped**.

2003: **SARS** came to Canada; intensive infection control stopped spread.

Microbiology–General Introduction

A. SIZE OF MICROORGANISMS

Large microorganisms (i.e., lice, worms) >1000 microns (1 mm)

-visible with naked eye

Medium microbes (i.e., amoeba, algae, bacteria, large viruses) 1–100 microns

-visible with light microscope

-most of the disease-producing (pathogenic) bacteria encountered in infectious diseases are in this category (e.g., Streptococcus, Staphylococcus, Salmonella, etc.)

Small microbes (i.e., virus, certain special bacteria such as mycoplasma and chlamydia) 30–100 nanometers (.01–.1 micron)

-visible with electron microscope

Extremely small microbes: prions—infectious protein molecules that have been misfolded and do not function properly (e.g., Mad Cow Disease)

B. NAMING

Naming of bacteria:

Most commonly, organisms are classified into families on the basis of the relatedness of their ribosomal RNA or rRNA (which is a stable sequence appropriate to use for classifying organisms).

Organisms are classified as per:

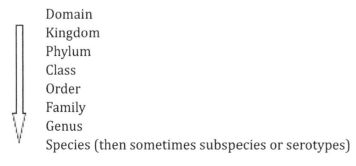

Domain
Kingdom
Phylum
Class
Order
Family
Genus
Species (then sometimes subspecies or serotypes)

The names we will use in this course are: **Genus, species**

Bacteria:

Examples of bacterial names (note that genus is always uppercase and species is always lowercase):

Staphylococcus aureus	*S. aureus*
Staphylococcus epidermidis	*S. epidermidis*
Salmonella typhi	*S. typhi*
Salmonella enteritidis	*S. enteritidis*
Streptococcus pyogenes	*S. pyogenes*
Stenotrophomonas maltophilia	*S. maltophilia*

Naming of parasites: use genus and species

Parasites: example of names

Taenia saginata	*T. saginata*
Taenia solium	*T. solium*
Trichinella spiralis	*T. spiralis*
Trichomonas vaginalis	*T. vaginalis*
Entamoeba histolytica	*E. histolytica*
Enterobius vermicularis	*E. vermicularis*
Echinococcus multilocularis	*E. multilocularis*

Naming of fungi: use genus and species

Fungi: example of names

Candida albicans	*C. albicans*
Cryptococcus neoformans	*C. neoformans*
Aspergillus niger	*A. niger*
Alternaria blumeae	*A. blumeae*

*Note that the organisms may have the same genus abbreviation yet are very different species; this is why it is important to know the species name. Also note the writing conventions where the genus is capitalized and the species is never capitalized. Italics are used.

Naming of viruses

Viruses are grouped into families depending on:

a. Type of nucleic acid

b. Strategy for replication

c. Morphology

The characteristics of the genome are used for classification of viruses into a scheme called the Baltimore System. This new system coexists side by side with the traditional ICTV scheme, devised by the International Committee on Taxonomy of Viruses, which is probably still more widely used.

A viral species is a group of viruses sharing the same genetic information and ecological niche.

For this course, we will focus on identifying viruses as DNA containing or RNA containing viruses.

*examples of DNA viruses

Herpes simplex virus 1

Herpes simplex virus 2

Human herpesvirus 3   (Varicella virus)

Human herpesvirus 4   (Epstein Barr virus)

Human herpesvirus 5   (Cytomegalovirus)

- All herpes viruses share a common characteristic: ability to remain latent in host cells.

*examples of RNA viruses:

Human immunodeficiency virus (HIV)-1

Human immunodeficiency virus (HIV)-2

Influenza A virus

Parainfluenza virus

Respiratory syncytial virus

Microbiology

We will study five major categories in this course and applications for infection control and patient care:

1. **Bacteriology**: study of bacteria

2. **Virology**: study of viruses

3. **Mycology**: study of fungi and yeast

4. **Parasitology**: study of protozoa (amoeba, etc.) and worms

5. **Immunology**: study of immunity (resistance to infection)

An important classification of living cells to know is whether the organism is a **prokaryote** or **eukaryote.**

Prokaryote: bacteria: small, unicellular organisms—genetic material dispersed through the cell, no "nuclear membrane"

Eukaryote: fungi, plant cells, human cells—genetic material collected in a nucleus with a surrounding nuclear membrane

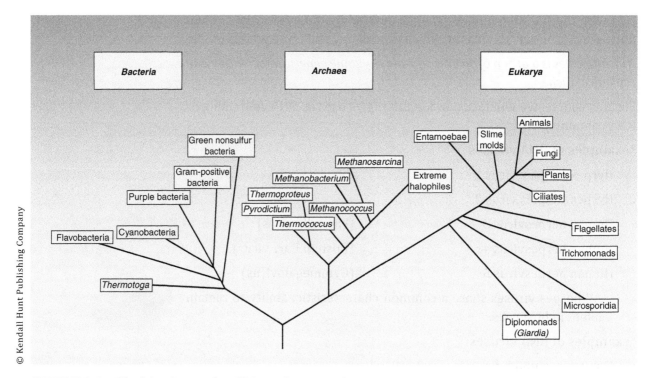

FIGURE 1.1   *The big picture classifying microorganisms*

Prokaryote means pre or before nucleus in Greek:

1. DNA not in enclosed envelope
2. DNA not associated with histones
3. Lack membrane-enclosed organelles (e.g., Golgi apparatus)
4. Cell walls almost always contain peptidoglycan
5. Divide by binary fission
6. All proteins start with the amino acid formylmethionine

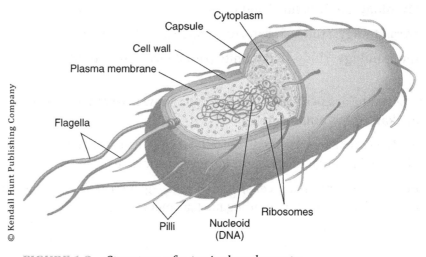

FIGURE 1.2   *Structure of a typical prokaryote*

Eukaryote means true nucleus in Greek:

1. DNA in cell nucleus, bounded by a nuclear membrane

2. DNA in nucleus found in multiple chromosomes

3. DNA associated with histones (chromosomal proteins)

4. Number of membrane enclosed organelles (e.g., Golgi apparatus, mitochondria, etc.)

5. Cell walls, if present, are very simple

6. Usually divide by mitosis

7. All proteins start with the amino acid methionine

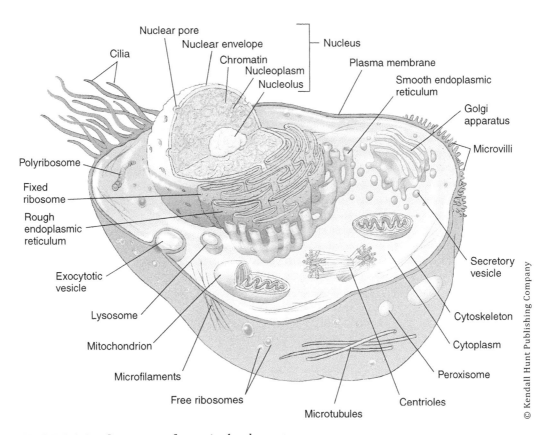

FIGURE 1.3   Structure of a typical eukaryote

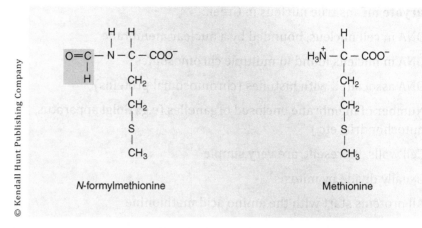

FIGURE 1.4   *N-formylmethionine and methionine*

Basic Bacteriology

1. Describe Gram staining: the procedure and the reactions, and give an example of bacteria that stain Gram positive, bacteria that stain Gram negative, and bacteria that must be visualized with other stains (i.e., acid-fast).

2. Differentiate between different bacterial morphologies.

3. Describe the major components of the prokaryote and its functions.

4. Understand how bacteria metabolize nutrients and the types of respiration involved.

5. Categorize organisms according to their growth characteristics; understand how different media can support growth and identification of organisms, and define plasmolysis.

6. Identify how common biofilms are formed, and describe their roles in disease.

Prokaryotes (Bacteria)

A. DIFFERENTIATION OF BACTERIAL ORGANISMS:

-Differentiation of organisms is important for the classification of bacteria into functional groups.

-Structures associated with prokaryotes determine the characteristics of bacteria with respect to staining reactions such as **Gram's stain**, mechanisms of pathogenesis (how bacteria exert deleterious effects on the host), and choice of antimicrobial drugs.

-The most important practical distinction to know about bacteria is the staining characteristic—that is, Gram's stain.

Gram's stain: developed in 1884 by Hans Christian Gram.

-It is still used as one of the major diagnostic tests used to identify disease-causing bacteria.

-It is based on cell wall structure.

*examples:

Streptococcus pneumoniae: Gram positive diplococci

Escherichia coli: Gram negative bacilli

***You must know the gram staining characteristics of all bacteria on the Top Bacteria to Know list for the final exam in the course.

Steps in Gram Staining

1. **Fix specimen** on slide (cells must adhere to the glass slide before starting staining). This is done by flooding the slide with methanol or by passing the slide with the specimen through a flame.

2. Add **crystal violet** (also called gentian violet) to the surface of the slide. The crystal violet penetrates into all cells. This is the **primary stain**.

3. Add **iodine** to the slide, washing away the excess crystal violet stain. The iodine is called a **mordant**—it helps the stain stay in the cells. It does this by combining with the crystal violet, and a large complex molecule is formed. This molecule is now unable to leave the cell through the cell wall containing the peptidoglycan mesh and is trapped in the cell.

4. Apply **decolorizer** (acetone/alcohol) rinse, and rinse away all remains of purple–brown color. This solvent is thought to be able to dissolve some of the lipid in the Gram negative cell membrane and make the cell leaky. Alcohol also dehydrates the peptidoglycan and shrinks it, so if there are many layers, it becomes very dense with very small passageways through it. **This is the differentiation step**. Gram positives retain the stain and are purple, and Gram negatives lose all stain and are colorless.

5. To enable visualization in the microscope, add **safranin** (pink/red dye) to the slide. This will **counter stain** the Gram negative bacteria so that

we can see them in the microscope. It does not affect the Gram positive bacteria because they are already strongly blue–purple colored.

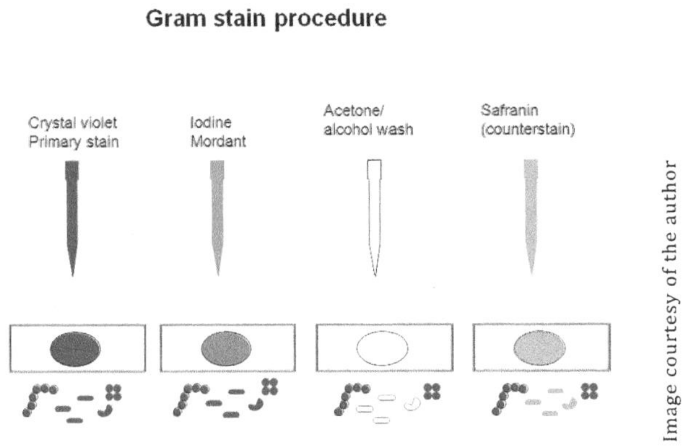

FIGURE 2.1   *Gram stain procedure*

Gram's Stain: Concept

-Inside the bacterial cell, crystal violet and iodine bind together to make a larger molecule. This large, complex molecule will be trapped inside of Gram positive organisms because they have a thick peptidoglycan layer in their cell walls. The thick peptidoglycan is made of many layers of n-acetyl muramic acid and n-acetyl glutamic acid joined by peptide bonds. A mesh forms, which has channels throughout, but the channels are very twisted and the mesh is tight. It is not easy for large molecules to get back through the mesh and out of the cell when the decolorization reagent is added.

-Gram negative organisms do not have this thick peptidoglycan layer (although they do have thin layers of peptidoglycan), and shrinkage is minimal, which allows the large CV-I complex to exit the cell walls when decolorizer is added.

-It is also thought that acetone–alcohol decolorizer is able to wash the CV-I complex out of Gram negative organisms easily because of the destruction of the phospholipid layer in the outer membrane of their cell walls by action of the acetone/alcohol on the phospholipid membrane.

-Gram negative organisms will have all stain removed after decolorization. In order for us to see them in the microscope, a counter stain (i.e., safranin) is applied, coloring them pink. Gram positive organisms remain dark purple throughout the procedure.

Important Exceptions to the Gram's Stain Rules

1. Bacteria that cannot be stained by Gram's stain:

    Mycobacterium species: for example, *Mycobacterium tuberculosis* (waxy cell wall prevents stain penetration)

    Mycoplasma species: for example, *Mycoplasma pneumoniae* (no cell wall)

    Dead or old bacteria (cannot retain cell wall integrity and become leaky)

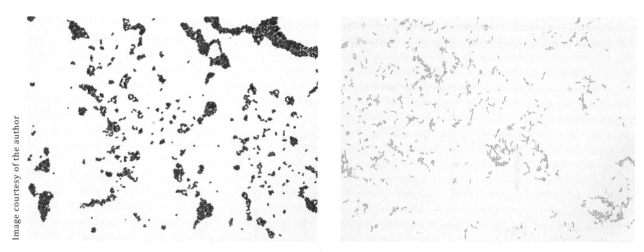

FIGURE 2.2   Photomicrographs demonstrating Gram positive and Gram negative reactions

2. Bacteria that can be stained but cannot be seen with light microscopy due to small size:

    Chlamydia species: elementary bodies too small to be seen with Gram's. stain and reticulate bodies found only inside of host cells

    Rickettsia, Erlichia species: intracellular bacteria

    Treponema pallidum: spirochaete, too slender to see in the microscope, cannot identify by Gram's stain

Other Important Differential Stains for Further Identification of Bacteria

1. **Acid-fast stain (Ziehl-Neelson)**: used for Mycobacterium, Nocardia, and a few other organisms like a parasite called Cryptosporidium.

    -Based on the fact that these bacteria have waxes in their cell walls. Carbol fuchsin is added to smear and heated—this enhances the penetration of the dye through the wax. Decolorization is done by exposing the smear to acid alcohol—this removes the red stain from the organisms that are *not* acid-fast. The counter stain, methylene blue, then colors the background so that it is easier to see the red-stained organisms.

2. **Negative staining for capsules**: some organisms have a polysaccharide capsule surrounding the cell walls, which are important for virulence. These capsules cannot be stained, so we use a negative stain, where the background is stained and the organism appears as a particle with a halo around the cell where the stain has been excluded (e.g., India ink staining for a yeast called Cryptococcus).

Other special stains: not done routinely;for visualization of special structures.

*examples:

- Stains for spores and flagella

- Acridine orange stain binds to DNA and fluoresces under UV light, allowing us to see even a few bacteria in a clinical specimen.

B. BACTERIAL MORPHOLOGY

-Most bacteria are monomorphic (all the same shape if the same species), but some are pleomorphic (may have slightly different shapes, like a short rod and a long rod in the same culture or specimen).

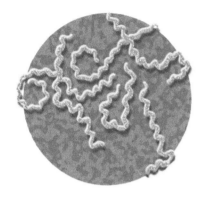
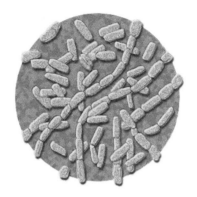
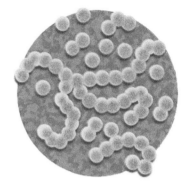

Spirillum
(corkscrew-shaped)

Bacillus
(rod-shaped)

Coccus
(spherical)

FIGURE 2.3   Bacterial shapes

Coccus (sing) (spherical): plural "cocci"

   -Round, sometimes slightly elongated or flattened on one side

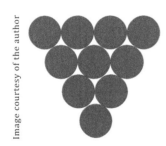

FIGURE 2.4   staphylococci: remain in clusters like grapes

FIGURE 2.5   diplococci: remain in pairs after dividing

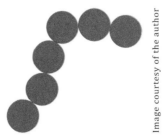

FIGURE 2.6   streptococci: remain in chains after dividing

Bacillus (sing) (rod-shaped): plural "bacilli"

-Can have tapered ends; some have blunt ends

Image courtesy of the author

FIGURE 2.7   coccobacilli: short, oval cells; usually small size

Image courtesy of the author

FIGURE 2.8   diplobacilli: remain in pairs after dividing

Image courtesy of the author

FIGURE 2.9   streptobacilli: remain in chains after dividing

Spiral bacteria various degrees of curving

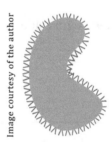

Image courtesy of the author

FIGURE 2.10   vibrio: short, curved rods; comma-like

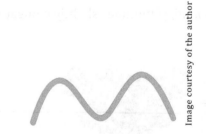

Image courtesy of the author

FIGURE 2.11   spirilla: wavy shape, loose curves, rigid

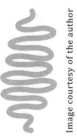

Image courtesy of the author

FIGURE 2.12   spirochaete: helical, tightly coiled but flexible

C. BACTERIAL CELL STRUCTURE

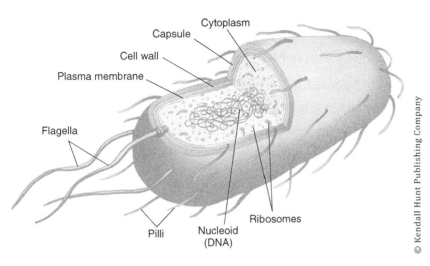

FIGURE 2.13   *The prokaryotic cell*

Structures Outside the Cell Wall:

Glycocalyx (sugar coat): polymer of polysaccharide or polypeptide. This can have several forms:

capsule: substance is organized and firmly attached (e.g., *Klebsiella pneumoniae, Streptococcus pneumoniae*)

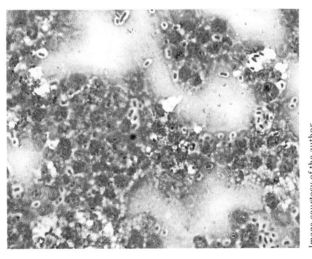

FIGURE 2.14   *Photomicrograph showing the capsule around K. pneumoniae*

<u>**or**</u> slime layer: loosely organized and loosely attached (e.g. *Pseudomonas aeruginosa*)

Flagella: long, filamentous appendages that function to propel bacteria. Four arrangements are possible on bacterial cells—this is characteristic of the species of the individual bacterium:

    monotrichous: single polar flagellum

    amphitrichous: tuft of flagella at each end

    lophotrichous: two or more flagella at one pole

    peritrichous: flagella evenly over entire cell

-Some flagella proteins can be used to subtype bacteria. For example, *E. coli* 0157:H7—the "**H**" antigen is from the flagella protein (*E. coli* has at least 50 different H antigens)

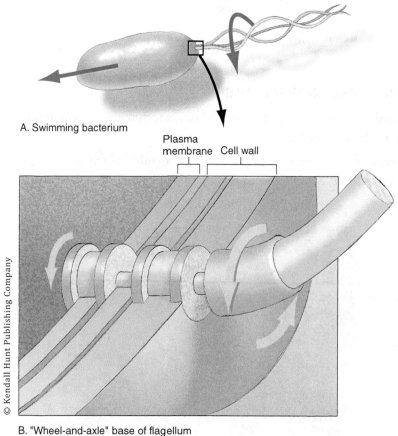

A. Swimming bacterium

Plasma
membrane   Cell wall

© Kendall Hunt Publishing Company

B. "Wheel-and-axle" base of flagellum

FIGURE 2.15   Flagella

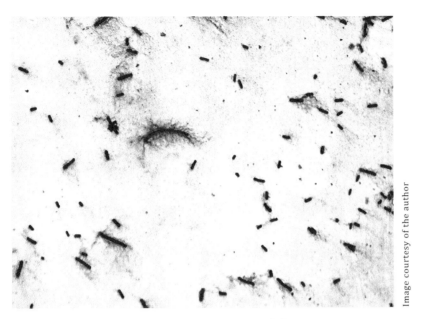

Image courtesy of the author

FIGURE 2.16 Flagella stain, Proteus mirabilis

Axial filaments: "internal flagellum"—used for motility by spirochaetes

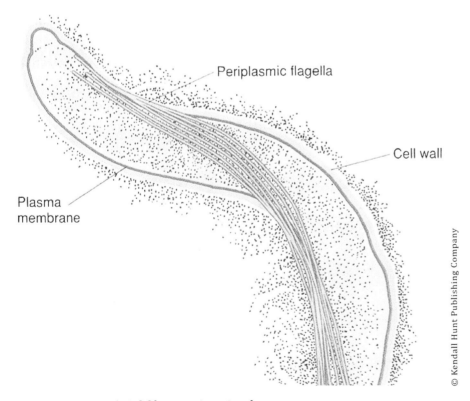

Periplasmic flagella

Cell wall

Plasma membrane

© Kendall Hunt Publishing Company

FIGURE 2.17 Axial filament in spirochaetes

For example, *Treponema pallidum* (cause of syphilis): bundles of fibrils arise at ends of cells and wind around beneath an outer sheath (internal flagella).

Fimbriae and pili: hair-like appendages on Gram negative bacteria—used for attachment and sometimes transfer of genes from one bacteria to another

> **Fimbriae**: used for adherence (e.g., *Neisseria gonorrhoeae*) to mucosal membranes

> **Pili**: used for attachment to host cells. An F-pilus is a special pilus used for joining bacterial cells for transfer of DNA from cell to cell. This transfer is called conjugation.

Cell Wall Structures

-The cell wall is a complex, semirigid structure responsible for the shape of the cell. It protects the interior of the cell. The major function is to protect cells from rupturing if the outside environment has lower osmolarity than the inside of the cell (fewer solute particles than inside the cell).

-The cell wall is an important site for action of some antibiotics and is constructed differently in Gram negative and Gram positive bacteria.

-Gram negative cell walls have an extra "outer membrane" external to the peptidoglycan layer. This outer membrane is studded with porin channels that restrict the movement of molecules in and out of the cell.

> **Peptidoglycan**: also called murein, major component of Gram positive cell walls

> -Repeating units of disaccharide attached by polypeptides that form a lattice structure or a 3D mesh. Gram positive cells have many layers of peptidoglycan.

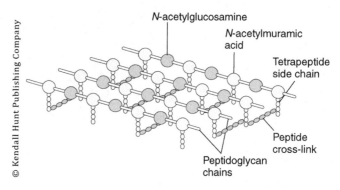

N-acetylglucosamine

N-acetylmuramic acid

Tetrapeptide side chain

Peptide cross-link

Peptidoglycan chains

© Kendall Hunt Publishing Company

FIGURE 2.18   Structure of one single layer of peptidoglycan

-The antibiotic penicillin interferes with final cross-linking of molecules in peptidoglycan and weakens it, so the cell easily bursts because of osmotic pressure.

-Gram positive cells are usually more susceptible to the action of penicillin because unlike Gram negatives, their cell walls do not have an outer membrane layer that prevents penicillin from entering the cell wall.

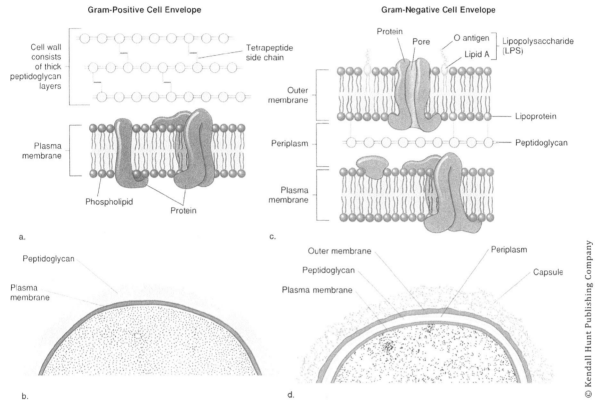

FIGURE 2.19   Gram positive cell wall

Teichoic and lipoteichoic acids: only found in Gram positives

-These molecules may function to increase adherence of the bacteria to the host cell, a prerequisite for infection. They may do this by changing the net charge on the bacterial surface, allowing it to more easily adhere to the target cell.

Lipopolysaccharide

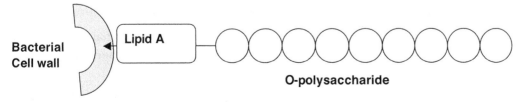

*FIGURE 2.20   **Lipopolysaccharide:** Only in Gram negatives, which have an outer membrane composed of lipopolysaccharide (LPS), lipoproteins, and phospholipid.*

LPS is important in two ways:

-Polysaccharide portion (called "**O**" antigen or polysaccharide) is used for typing bacteria (e.g., *E. coli* O157:H7).

-The lipid portion of LPS, **lipid A**, is referred to as an **endotoxin** and

is toxic in the blood causing systemic effects like fever and shock.

Plasma or cytoplasmic membrane

-Thin membrane lying inside of the cell wall, enclosing the cytoplasm of the cell

-Prokaryotes' plasma membranes are composed mainly of a bilayer of phospholipids, with the polar heads facing out and the non-polar fatty acid tails inside, and proteins.

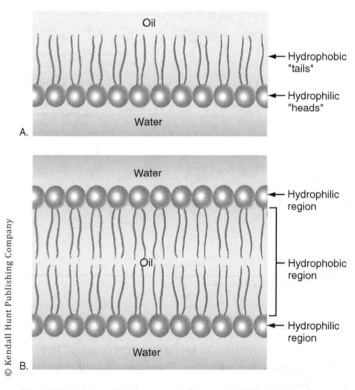

FIGURE 2.21   Plasma membrane: double layer of phospholipids

-Eukaryotes' plasma membranes are composed of phospholipids, proteins, carbohydrates, and sterols like cholesterol and are usually more rigid.

-Proteins associated with plasma membranes can be external to the bilayer or can be transmembrane structures that allow the movement of molecules through the phospholipid bilayer.

-Membranes have selective permeability, both active (energy requiring) and passive movement of molecules (diffusion) through protein channels.

-This is the location of enzymes for production of ATP (energy) in prokaryotes.

-Some disinfectants (e.g., alcohols and quaternary ammonium compounds) and antibiotics (e.g., polymixin) disrupt bacterial cell plasma membranes.

Cytoplasm

-Substance of the cell inside the plasma membrane

-80% water

-Major structures are nucleoid area, ribosomes, and reserve deposits called inclusions. No cytoskeleton is present in prokaryotic cells.

Nucleoid

-Single long, continuous thread of double-stranded DNA anchored in the plasma membrane. This is the bacterial chromosome, and it is attached to the plasma membrane.

-It contains the genetic information for the cell structures and functioning.

-Unlike eukaryotic cells, there is no bounding membrane around the nuclear material.

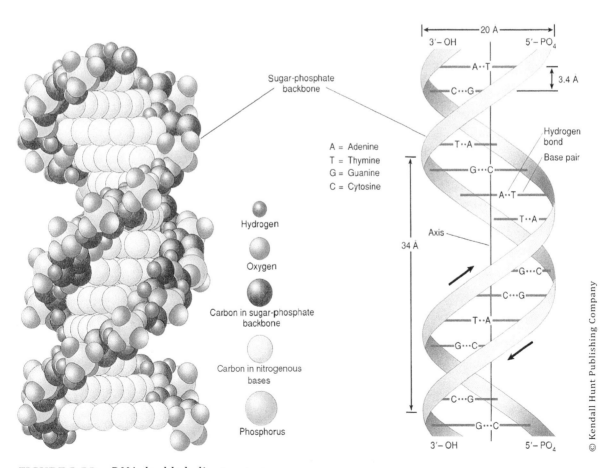

FIGURE 2.22   *DNA double helix structure*

Plasmid

-Some bacteria have a separate small circular piece of DNA, which codes for a restricted number of genes.

-Plasmids can mediate resistance and production of virulence factors. They are independent of the chromosome and reproduce separately.

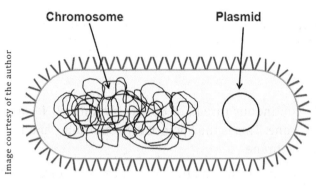

FIGURE 2.23   *Plasmid*

Ribosomes

-These are the site for protein synthesis. Two subunits are composed of protein and RNA. Prokaryotic ribosomes are smaller and less dense than eukaryotic ribosomes.

-Prokaryotic ribosomes are classed by density centrifugation as 70S ribosomes, whereas eukaryotic ribosomes are 80S.

-Proteins are coded for by RNA made in the cell nucleus from DNA.

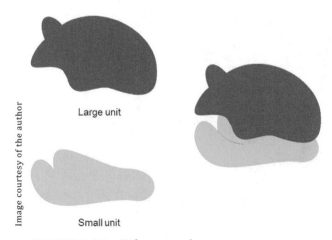

FIGURE 2.24   *Ribosomes have two components*

Inclusions

-Reserve deposits of nutrients

   *examples: lipid inclusions in Mycobacterium

   metachromatic granules in *C. diphtheriae* contain phosphates for synthesis of ATP

   polysaccharide granules contain glycogen and starch

Endospores

-Some Gram positive bacteria (e.g., Clostridium, Bacillus) form resting cells called endospores. These are a survival mechanism for the bacteria that can form them. Endospores are extremely resistant to heat, chemicals, and drying.

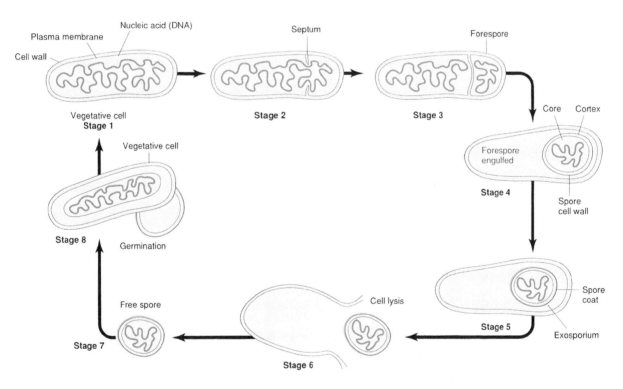

FIGURE 2.25   Steps in endospore formation

-Endospores consist of a thick layer of peptidoglycan and protein that form a coat outside of the cell membrane to protect the genetic information for the cell. They are metabolically inert until the spore becomes active, germinates, and becomes a growing, metabolizing vegetative cell.

-These are located terminally, subterminally, or centrally in cells, depending on the species (this positioning can be used to help speciation).

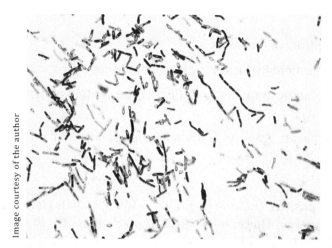

FIGURE 2.26   *Clostridium botulinum with subterminal endospores*

C. BACTERIAL METABOLISM

Metabolism: the sum of all chemical reactions within an organism, including those that release (catabolic) and those that produce energy (anabolic). Enzymes for metabolism are located in the plasma membrane of the bacterial cell.

Catabolism: chemical reactions that release energy and break down organic compounds to simpler compounds (e.g., breakdown of glucose to carbon dioxide and water).

Anabolism: chemical reactions that require energy and build complex organic molecules from simpler compounds (e.g., formation of polysaccharides like glycogen from simple sugars like glucose).

Metabolism:

-Efficient metabolism depends on ensuring that the chemical reactions in the metabolic pathways are functioning optimally.

-Reaction rates are temperature dependent: the higher the temperature, the higher the metabolic rate, but living organisms have restrictions, and high temperatures may kill cells.

-Solution: **enzymes**

Enzymes:

-Large protein molecules that serve as biological catalysts to power chemical reactions

-Efficient reactions are at least 100,000,000 times faster than reactions without enzymes

-Specific for certain substrates

-Have suffix "ase"

-May need cofactors (i.e., metal ions like zinc)

-Recyclable; unchanged during reaction

-Mechanism of enzyme action:

1. Surface of substrate comes in contact with the "active site."
2. Temporary complex forms.
3. Substrate structure is transformed by the enzyme.
4. Enzyme releases transformed substrate.
5. Unchanged enzyme can now react in another reaction.

Enzymes: activity is regulated by cellular controls:

1. **Temperature**: enzymes have optimal temperature ranges in which they have the best activity. If the temperature is too high, they will denature, and if the temperature is too low, they will not function.

2. **pH**: enyzmes all have an optimal pH for activity that is neither too high nor too low.

3. **Substrate concentration**: if the enzyme is saturated (all binding sites on enzymes are occupied), then the enyzme reaction is rapid.

4. **Inhibitors**: some poisons will prevent enzymes from functioning (e.g., mercury, silver)

Enzyme inhibition: "competitive" and "noncompetitive" inhibitors

-**Competitive** enzyme inhibitors compete with the natural substrate for the active site and prevent binding of the enzyme to substrate.

-**Noncompetitive** enzyme inhibitors interact with another part of the enzyme, which causes the active site to change shape and be nonfunctional.

Metabolic Reactions

Oxidation: produces energy, removal of electrons

-All oxidation reactions are paired with reduction reactions—these reactions are called **REDOX** reactions.

-Energy released by oxidation is trapped by ADP (adenosine diphosphate) to form ATP (adenosine triphosphate), which can then be used as an energy source for cellular functions.

-Microbes use redox reactions to break down nutrients for energy.

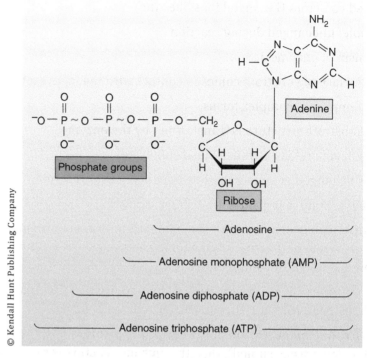

FIGURE 2.27   *Structure of the energy molecule: ATP*

Carbohydrates: most microorganisms use carbohydrates as their primary source for production of energy or ATP.

-Glucose is the most common nutrient (carbohydrate) source.

-Two processes by which glucose can be used:

    A. Cellular respiration

        i.   Aerobic

        ii. Anaerobic

    B. Fermentation

-Both processes use glycolysis (e.g., Embden-Meyerhof pathway) where the final product is pyruvate.

Aerobic cellular respiration (large amount of ATP generated)*

    (aerobic respiration needs O_2; anaerobic doesn't)

    Glycolysis produces pyruvic acid and some ATP.

    Krebs cycle (or TCA cycle) takes a derivative of pyruvic acid and breaks it down to CO_2, producing more ATP.

    Electron transport chain becomes activated and much more ATP is produced.

    -Carrier molecules of electron transport chain:

        flavoproteins (derived from vitamin B_2)

cytochromes (contain iron)

ubiquinones or coenzyme Q (nonprotein)

Net energy possible from one molecule of glucose is ~38 ATP.

Anaerobic cellular respiration (small amount of ATP generated)

-This is the only part of the Krebs cycle that functions without O_2, and the number of electron transport carriers is less; therefore, there is less ATP, and bacteria using anaerobic respiration grow more slowly than aerobic bacteria.

-In anaerobic respiration, the final electron acceptor is an inorganic molecule rather than O_2.

*examples: nitrate ion to nitrite, nitrous oxide, N_2

sulfate ion to H_2S

carbonate ion to CH_4 (methane)

Net energy possible from one molecule of glucose is ~4 ATP.

Fermentation (small amount ATP generated):

-First stage is glycolysis.

-Pyruvate is converted to other compounds (i.e., alcohol or lactic acid).

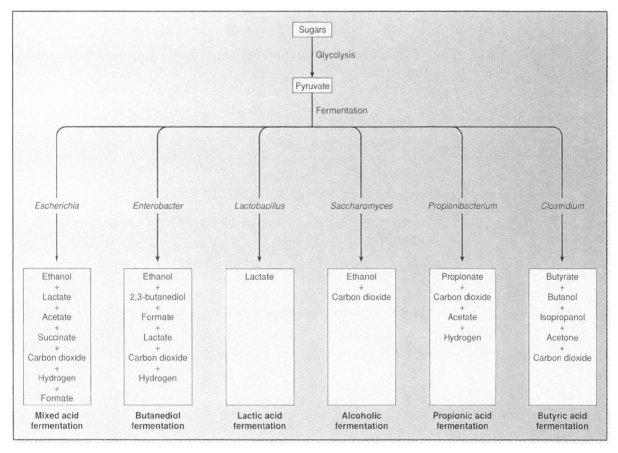

FIGURE 2.28   Fate of pyruvate in bacteria

Net energy possible from one molecule of glucose ~1–2 ATP.

Fermentation: important biological process (production of wine, yogurt, bread, etc.)

-Process does not need oxygen.

-It does not use Krebs cycle or electron transport chain.

-It produces very small amounts of ATP because the energy is not released in the end product but remains in the bonds.

-Lactic acid and alcohol are important products of fermentation (Saccharomyces yeast produces ethanol as a final product—important in wine and beer industries).

-Different microorganisms can ferment different substrates; this is dependent on the type of enzyme present.

-Chemical analysis of the fermentation end products can be used to identify bacteria biochemically.

Lipid and protein catabolism

Lipids: broken down by lipases to fatty acids and glycerol—this can then be taken care of by the Krebs cycle

Proteins: broken down extracellularly by proteases eventually enter Krebs cycle

D. BACTERIAL GROWTH

-Two main categories of factors influence bacterial growth: physical and chemical.

Physical

1. **Temperature**:

pyschrophiles (cold-loving)

psychrophiles opt. 15 °C

psychrotrophs opt. 20°–30° C

-usually responsible for food spoilage because they can grow at refrigerator temperatures (i.e., Listeria)

mesophiles (moderate temp) opt. 25°–40° C

-human pathogens 37°C

thermophiles (heat-loving) opt. 50°–60°C

-hyperthermophiles (i.e., hot springs, 100°C)

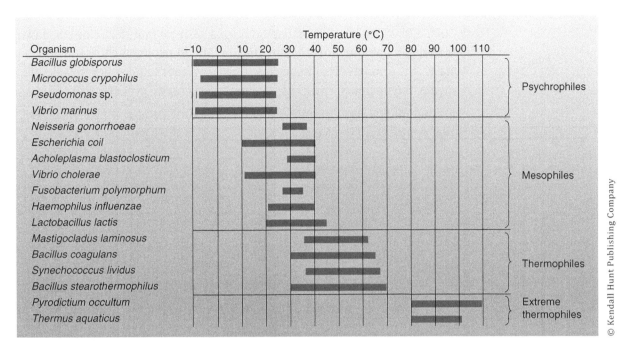

FIGURE 2.29   Temperature preferences of organisms

Why is it important to know the optimal growth for human pathogens?

Listeria monocytogenes: Facultative Gram positive non-spore forming bacillus, motile and a food pathogen, growing at refrigerator temperatures. Also grows well over a wide pH range (<5.5–9.5) and in high salt concentrations. Great opportunity for a food pathogen!

Normally exists in soil and water and is found in animal intestines. Causes significant disease in humans and animals. In animals: CNS (central nervous system) infections in goats and cattle "circling disease;" also septic abortion. In humans: food-borne disease with nausea and diarrhea, CNS infections, which may lead to death and abortion.

Pathogenesis: acquired by ingestion of contaminated food (fecal–oral). Bacteria invade through infecting macrophages (an immune cell that "eats" bacteria), freeing itself from the internal compartment the macrophage imprisons it in with an enzyme, listeriolysin, and multiplies freely in the cytoplasm of the macrophage. It infects nearby cells by rearranging the actin in the host cell to make a "tail" on the bacterium, which can then shoot from one cell to the next like a rocket. The intracellular growth increases its pathogenicity and enables it to evade the immune system.

Human infections: meningitis, encephalitis, septicemia, and spontaneous abortion in pregnant women. Mortality of CNS infections is about

Continued

20%–50%. The incubation period is long, several months before disease is noticed. Lab diagnosis can be difficult. Food products at risk are coleslaw, soft unpasteurized cheeses, turkey wieners and other sliced cold meats, mushrooms, and prepackaged salads (even prewashed!)

Epidemiology: hard to track due to long incubation period. 1700 cases/year reported in the United States, but this is the tip of the iceberg.

2. **pH** (6.5–7.5 usual for human pathogens)

Alkophiles like to live in high pH; acidophiles like to live in low pH.

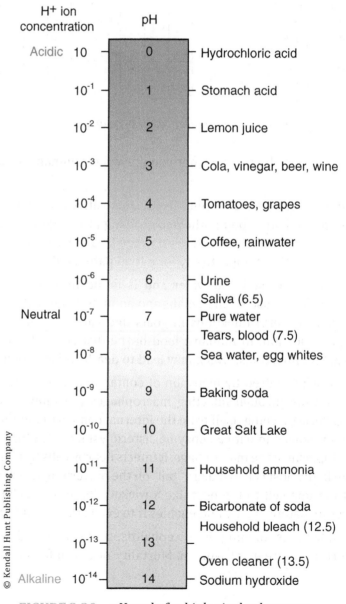

FIGURE 2.30   *pH scale for biological substances*

3. Osmotic pressure

-Nature always wants to be in balance with equal osmotic pressures or numbers of particles per unit of fluid on both sides of a membrane (isotonic).

-When the bacterial cell is put into a hypertonic solution, the water from the cell will leave the cell through the plasma membrane in an attempt to equalize osmotic pressure. This causes the phenomenon we call **plasmolysis.**

-Cell growth is inhibited as the plasma membrane detaches from the cell wall. This is why salt and sugar solutions prevent bacterial growth in foods.

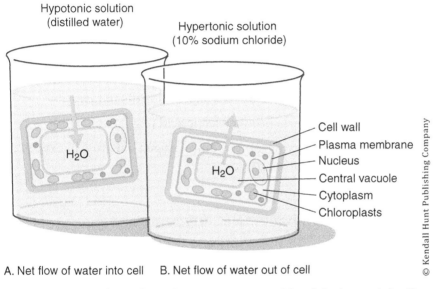

A. Net flow of water into cell   B. Net flow of water out of cell

FIGURE 2.31   Plasmolysis: hypertonicity outside of the bacterial cell

-Bacteria that like to grow in higher salt concentrations than normal body concentrations are called **halophiles**. Some bacteria that live on the skin, salty from sweat, or in the intestine, salty due to bile, are called **facultative halophiles**—they can live in normal or slightly higher salt concentrations (usually tolerate between 2% and 15% salt).

-**Obligate halophiles** grow well in high salt concentrations (e.g., Dead Sea halophiles need 30% salt for growth). These are not human pathogens.

Chemical

-**Carbon** is one of the most important requirements for growth in living organisms.

-Bacteria that cause disease in humans are **chemoheterotrophs.**

-They use carbon from organic compounds to obtain energy for cellular processes and growth.

-They need other elements to synthesize cellular molecules: N, S, P, O (e.g., synthesis of DNA requires nitrogen and phosphorus).

-Trace elements are often required as cofactors for enzyme activity.

-**Oxygen**: bacteria can be classified on the basis of their relationship with oxygen:

1. **Obligate aerobes**: need oxygen for growth
2. **Facultative anaerobes:** can use oxygen for growth but can grow using fermentation or anaerobic respiration when oxygen is not available
3. **Obligate anaerobes**: cannot use oxygen and are harmed by its toxic properties (e.g., superoxide radicals, hydroxyl radicals, etc.)
4. **Aerotolerant anaerobes**: do not use oxygen for growth but tolerate it because they produce enzymes that can break down the oxygen radicals (e.g., catalase, superoxide dismutase)

-Many of these bacteria produce lactic acid (e.g., lactobacilli).

5. **Microaerophiles**: aerobic, require oxygen but grow in oxygen concentrations lower than in air

Growth of bacteria in different gaseous conditions

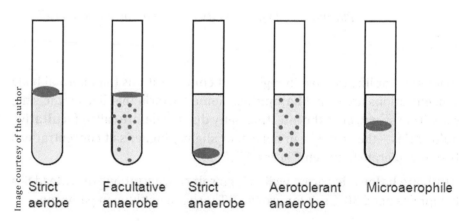

FIGURE 2.32   *Gaseous requirements of bacteria*

-Organic factors:

> *examples: amino acids, purines, etc.

Habitats for Human Pathogens: Extracellular vs. Intracellular Organisms

-**Intracellular organisms**: evade white blood cells by hiding in host cells, can only be affected by antibiotics that penetrate through host cell membranes (e.g., tetracycline). Can grow in host cells; usually dependent on host cell for energy

> -Usually cannot be grown in the laboratory on artificial culture media (e.g., *Chlamydia trachomatis*)

-**Extracellular organisms**: can be grown on artificial media. Possess machinery for production of own energy (e.g., *Staphylococcus aureus*)

-**Facultative intracellular organisms**: can invade and grow inside of host cells or outside of host cells (e.g., *Mycobacterium tuberculosis*)

Biofilms: Bacteria are NOT "Loners"

-It is now estimated that about 70%–80% of all human infections are associated with the production of "biofilms" in the body.

-Biofilms are communities of bacteria that are usually held together with a polysaccharide slime. Bacteria living in such a community produce chemical signals to communicate with other bacteria. This is called **quorum sensing**. A biofilm is a constantly changing structure—bacteria can leave the biofilm and go to seed a new infection somewhere else in the body.

-Bacteria in a specific biofilm can be all of the same kind or a mixture of many types of bacteria. Sometimes the makeup of a biofilm can change; a good example is dental plaque, where the early colonizers are Streptococci, and then later the anaerobic Gram negative bacteria enter the biofilm.

-Any artificial device implanted in the body is susceptible to biofilm formation and, if this occurs, presents a difficult situation for treatment that is usually resolved by removing the device surgically.

-It is thought that bacteria, by living in a community, reap benefits for their survival. They are resistant to white blood cells and antibiotics while in this biofilm. This presents challenges for treatment of infection.

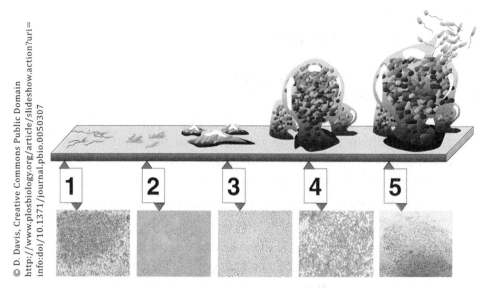

FIGURE 2.33   *Development and dynamics of a biofilm*

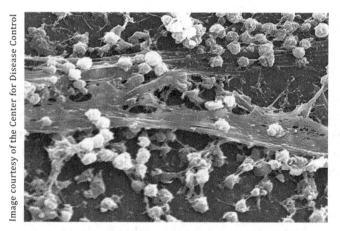

FIGURE 2.34   *Staphylococcus aureus biofilm on a catheter*

E. BACTERIAL REPRODUCTION AND GROWTH PHASES

-Bacteria normally reproduce by binary fission, where one cell divides into two identical clones.

Bacterial reproduction = binary fission

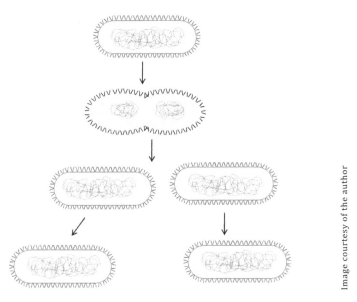

FIGURE 2.35   *Bacterial reproduction = binary fission*

-The factors affecting bacterial growth will have the same effect on bacterial reproduction:

E. coli generation time is ~20 minutes on optimal complex media at 37' °C, but ~60 minutes on simple media. *E. coli* is a member of the Enterobacteriaceae, also known as "coliforms."

TABLE 2.1   *Typical generation times in optimal conditions*

Bacterium	Growth Medium	Temperature (°C)	Generation Time (min)
Bacillus subtilis	Complex medium	36	35
Clostridium botulimum	Glucose broth	37	35
Eschrichia coli	Broth	37	17
Lactobacillus acidophilus	Milk	37	66
Mycobacterium tuberculosis	Synthetic medium	37	792
Pseudomonas aeruginosa	Glucose broth	37	31
Pseudomonas aeruginosa	Lactose broth	37	34
Pseudomonas aeruginosa	Tryptic meat broth	35	32
Shigella dysenteriae	Milk	37	23
Staphylococcus aureus	Glucose broth	37	32
Streptococcus latis	Lactose broth	30	48
Streptococcus latis	Glucose milk	37	26
Streptococcus latis	Peptone milk	37	37
Streptococcus pneumoniae	Glucose broth	37	30
Xanthomonas campestris	Glucose broth	25	74

From Philip L. Altman and David S. Dittmer, *Biology Data Book,* Volume 1. Copyright © 1972 Federation of American Societies for Experimental Biology. Reprinted by permission.

-Bacteria multiply so quickly that we have to use the logarithmic expression. For example, *E. coli* has a generation time of 20 minutes. In 24 hours. one cell would be 100,000,000,000,000,000,000,000 (1×10^{23}).

Bacterial Growth Phases

-The kinetics of bacterial growth in optimal conditions is known as the bacterial growth curve.

-This is important because the most rapidly dividing growth phase is the phase most susceptible to antibiotics.

-Growth phases are: lag, log, stationary, and death phase.

1. **Lag phase**: bacteria do not immediately start replicating; little or no cell division.

2. **Log phase**: cells begin to divide and enter logarithmic growth; most active metabolically in this phase.

3. **Stationary phase**: reproduction and number of cells slows.

4. **Death phase**: number of deaths exceeds the number of cells formed. Also called logarithmic decline phase.

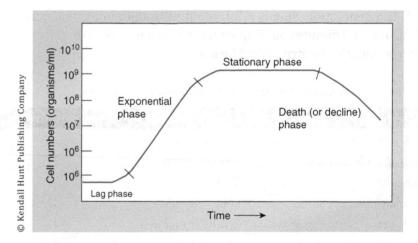

FIGURE 2.36   *Bacterial growth phases*

Culture of Microorganisms

-Need nutrient material; this may be solid, semisolid, or both.

-For culture of specimens, the nutrient medium should be sterile initially so growth of the applied specimen (inoculum) can be detected.

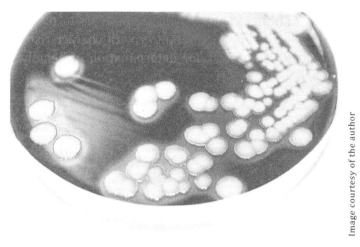

Image courtesy of the author

FIGURE 2.37 *Photomicrograph of Staphylococcus on blood agar*

-Usually use agar, a complex polysaccharide from algae, to provide the solid culture matrix in a small plastic dish called a Petri dish.

-Bacteria usually grow on agar surfaces as "colonies" or heaps of bacteria that originate from one bacterial cell.

-We have to know the growth requirements in order to successfully cultivate the bacteria we are interested in (e.g. *Haemophilus influenzae* needs haemin and nicotinamide adenine dinucleotide or NAD in the media before it will grow).

-In general, complex media with many nutrients, like Sheep Blood Agar (SBA), is used as a routine culture media in the routine hospital laboratory because most human pathogens grow best on this.

-Media for growth of anaerobic bacteria must be "reduced" (i.e., the oxygen removed) in order for the bacteria to grow (e.g., addition of sodium thioglycollate to the media). Culture must also be done in the absence of oxygen.

-Some bacteria need increased levels of CO_2 in order to grow (e.g., *Neisseria gonorrhoeae, Haemophilus influenzae*). The incubators used in the lab are perfused with 5% CO_2 and are usually kept at 37 °C.

Choosing a Medium for Isolation of Bacteria from a Clinical Specimen

-**Selective media**: suppress growth of unwanted bacteria and support growth of desired bacteria (e.g., bismuth sulfite agar for Salmonella from feces). This type of media is necessary when looking for a disease-producing bacterium (a pathogen) in a sample also containing a high number of normal bacterial species (normal flora).

-Differential media: ingredients in media allow us to tentatively identify bacterial species based on different growth characteristics with the medium (e.g., sheep blood agar for determination of hemolytic activity (*S. pyogenes* – beta-hemolysis)).

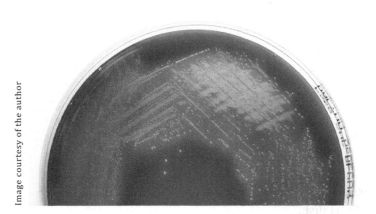

FIGURE 2.38a: Beta-hemolysis on blood agar

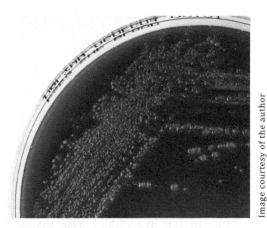

FIGURE 2.38b: Alpha-hemolysis on blood agar

-Laboratory media is often **both selective** and **differential** (e.g., xylose lysine deoxycholate agar for Salmonella—Gram positives are inhibited from growing, and Salmonella turn black on the agar while other bacteria do not).

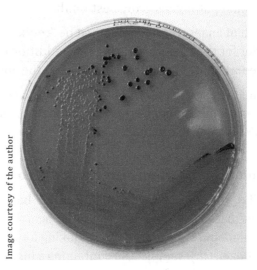

FIGURE 2.39   Salmonella on XLD agar

Interested? Want to learn more?

For more reading, several texts online at the U of A library are recommended:

1.   Brooks, GF, Carroll KC, Butel JS, Morse SA, editors. Jawetz, Melnick, and Adelberg's Medical Microbiology, 24th ed. Blacklick OH-McGraw Hill; 2007.

2.   Ryan KJ, Ray CG, editors. Sherris Medical Microbiology, 5th ed. New York – McGraw-Hill, 2010.

3.   Todar's Online Textbook of Bacteriology

http://www.textbookofbacteriology.net/

Chapter 3

Basic Virology

Learning Objectives:

1. Differentiate among bacteria, virus, and prions.
2. Describe the general structure of an enveloped and nonenveloped virus.
3. Understand how a virus replicates using a host cell.
4. Explain how a virus can be a causative agent for cancer.
5. Discriminate between active, latent, and chronic infections with virus.
6. Understand the pathogenic mechanism for prions, and give examples of prion diseases.

Introduction

VIRUSES ARE NOT LIVING CELLS!

-But they are infectious and can cause disease. Everyone has heard of viruses and viral diseases, but not everyone realizes that they are **different** from bacteria and their diseases, and that they must be treated with different types of chemotherapeutic agents.

-Most of the visits to the family practitioner for infectious disease are due to viral infections; it is important to be able to distinguish between viral and other infections in order to choose an appropriate treatment modality.

-Viruses are featured in the news on an almost daily basis, be it due to outbreaks of flu-like disease or pneumonia (Influenza, SARS), outbreaks of gastroenteritis (Norwalk, rotavirus), or the feared viral hemorrhagic fevers (Ebola, Lassa, dengue hemorrhagic fever).

-Viruses can be transmitted many different ways; the "mode of transmission" depends on the individual virus, its structure, and its ability to cause disease (pathogenicity). For example, poliovirus: its transmission is by the fecal–oral route from contaminated water as a reservoir or source. This virus is resistant to environmental conditions, and it can survive in an infectious state for extended periods of time.

-Hepatitis B and HIV, on the other hand, are easily inactivated by many disinfectants, by drying, and by adverse environmental conditions. The transmission of these latter two viruses is mainly by direct transfer from one person to another via blood transfusions or sexual contact.

-Many viruses are feared because they are easily transmitted to large groups of people (e.g., Influenza, SARS) and because the number of antiviral drugs that exist for treatment is limited. We do not yet have drugs available that are effective against all types of viral infections.

-Viruses are normally quite species specific. For example, the virus that causes the common cold can be fatal for other primates, yet a herpes virus that causes only mild disease in primates is deadly for humans (Herpes B). Dogs may contract distemper and parvovirus, which are not communicable to humans. On the other hand, there are viruses that can infect many different species. One example is rabies, an extremely fatal disease for humans as well as for animals.

-Some viruses can mutate quickly and, by mutating, adapt to other host species. World Health experts are always on the lookout for viruses that can "jump the species barrier" and quickly spread in the new hosts because the hosts lack effective immunity to these "new" viruses.

-Some viruses are **oncogenic** and can cause tumors by initiating cell transformation. Examples are EBV (Epstein-Barr virus), papillomavirus (wart virus), Hepatitis B (serum hepatitis), and HTLV-1 (a retrovirus). Transformation is the induction of inheritable changes in the way the cell grows and immortalization of the cell. This occurs when viruses disturb the normal cell control mechanisms involved in normal cell growth and replication.

In this chapter, we first address the basic biology of viruses (individual viruses can also be called **virions**) and use this knowledge to understand the mechanisms by which various viruses can cause disease, how some antiviral chemotherapeutic agents work, and in some cases why they do not work.

Comparison of Viruses and Bacteria

Virus	Bacteria
-10–500 nm	- ~500–2000 nm (much larger!)
-Multiply only inside of cells	-Most are free-living, multiply in the absence of other cells
-Contain DNA or RNA, never both	-Always contain DNA and RNA
-Few enzymes	-Many enzymes
-No ribosomes or enzymes for metabolizing nutrients	-Contain ribosomes and enzymes for metabolism of nutrients

Basic Structure of the Virus

1. **Size**

-Viruses are smaller than most bacteria. Electron microscopy is usually necessary to achieve the proper resolution to visualize these small particles.

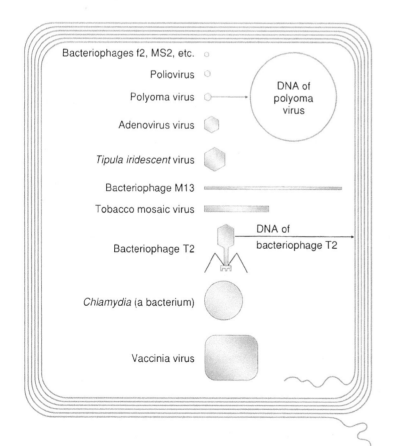
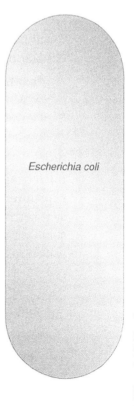

FIGURE 3.1   Relative sizes of different virions as compared to a bacterium

-Range in size: ~10 nm to 300 nm in diameter (1/10 of the size of most medically important bacteria).

2. **Composition of viruses**

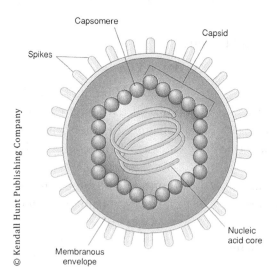

FIGURE 3.2   Basic structure of an enveloped virus

-Viruses have a core consisting of **RNA** or **DNA**, never both! Viruses can be divided into two major groups according to their nucleic acid composition.

-RNA or DNA in a virion can be either single stranded or double stranded; it can be in one piece or divided into many pieces or segments; it can be circular or linear.

> *example**: An example of a DNA virus is the Herpes simplex virus, which has a double strand of DNA (HSV-1 causes cold sores; HSV-2 causes genital herpes). An example of an RNA virus is the measles virus, which has a single strand of RNA.

-Viruses have a protein layer enclosing the RNA or DNA called a **capsid** or **nucleocapsid.** This protective coat is composed of protein molecules called **capsomeres**. The number of capsomeres can be used to classify viruses. The symmetrical arrangement of the proteins determines the shape of the virus—some are bullet shaped like the rabies virus, some are spherical like the Norwalk virus, some are helical like the Influenza virus, and some are icosahedral (20 sides or facets) like the Adenovirus.

-Shape can be used to identify viral entities because it is characteristic of individual viruses.

> *example**: An outbreak of a diarrheal disease on a cruise ship necessitates that fecal specimens be examined by electron microscopy to determine the cause of the outbreak. Often, caliciviruses, of which Norovirus is a well-known member, are responsible and appear as small icosahedral viral particles.

-Viruses may have an **"envelope"** surrounding the capsid. This envelope is usually comprised of a bilayer of phospholipids acquired from the host

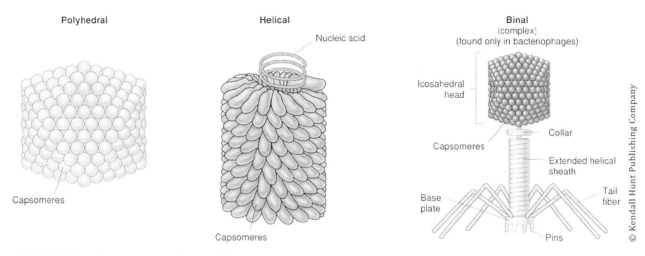

FIGURE 3.3   Common nucleocapsid structures

cell membrane when the newly formed viruses cleave off from the host cell. Envelopes can be altered by the virus and may contain spikes or glycoprotein projections that function in cellular attachment and recognition of binding sites on host cells. A nonenveloped virus will also have "spikes" or glycoprotein projections, but they will be anchored in the capsid.

> ***example**: Influenza A virus has two types of protein projections protruding out from its envelope: the **HA or haemagglutinin**, which attaches to the sialic acid receptors on red blood cells and cells lining the mucous membranes, and the **NA or neuraminidase**, which helps the virus exit from the host cell after replication. Influenza viruses can be typed according to the subtype of H and N antigens. The flu epidemic of 1918 that killed millions of people was due to a H1N1 strain of Influenza A.

Nomenclature

Viruses are grouped into families depending on:

a) Type of nucleic acid
b) Strategy for replication
c) Morphology

The characteristics of the genome are used for classification of viruses into a scheme called the Baltimore System. This new system coexists side by side with the traditional ICTV scheme, which was devised by the International Committee on Taxonomy of Viruses and is probably still more widely used.

A viral species is a group of viruses sharing the same genetic information and ecological niche.

> ***examples**: Herpes simplex virus 1   Human immunodeficiency virus (HIV)-1
>
> Herpes simplex virus 2   Human immunodeficiency virus (HIV)-2

There are 24 virus families that are recognized presently to infect vertebrates. You will not be expected to know all of the families, but you should be familiar with the viruses that are most important for human medicine. These will be highlighted in subsequent lectures.

The following table lists the viruses that most commonly cause infection in humans. *It is added for your reference and does not have to be memorized, but you should be able to recognize and identify the DNA viruses.*

Medically Relevant Viruses

DNA-CONTAINING

TABLE 3.1   *DNA-Containing Viruses*

DNA viruses	Genome	Enveloped?	Examples
Herpesviridae	DS DNA (icosahedral)	Yes	Herpes simplex
			Varicella zoster (chickenpox)
			Cytomegalovirus
			Epstein-Barr virus
Poxviridae	(ovoid)	Yes	Vaccinia (cowpox)
			Variola (smallpox)
			Molluscum contagiosum
Adenoviridae	DS DNA (icosahedral)	No	Upper respiratory tract and eye infections
Papovaviridae	DS DNA (icosahedral)	No	HPV (human papilloma virus = wart virus)
			Polyomavirus (JC virus)
Parvoviridiae	SS DNA (isosahedral)	No	B19 (Fifth Disease)
Hepadnavirus	Partially DS DNA (icosahedral)	Yes	Hepatitis B virus

TABLE 3.2   *RNA-containing viruses*

RNA viruses	Genome	Enveloped?	Examples
Picornaviridae	SS RNA + sense (icosahedral)	No	Enteroviruses such as poliovirus, Hepatitis A
			Rhinoviruses (colds)
Caliciviridae	SS RNA + sense (icosahedral)	No	Norwalk virus (gastroenteritis)
Astroviridae	SS RNA + sense (icosahedral)	No	Gastroenteritis
Togaviridae	SS RNA + sense (spherical)	Yes	Rubella

TABLE 3.2 *RNA-containing viruses—cont'd*

RNA viruses	Genome	Enveloped?	Examples
Flaviviridae	SS RNA + sense (spherical)	Yes	Hepatitis C Yellow fever and Dengue fever
Coronaviridae	SS RNA + sense (pleomorphic)	Yes	Common cold SARS
Paramyxoviridae	SS RNA, − sense (spherical)	Yes	Measles, mumps
Rhabdoviridae	(bacilliform)	Yes	Rabies
Filoviridae	(bacilliform)	Yes	Ebola virus
Orthomyxoviridae	SS RNA − sense (spherical, segmented)	Yes	Influenza A, B, C
Bunyaviridae	(amorphic, segmented)	Yes	Hantavirus
Arenaviridae	(spherical, segmented)	Yes	LCV (lymphocytic choriomeningitis virus)
Reoviridae	DS RNA (icosahedral, segmented)	No	Rotavirus
Retroviridae	SS RNA + sense (spherical)	Yes	HIV HTLV-1, HTLV-II

Why is it important to know if a virus is enveloped or nonenveloped?

Answer: Enveloped viruses are more easily inactivated by disinfectants than "naked" viruses (e.g., Hepatitis B and HIV are both enveloped viruses and can be easily inactivated by alcohols or bleach).

PROCESS OF VIRAL INFECTION

1. **Attachment and penetration**

-Attachment is often initially nonspecific, then followed by specific attachment to receptors on host cell. The affinity for specific cells or tissues can be called **"tropism."**

*example: Influenza virus attaches specifically to sialic acid residues on mucous membranes or red blood cells by means of its "hemagglutinin glycoprotein."

-Penetration into the host cell:

-Viral particles must either fuse with or cross the host cell membrane and are either phagocytosed or endocytosed by the host cell.

-Virus is carried into the cytoplasm of the host cell.

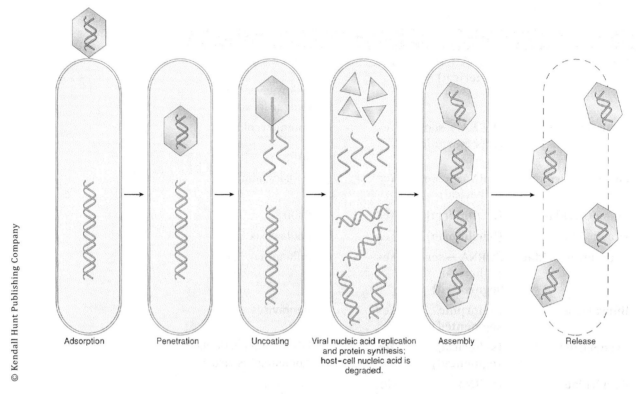

| Adsorption | Penetration | Uncoating | Viral nucleic acid replication and protein synthesis; host-cell nucleic acid is degraded. | Assembly | Release |

FIGURE 3.4   Generalized process for viral infection

-The envelope and/or capsid can either be removed during penetration of host cell membranes or after entry of the virus into a membrane-bound inclusion.

-Viral nucleic acids are released into the cell cytoplasm. Some viruses can replicate in the cytoplasm, but others dependent on using the host cell's enzymes will be transported into the nucleus for replication.

2. Replication of viruses in host cells

-Different viruses may have slightly different methods by which they replicate, according to their nucleic acid makeup.

Transcription

- Viral mRNA is produced unless the viral genome acts as mRNA directly (+ sense).

Translation

- Proteins are synthesized for the new virions from the mRNA.

Genome Replication

-Many copies of the genome are produced.

Assembly

New virus particles: nucleocapsids form around the DNA or RNA. The "instructions" for this procedure are contained in the genetic material of the virus itself.

Release

-Newly replicated virions are released by the cell. If virions are nonenveloped, they usually lyse the cell. Some enveloped viruses lyse the cell, but others do not and can cause chronic infections with a minimum of inflammation.

3. Transcription of viral genomes

-Different if DNA or RNA virus; DNA or RNA polymerases work to put together copies of the DNA or RNA.

-If DNA virus, host cell DNA polymerase is used directly to make more virus DNA. Replication usually happens in the host cell nucleus because this is where the DNA polymerase needed to produce a copy of the DNA is located. **Uses DNA-dependent DNA polymerase (usually provided by the host cell).**

-If RNA virus, virus must carry its own polymerase enzyme to produce mRNA, and this can happen in the cytoplasm of the host cell. **Uses RNA-dependent RNA polymerase (carried by the virus).**

-RNA retrovirus (e.g., HIV) carries its own reverse transcriptase enzyme in capsid, ss RNA is first made to ss DNA, then ds DNA is formed and integrates with host DNA in the chromosome.

Integrated viral DNA is then transcribed by the host cell polymerase and makes more virus mRNA. **Uses RNA-dependent DNA polymerase for making DNA from RNA.**

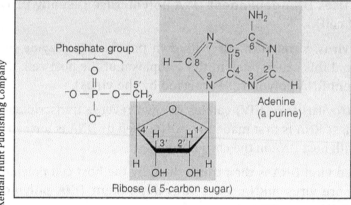

a. Pyrimidines

b. Purines

© Kendall Hunt Publishing Company

c. Nucleotide

FIGURE 3.5   *Nucleic acids involved in the structure of DNA and RNA*

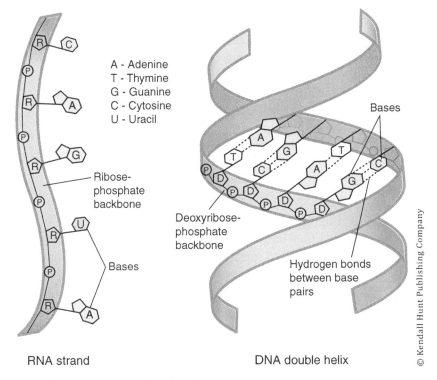

A - Adenine
T - Thymine
G - Guanine
C - Cytosine
U - Uracil

Ribose-
phosphate
backbone

Bases

Deoxyribose-
phosphate
backbone

Bases

Hydrogen bonds
between base
pairs

RNA strand

DNA double helix

© Kendall Hunt Publishing Company

FIGURE 3.6   *RNA vs. DNA molecules*

Generation of mRNA by viruses

-mRNA is the molecule responsible for the synthesis of proteins in the cell.

*   **DNA viruses**

    DNA viruses (ss and ds) replicate their DNA genome using **DNA-dependent DNA polymerase**.

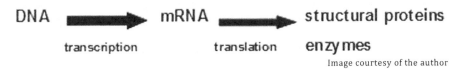

DNA ⟶ mRNA ⟶ structural proteins
      transcription   translation   enzymes

Image courtesy of the author

FIGURE 3.7   *DNA-directed protein synthesis*

- **DNA reverse transcribing viruses (e.g., Hepatitis B)**

  -These viruses have a partially double-stranded DNA genome. First, a completely double-stranded DNA genome is made then transcribed by host cell DNA-dependent RNA polymerase to generate both mRNA and an RNA replicative intermediate. The RNA copy of the genome is then reverse transcribed to DNA by a *virally encoded reverse transcriptase.* The scheme for replication can be simplified to **DNA → RNA → DNA**.

- **RNA viruses**

  Viruses with ds RNA (double-stranded RNA) transcribe their genomes into mRNA in much the same way that the ds DNA viruses do except that they use an **RNA-dependent RNA polymerase**. This enzyme is also used to replicate the RNA genome.

  Viruses with ss RNA are either "positive" or "negative" sense. Positive sense ss RNA can be used as mRNA and directly translated to produce viral proteins. Negative sense ss RNA must first be transcribed to yield positive sense mRNA by RNA-dependent RNA polymerase before any viral proteins can be translated.

  In all RNA viruses, the genomes are transcribed by use of **RNA-dependent RNA polymerase**, which is always encoded for by the virus itself.

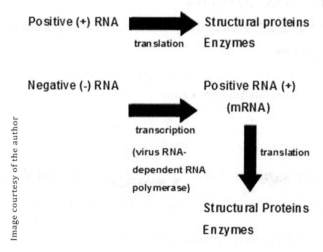

FIGURE 3.8   Protein synthesis pathways in positive and negative sense viruses

- **RNA reverse transcribing viruses**

  These viruses are called "retroviruses," and a very well-known example is HIV (Human Immunodeficiency Virus) replicate through a DNA intermediate. After entry into the host cell, the ss RNA virus is transcribed to generate a DNA–RNA hybrid intermediate using a virally coded **RNA-dependent DNA polymerase (reverse transcriptase).** The RNA is then digested away and is replaced by a DNA copy. Viral mRNAs and progeny genomes are generated using DNA-dependent RNA polymerase. Retroviruses can incorporate the viral DNA into the host cell chromosome, thereby ensuring that every time the DNA is transcribed in the host, copies of the virus will also be transcribed. Virus in this form is usually called a "**provirus**" and is a latent form.

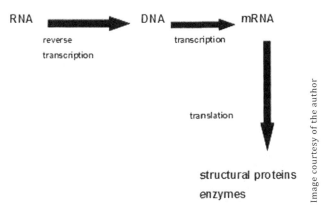

FIGURE 3.9 *Protein synthesis directed by RNA retroviruses*

Summary of viral genome replication:

DNA viruses use **DNA polymerase,** either host derived or virally derived for replication of genome.

DNA → DNA

RNA viruses use **RNA-dependent RNA polymerase** for replication of genome.

RNA → RNA

Viruses using reverse transcription:

DNA viruses (e.g., Hepatitis B)

DNA → RNA → DNA

RNA viruses (e.g., HIV)

RNA → DNA → RNA

4. **Translation (protein synthesis)**

Translation of mRNA to Proteins

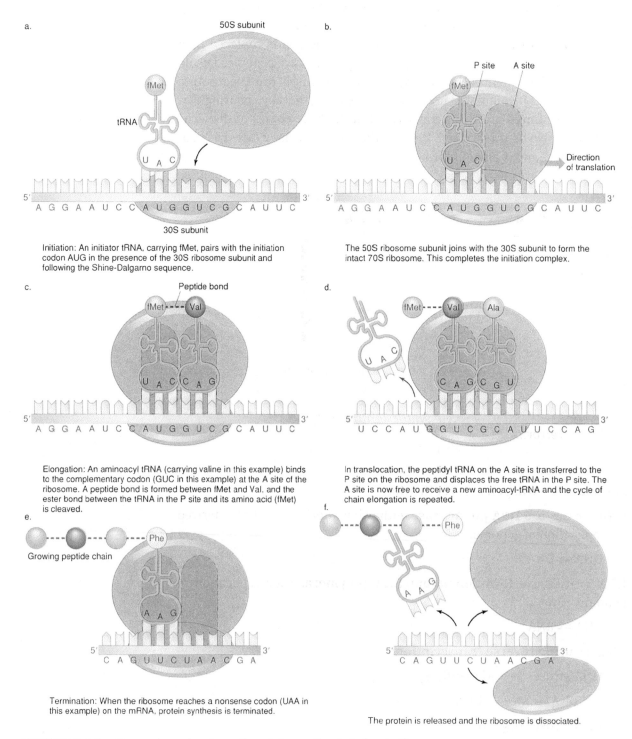

a. **Initiation:** An initiator tRNA, carrying fMet, pairs with the initiation codon AUG in the presence of the 30S ribosome subunit and following the Shine-Dalgarno sequence.

b. The 50S ribosome subunit joins with the 30S subunit to form the intact 70S ribosome. This completes the initiation complex.

c. **Elongation:** An aminoacyl tRNA (carrying valine in this example) binds to the complementary codon (GUC in this example) at the A site of the ribosome. A peptide bond is formed between fMet and Val, and the ester bond between the tRNA in the P site and its amino acid (fMet) is cleaved.

d. In translocation, the peptidyl tRNA on the A site is transferred to the P site on the ribosome and displaces the free tRNA in the P site. The A site is now free to receive a new aminoacyl-tRNA and the cycle of chain elongation is repeated.

e. **Termination:** When the ribosome reaches a nonsense codon (UAA in this example) on the mRNA, protein synthesis is terminated.

f. The protein is released and the ribosome is dissociated.

FIGURE 3.10   *General mechanism of protein synthesis in host ribosomes*

-Vertebrate viruses generally follow the rule of "one mRNA = one protein" (**monocistronic**), and many of the viruses produce several mRNAs, depending on the number of proteins that need to be synthesized. In order for translation to occur from mRNA, poly A (AAA) must be added to the 3' end of the molecule, and a cap to the 5' end.

-A few viruses produce only one mRNA but translate a large polyprotein with embedded **protease** enzymes allowing the cleavage of the larger protein to separate into fully functional smaller proteins. Viruses like HIV and herpes use both strategies and produce both polyproteins and single proteins. These protease enzymes, as well as reverse transcriptase enzymes, have been used as targets for antiviral agents.

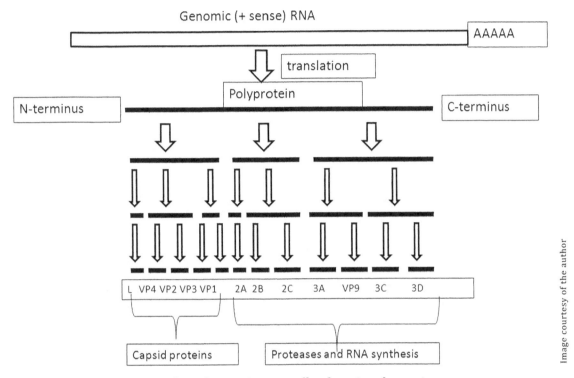

FIGURE 3.11   *Cleavage of a polyprotein to smaller functional proteins*

Why are some viruses more prone to mutation than others?

-Virally coded RNA polymerases have a much higher "error rate" than the host cell DNA polymerase because they lack the "proofreading ability" of DNA viruses and thus introduce more errors or mutations into the genome. (This results in a constantly changing viral genome and the production of "quasi"-species. This rapid mutation can be used as a strategy for evading immune defences because the immune system will not immediately recognize the new viral genome.)

Lytic and Persistent Infections

In persistent infections, the release of viruses (often enveloped) does not usually harm the host cell, and as a result, the host cell can produce or "shed" the virus for long periods of time (chronic infections; e.g., Hepatitis B).

In lytic infections, the outcome of viral infection is death of the host cell (e.g., poliovirus).

Latent Infection:

-Virus is present in cells but is not replicating until triggered by external factor. The host has earlier been infected with a virus, which, after the disease or infection was under control, hides in various body cells in an inactive form. This form can be reactivated by many stressors, and we do not understand the mechanism well.

> *****example**: Herpes simplex type 1 triggered by stress, sunlight, or other infections
>> Herpes simplex type 2 triggered by stress, hormone fluctuation, etc. HIV triggered by antigenic stimulation caused by an infection of another kind.

Virus–Host Interactions

1. **Productive**: the virus replicates and produces many copies. These infections often kill the host cell, and when this occurs, the infection is termed a **lytic** infection. An example is adenovirus.

2. **Latent**: the viral genome persists in the host cell in a nonreplicative form, so no infectious virus is present, but viral genomes can reactivate and produce infectious progeny. Herpes viruses are an example of viruses that can establish latency. An example is varicella zoster, which causes shingles.

3. **Chronic**: the virus replicates without causing massive cell lysis and persists in the host for extended periods of time, sometimes a lifetime. An example of a virus that can establish such a persistent infection is Hepatitis B.

Isolation and Identification of Virus in the Laboratory

-Grown in cell culture or in embryonated eggs

-Identified by structure using electron microscopy or by function (type of proteins produced), effect on cell culture also called cytopathic effect or **CPE** (lysis of cells, formation of "plaques"), or identification of the RNA or DNA by PCR (polymerase chain reaction)

-Some viruses do not grow "in vitro," only "in vivo"

Bacteriophages

-Viruses that infect bacterial cells and can transfer new genes from one bacteria to another (in the case of *C. diphtheriae*, a gene for toxin production is transferred from the harmless bacterium to the pathogen).

-These can be used for "genetic engineering."

> *****example**: production of porcine insulin from *E. coli* bacteria after insertion of a gene for insulin production using a bacteriophage to carry that gene from cell to cell

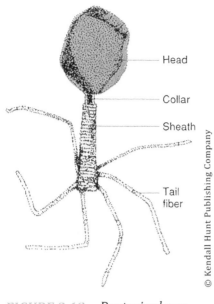

- Head
- Collar
- Sheath
- Tail fiber

© Kendall Hunt Publishing Company

FIGURE 3.12   *Bacteriophage structure*

Disease: The Effect of Viral Infection

-production of specific disease entities (e.g., chickenpox, herpes, measles, mumps, hepatitis)

-Transmission could be air-borne (hanging indefinitely on very tiny droplet nuclei), inhaled droplets from a cough or sneeze (large droplets—travel only about a meter, then drop), in food and water (fecal–oral), direct transfer from other infected hosts, or bites of arthropod vectors.

-Infection may be persistent and result in many asymptomatic carriers or can become latent and reactivate at a later time.

Cancer

-Some viruses can "transform" host cells to cancer cells (oncogenic).

-Not all "transformed" cells become cancerous (i.e., Human papillomavirus—benign tumour with cutaneous warts).

-Cancer-producing viruses can be RNA or DNA viruses.

Common Methods Used in the Clinical Virology Laboratory

1. EM (electron microscopy)

A direct method that has earlier been used extensively for the visualization or detection of viral particles in biological specimens such as stool uses electron microscopy. Viruses are identified by their structures and sizes.

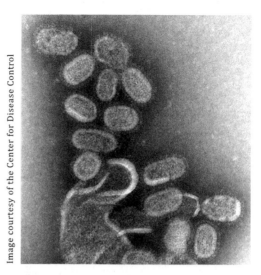

Image courtesy of the Center for Disease Control

FIGURE 3.13   Electron microscopic image of virus particles

2. Hemagglutination tests

a. For virus detection:

-This is based on the principle that certain viruses have H glycoproteins that attach to sialic acid moieties on cells. Red blood cells (RBC) have sialic acid residues. Mixing virus with red blood cells results in binding with a lattice structure forming. This web settles eventually as a diffuse layer in the bottom of a tube: the diffuse pattern represents a positive test.

-The same principle can be used directly on a cell culture that has been inoculated with a patient specimen thought to contain virus particles (of viruses with the H glycoprotein): RBC are added to the cell culture, and if the virus is present, then the RBC will clump on the host cells that contain the virus. This is a common way to tell if there is virus in a cell culture—the cell culture will, if positive, then be tested with other more specific tests to confirm the identity of the virus (like fluorescent antibody techniques).

b. For antibody detection:

-Virus is adsorbed to the surface of the indicator red blood cells. If antibodies are present in the serum, then a lattice structure forms, and the pattern is a diffuse one on the bottom of the tube.

c. For antibody detection (a neutralization assay):

-Patient serum is mixed with inactivated virus and then mixed with RBC. If the patient serum contains antibodies, then these antibodies will neutralize the virus, and there will be nothing to react with the RBC, so these plummet to the bottom of the tube in a button (no lattice structure is a positive test for the presence of antibody).

3. Growth in tissue cell culture

-Patient specimens are treated and incubated on a monolayer of immortalized cells, then observed for growth over a period of days to weeks. There is no one type of cell that can be used to detect all viruses; therefore, a variety of different cell types are generally used for each type of biological specimen according to the expected types of viral pathogens. Detection of viral growth can be done by visually inspecting the cell monolayer after an interval of time (usually not before 1–2 days of incubation). Each type of virus will have characteristic patterns of cell disruption or alteration—**CPE** or **cytopathic** effects (e.g., rounding of cells in the culture or the formation of giant cells).

-Suspected positive cultures may then be tested using a variety of methods to identify the viral type (e.g., hemagglutination, direct fluorescent antibody).

4. DFA (direct fluorescence antibody) test

-A rapid method often used in the clinical laboratory when a quick result is needed to determine patient care and/or infectiousness. With this method, a smear of the biological specimen (e.g., nasopharyngeal aspirate or material scraped from a blister) is spread on microscope slide. After fixation to ensure that the material will stays on the slide, the slide is stained with a monoclonal antibody conjugated with FITC (fluorescein isothiocyanate). If the monoclonal antibody specifically binds to the virus-infected cells and the virus particles, a green fluorescence is seen in the UV-microscope. This method is commonly used for the diagnosis of RSV in small children and

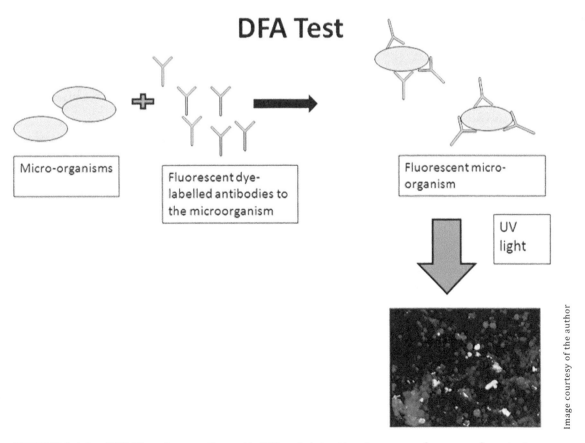

Image courtesy of the author

FIGURE 3.14   *RSV (Respiratory Syncytial Virus) detection in a nasopharyngeal aspirate*

can also be used for the presumptive diagnosis of Influenza, herpes, and other pathogens. It is rapid and **very** useful for the clinician.

-Areas where virus is located should be apple-green. Background cells are red.

4. EIA (enzyme immunoassay) (sometimes called ELISA or enzyme-linked immunosorbent assay)

-Several different types of EIA procedures can be used for detection of virus. In most of the analytical procedures, monoclonal antibodies are attached to the wells of 96 well plastic plates, specimen or culture supernatant is added, and the mixture is incubated. A reaction can be measured if a marker has been added to the system that will react with a substrate system if present and be read as a change in color. This type of system can be made more specific by employing a double-sandwich technique (e.g., monoclonal IgM antibodies specific for a virus are first bound on a plastic surface). This technique is called "IgM capture assay," Specimen is added and, if the virus is present, binds to the bound IgM antibody. Another antibody specific to the virus is added and will bind, creating a

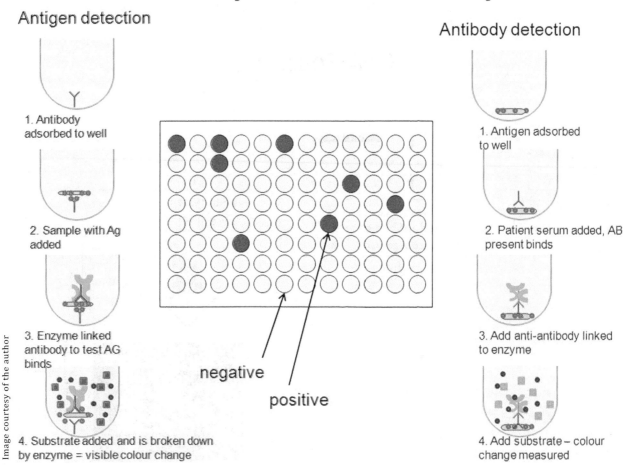

EIA = Enzyme Immunoassay

Antigen detection

1. Antibody adsorbed to well

2. Sample with Ag added

3. Enzyme linked antibody to test AG binds

4. Substrate added and is broken down by enzyme = visible colour change

negative

positive

Antibody detection

1. Antigen adsorbed to well

2. Patient serum added, AB present binds

3. Add anti-antibody linked to enzyme

4. Add substrate – colour change measured

Image courtesy of the author

FIGURE 3.15   EIA technique

"sandwich." This complex can be detected by labeling the second antibody with an enzyme, and upon the introduction of the specific substrate for this enzyme, a color reaction is produced. This can be read in a spectrophotometer and the relative concentration of virus particles in the original specimen calculated from the intensity of color development. These types of tests are commonly used to test for the presence of Hepatitis and HIV virus.

-EIA can also be modified for detection of patient antibodies to viruses. Virus is bound to the plastic, then patient sera are added to the system.

5. Nucleic acid assays

-There are many different types of nucleic acid assays on the market for the detection of microorganisms, and one of the most commonly used is the PCR or polymerase chain reaction. This test will detect the presence of the microbial genome if present in a sample. PCR is used to detect DNA genomes and RT-PCR is used for detection of RNA genomes. Advantages of these methods are that they are very sensitive and specific, although they detect both living and nonliving organisms. A further advantage is that if a virus such as Hepatitis C is detected, the genome can then further be sequenced to confirm the identity of the virus and to provide a subtype to the clinician, who can guide antiviral therapy (e.g., subtype 1 is less susceptible to antivirals).

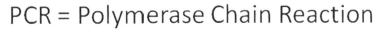

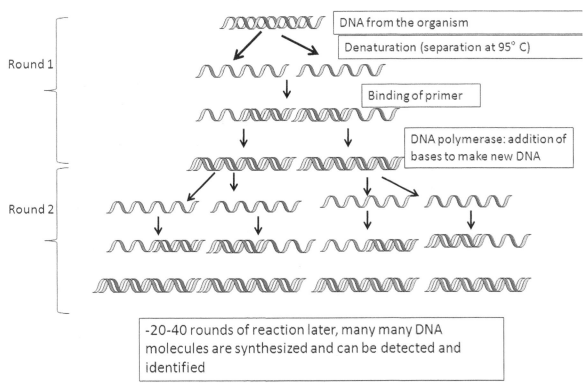

Image courtesy of the author

FIGURE 3.16   Polymerase chain reaction

6. **Western Blot confirmation of antibody specificity** (e.g., used in HIV diagnostics)

Protein antigens extracted from the virus are separated electrophoretically based on their molecular charge, and patient serum is allowed to react with the separated proteins. If the patient has specific antibodies to the viral proteins, a band will appear after staining.

*examples: HIV diagnostics

- Laboratory diagnosis of HIV infection is done by either testing for antibodies to the HIV-1 virus or by detecting the HIV-1 virus by nucleic acid detection (e.g., RT-PCR). Viral load is important for disease staging.

- Routinely, serum from patients is tested for antibodies to p24, a protein associated with the core of the virus, and if a positive result is obtained by EIA, then a confirmation is commonly done by doing "Western Blotting."

- Bands of HIV-antigen combined with anti-HIV-antibody at the p24, gp41, gp120, and sometimes the gp160 molecular weight positions are diagnostic of infection.

- Confirmation of a positive antibody test for HIV-1 usually requires the presence of three of these antigens in the patient sera.

PRIONS

-Prion = proteinaceous infectious particle

-Defined as late as 1982 by Stanley Prusiner

-Not virus—in separate class for itself—not a living organism or cell, just a protein molecule that is dysfunctional due to being improperly folded.

-Normal proteins are synthesized in long chains of amino acids, then they fold together to eventually produce a 3D structure where the binding sites are located. In prion proteins, the folding doesn't function properly, and the misfolded proteins are deposited as alpha-helixes instead of a 3D structure.

-These 'prion' protein molecules act as infectious agents in susceptible exposed animals and cause fatal disease (e.g., Mad Cow Disease or BSE (bovine spongiform encephalopathy), scrapie in sheep, kuru in N. Guinea as result of cannibalism).

-Mode of infection is direct transmission, often ingestion of foodstuffs contaminated with prion proteins.

-The prion protein is designated PrP^{sc} (normal cells have a similar protein, PrP^c).

-If an abnormal prion protein enters a cell, it changes a normal protein to an abnormal protein, resulting in the accumulation of abnormal protein.

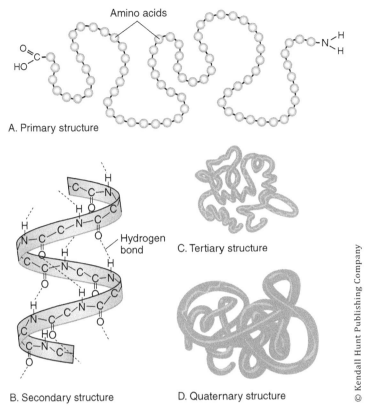

A. Primary structure

B. Secondary structure

C. Tertiary structure

D. Quaternary structure

Hydrogen bond

Amino acids

© Kendall Hunt Publishing Company

FIGURE 3.17   Normal folding of proteins

-These abnormal proteins get deposited in the brain of affected animals and can be used for diagnosis at postmortem (no test while animal is living).

-No treatment for the diseases is caused by prions.

-Prions are very hard to destroy and tolerate formalin and some autoclaving and chemicals.

Interested? Want to learn more?

For more reading, several texts online at the U of A library are recommended:

1. Brooks, GF, Carroll KC, Butel JS, Morse SA, editors. Jawetz, Melnick, and Adelberg's Medical Microbiology, 24th ed. Blacklick OH-McGraw Hill; 2007.

2. Ryan KJ, Ray CG, editors. Sherris Medical Microbiology, 5th ed. New York – McGraw-Hill, 2010.

3. Norkin C. Virology: Molecular Biology and Pathogenesis. ASM Press, 2010.

Chapter 4

Basic Mycology

Learning Objectives:

1. Differentiate fungi from bacteria; identify fungi as eukaryotes.
2. Identify fungal components that can be used as a target for antifungal therapy.
3. Describe the characteristics of dimorphic fungi.
4. Define three types of fungal infections (superficial, cutaneous, systemic).
5. Define opportunistic, and give examples of opportunistic infections.

Fungi That Cause Human Disease

Note that the treatment of septate and nonseptate fungi is different, and this is one of the details that clinicians think important when they choose an appropriate drug for treatment.

-Fungi are increasingly important as nosocomial (hospital-acquired) infections and as infections of immunocompromised. Only few are primary pathogens causing disease even in healthy immunocompetent individuals.

-Fungi have many beneficial functions in nature, decomposition of plant matter, symbiotic interactions with plant roots, breakdown of cellulose, and also some development into edible mushrooms. We can use certain yeast species as leavening agent for bread.

-Fungi differ from bacteria in that they are eukaryotes, contain sterols, and have no peptidoglycan in cell walls. They do have chitin in their cell walls, and we can use this to stain them with calcofluor white (fungi in a direct clinical specimen will fluoresce).

-Fungi contain sterols in the cytoplasmic membrane because they are eukaryotes but **ergosterol** instead of **cholesterol** like we have in our plasma membranes. This is important to know for the treatment of the microorganism. Amphotericin B is one of the main antifungal drugs—this forms a complex with the ergosterol in the plasma membrane and causes the formation of pores or channels, allowing cell lysis to occur.

-Identification in the laboratory: yeasts are routinely identified on the basis of biochemical tests in a similar manner to bacteria; multicellular fungi are identified on the basis of appearance and structure and how they grow. Molecular diagnostics have been slow to reach the mycology laboratory, but some molecular tests are now starting to be used (e.g., PCR or polymerase chain reaction where you search for a specific chunk of DNA that identifies the species).

Three types of fungi to remember

    a. **Molds**

    b. **Yeasts**

    c. **Dimorphic fungi**

A. MOLDS

-Body of fungus is called a **thallus**, consists of long filaments called **hyphae** joined together in a mass (may look like a white mat on moldy fruit).

-**Septa**: most hyphae have cross walls, which divide them into distinct cell units with a single nucleus. These hyphae are called **septate hyphae**.

-A few fungi have hyphae that are not septate; these are called **coenocytic hyphae**.

-**Vegetative hyphae**: portion of hyphae that absorbs nutrients.

-**Reproductive or aerial hyphae**: part that projects above the surface and may have structures responsible for reproduction.

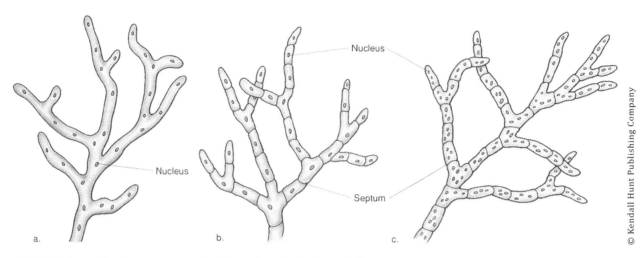

FIGURE 4.1   *Hyphae: coenocytic (a) and septate (b and c)*

B. YEASTS

-Nonfilamentous, unicellular fungi; usually oval or spherical

-Reproduce by budding (bud eventually breaks away from parent cell)

-If buds fail to detach, get formation of pseudohyphae (e.g., *Candida albicans* may attach to epithelial cells as a yeast but invades deeper through the tissues by means of pseudohyphae)

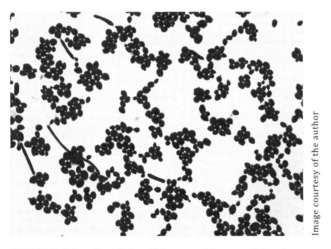

FIGURE 4.2   *Candida albicans with pseudohyphae*

-Most are capable of facultative anaerobic growth—important for invasiveness (e.g., *Saccharomyces* species produce ethanol for wine making)

-Some yeasts produce a polysaccharide capsule (e.g., *Cryptococcus neoformans*)

Cryptococcus neoformans: This yeast is often found in pigeon droppings and is dispersed in the environment. Individuals with leukemia and other immune disorders are at risk for chronic meningitis due to this organism.

The yeast produces a polysaccharide capsule useful for identification of the yeast in body fluids. A drop of cerebral spinal fluid is placed on a glass slide, and then a drop of India Ink is added. Examination in a microscope will show a halo around the yeast cell (where the capsule prevents the ink from penetrating to the cell wall).

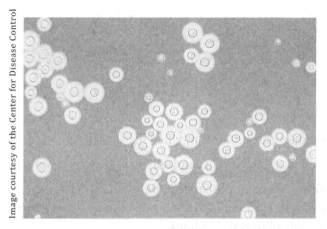

Image courtesy of the Center for Disease Control

FIGURE 4.3 *Cryptococcus neoformans in India Ink*

Recently a new species of Cryptococcus, *C. gatti,* has been found to cause serious disease, especially pneumonia on Vancouver Island and along the coastal mainland, over an area stretching from Oregon all the way up the BC coastline. This species of Cryptococcus has newly emerged in Canada as a pathogen. It was known to exist in Australia but has now made its way over the Pacific Ocean by unknown means.

C. DIMORPHIC FUNGI

-Two forms of growth can grow as a mold or as a yeast depending on temperature, so we say that dimorphism is temperature dependent (e.g., *Histoplasma capsulatum, Coccidioides immitis, Blastomyces dermatiditis, Sporothrix schenkii,* etc.)

Sporothrix schenckii is a dimorphic fungus that causes "Rose Gardener's Disease." It lives on rose thorns and in hay, moss, and wood and infects the skin when a puncture occurs (hence the name of the disease). A black necrotic lesion often develops at the site of inoculation, and the inflammation often progresses along the lymphatics, causing lymphangitis.

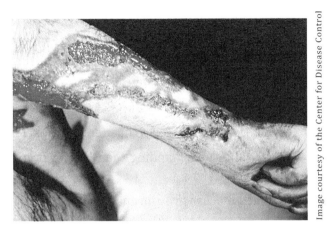

Image courtesy of the Center for Disease Control

FIGURE 4.4   Lymphangitis caused by Sporothrix

The geographical distribution of this dimorphic is widespread, and epidemics have occurred in the United States (in 1988 there were 84 people in 15 different states that were infected after handling sphagnum moss).

Fungal Reproduction

-Both sexual and asexual reproduction occur.

-Most filamentous fungi reproduce asexually by fragmentation of hyphae.

-Spore appearance is often used as a method of visually identifying the filamentous fungi.

-Fungal spores are very different from bacterial spores—bacterial spores are only for the protection of the organism from adverse environments, but fungal spores are for reproduction.

-Spores can be asexual or sexual.

-Asexual spores are formed by hyphae.

-Sexual spores result from the fusion of two spores to form a zygote.

Asexual Spores

*example: conidiospore of Aspergillus species

Sexual Spores

-Three phases of sexual reproduction:

1. Plasmogamy: haploid nucleus of one cell penetrates the cytoplasm of the recipient cell.

2. Karyogamy: nuclei fuse to form a diploid zygote nucleus.

3. Meiosis: diploid nucleus gives rise to haploid nuclei.

Fungal Nutrition

-Fungi are chemoheterotrophs—absorb nutrients like bacteria.

-Fungi are less nutritionally demanding than bacteria; grow better than bacteria in extreme conditions.

-Most are aerobic, but some can grow in anaerobic conditions (e.g., *Candida albicans*).

-Most grow best at 25°–30 °C

Fungal Diseases

-All fungal infections are called mycoses (plural) or mycosis (singular).

Types of mycoses:

A. **Superficial mycoses**: fungal infection along surface of hair shafts and outer layer of skin

   - Mild infections

   *examples: Black and white piedra (hairs of scalp)

   Tinea versicolor caused by *Malezessia furfur* (yeast)

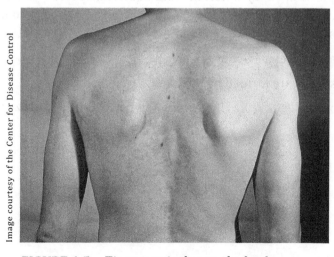

Image courtesy of the Center for Disease Control

FIGURE 4.5   Tinea versicolor on the back

B. **Cutaneous mycoses**: fungal infection of deeper layers of the epidermis (e.g., ringworm and athlete's foot. **Note: ringworm is not a worm!**)

-Caused by fungi called dermatophytes (produce keratinase and degrade keratinocytes in the outer layer of skin).

-Clinical diseases are called the "tineas" (i.e., tinea cruris = ringworm of the groin; tinea pedis = ringworm of the feet).

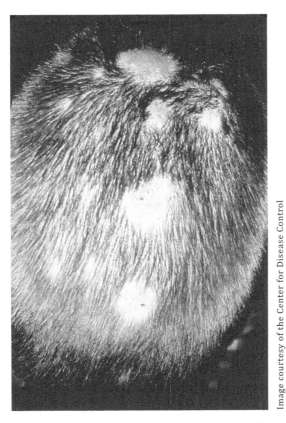

Image courtesy of the Center for Disease Control

FIGURE 4.6 **Tinea capitis:** *ringworm of the head and scalp*

Tinea pedis:	athlete's foot
Tinea corporis:	ringworm on the body surface
Tinea barbae:	ringworm of the hair follicles in the beard
Tinea cruris:	ringworm of the groin (also called jock itch)
Tinea unguium:	ringworm of the nails

-Causative fungi for the dermatophytic infections can belong to any of the following three genera:

    a. Microsporum

    b. Trichophyton

    c. Epidermophyton

C. **Systemic mycoses**: infections in deep tissues (organs)

-Caused by primary pathogens (e.g., *Histoplasma capsulatum, Coccidioides immitis, Sporothrix schenckii, Penicillium marneffei, Paracoccioides brasiliensis,* etc.)

or by opportunistic fungi (e.g., *Candida albicans* and *Aspergillus species*)

Fungi as Opportunistic Pathogens:

-Opportunistic pathogens are common causes of infections in immuno-compromised individuals

1. **Aspergillosis**: often caused by *Aspergillis niger*, infects people with debilitating lung diseases and immunocompromised individuals. Often cause granulomas and may appear as fungal "balls" in the lung tissue

2. **Candidiasis**: *Candida albicans* causative agent; vulvovaginal candidiasis and thrush; occurs in newborns, the immunocompromised, or people who have been treated with antibiotics. This yeast is part of the normal flora of the intestines.

3. **Mucor** infection: often associated with diabetes

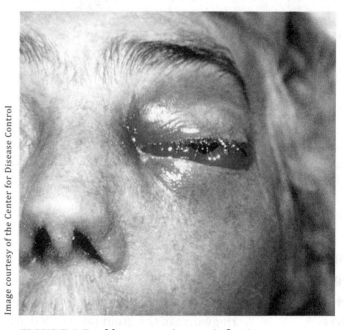

Image courtesy of the Center for Disease Control

FIGURE 4.7   Mucor species eye infection

Treatment of Fungal Infections:

-Antifungal agents have some problems with toxicity due to the fungi being eukaryotes. Amphotericin B has been the most commonly used systemic drug due to relatively minor side effects.

-The major problem with treatment of fungal infections is to ensure adequate penetration of the antifungal drug to the site of infection. Lengthy treatment is often necessary (months rather than days).

-Immunocompromised individuals are a special problem for treatment because unless you have a good functioning immune system, you will not be able to clear an infection easily. It is the combined actions of the immune system and the antimicrobial agent that cure a disease.

Interested? Want to learn more?

For more reading, several texts online at the U of A library are recommended:

1. Brooks, GF, Carroll KC, Butel JS, Morse SA, editors. Jawetz, Melnick, and Adelberg's Medical Microbiology, 24th ed. Blacklick OH-McGraw Hill; 2007.

2. Ryan KJ, Ray CG, editors. Sherris Medical Microbiology, 5th ed. New York – McGraw-Hill, 2010.

Chapter 5

Basic Parasitology

Learning Objectives:

1. Differentiate between protozoa and metazoa.

2. Describe how different parasitic organisms cause disease in humans, and list the organisms causing specific diseases.

3. Identify some commonly occurring ectoparasitic infections and their causes.

4. Describe the epidemiology of parasitic infections.

Three major categories of human parasites:

Protozoa

Metazoa

Ectoparasites

TABLE 5.1   *Medically Important Protozoa*

Site	Species	Transmission	Disease
Intestinal tract	1. *Entamoeba histolytica*	Ingestion of cysts in food, water	1. Amoebiasis
	2. *Giardia lamblia*		2. Giardiasis
	3. *Cryptosporidium* sp.		3. Cryptosporidiosis
Eye	Acanthamoeba	Cysts in dust, invade damaged eye	Acanthamoebiasis
Urogenital tract	*Trichomonas vaginalis*	Sexual (direct)	Trichomoniasis
Blood and tissue	1. Trypanosoma spp.		
	a. *T. cruzi*	a. reduviid bug	a. Trypanosomiasis, Chaga's disease
	b. *T. gambiense*	b. tsetse fly	
	c. *T. rhodesiense*	c. tsetse fly	b. + c. Sleeping sickness
	2. Leishmania spp.	a. sand fly	a. Visceral leishmaniasis (kala-azar)
	a. *L donovani*	b. sand fly	
	b. *L. tropica, L. mexicana*	c. sand fly	b + c. Cutaneous and mucocutaneous leishmaniasis
	c. *L. braziliensis*		
Blood and tissue	*Toxoplasma gondii*	Ingestion of cysts in raw meat, soil with cat feces	Toxoplasmosis
Blood and tissue	Plasmodium spp.	Anopheles	Malaria
	P. vivax P. malariae	Mosquito	
	P. ovale P. falciparum		
	P. knowlesii		

1. Medically Important Protozoa

Protozoa: one-celled eukaryotes

-Four categories of protozoa according to their appearance and structure:

1. Archaezoa (e.g., Giardia)
2. Microspora (e.g., Cryptosporidium)
3. Ameobozoa (e.g., Entamoeba)
4. Apicomplexa (e.g., Plasmodium)

- Most reproduce asexually by fission, budding, or schizogony (multiple fission where the nucleus undergoes several divisions before the cell divides).
- Some can reproduce sexually, by formation of gametes (haploid sex cells) (i.e., Plasmodium sp.).
- Some protozoa have a **cyst** form, used to protect the organism from inhospitable environments. Growing form: **trophozoite.**
- Cyst form may also be called an **oocyst** in apicomplexa (e.g., crypto-sporidium).
- Protozoans are mostly aerobic, but some can metabolize anaerobically.

Entamoeba histolytica: causative agent of amoebic dysentery; invasive

-Fecal–oral transmission; ingestion of cysts (cyst wall breaks down in the cut, releasing the trophozoite form, which is actively invasive and can penetrate the intestine)

-Can also be transmitted sexually by trophozoite form, from mucous membrane to mucous membrane

-Only pathogenic amoeba found in the human intestine; need to differentiate from apathogenic species, which may look the same

-Primary food is the red blood cell; feeds on mucus (intestine), which causes ulcer formation

-Known to cause "flask-shaped ulcers",—broad based with small top portion

-Can exist as both trophozoite and cyst in humans

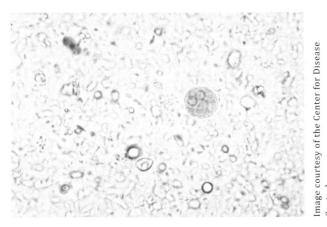

Image courtesy of the Center for Disease Control

FIGURE 5.1   Entamoeba histolytica cyst in a fecal concentrate

-Relatively resistant to chlorine

-Treat with metronidazole or antiparasitic drugs

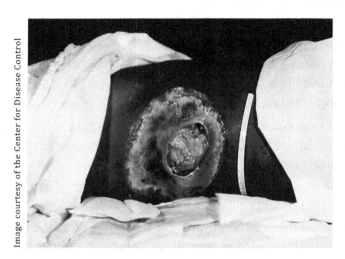

FIGURE 5.2   *Entamoeba histolytica ulcer on a flank*

Giardia lamblia: causative agent of giardiasis or "beaver fever"

-Flagellate (motile by whipping of flagella)

-Fecal–oral transmission (or sexual transmission)

-Found in small intestine of many animals (cyst dissolved by stomach acid and the trophozoite attaches to the mucous membranes in the duodenum and small intestine, covering the surface and not allowing any reabsorption of nutrients)

-Causes intestinal upsets, flatulence, nausea, abdominal pain, and diarrhea

-Exists as both trophozoite and cyst

-Cysts survive well in environment and have increased resistance to chlorine

-Treat with metronidazole or antiparasitic drugs

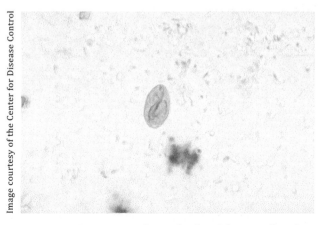

FIGURE 5.3   *Cyst of Giardia lamblia in a fecal concentrate*

Acanthamoeba species

-Causes inflammatory eye infections, especially in contact lens wearers

-Found in water and dust; exists as both cyst and trophozoite form

-Important for contact lens wearers: eye loss is a possible outcome; important to use sterile solutions for contact lens cleaning, NOT tap water

-Difficult to treat; may need surgical interventions (like cornea transplants)

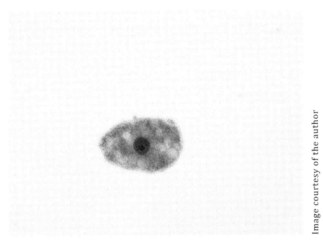

Image courtesy of the author

FIGURE 5.4   *Trophozoite of Acanthamoeba in a bronchial wash specimen*

Trichomonas vaginalis: causes an STI

-Flagellate, motile

-No cyst stage, dries out easily; therefore, must be transferred from person to person quickly: mucous membrane to mucous membrane

-Found in vagina and male urethra

-Causes intense itching and inflammation of the genitals

-Can be treated with metronidazole

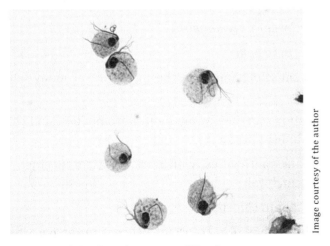

Image courtesy of the author

FIGURE 5.5   *Trophozoites of Trichomonas vaginalis*

Microsporidia: obligate intracellular parasites, very small

-From cows, rats, dogs, and cats

-Humans ingest the oocysts, which then release sporozoites

-Cause chronic diarrhea, keratoconjunctivitis, gall bladder infections, and respiratory infections in immunocompromised

-Can cause severe diarrhea in immunocompetent individuals

-Fecal–oral transmission

-Often implicated in outbreaks, swimming pools, and contaminated water ingestion

-Relatively resistant to chlorine

-No good treatments available

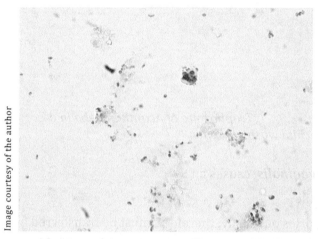

Image courtesy of the author

FIGURE 5.6   *Microsporidia spores in a fecal concentrate*

Cryptosporidia: common agent of waterborne diarrhea

-Three types: *Cryptosporidium parvum*** (most pathogenic)

   Cyclospora cayetanensis

   Isospora belli

-Fecal–oral transmission; found in the intestines of many animals (e.g., cows and pigs)

-Causes long-lasting diarrhea in the immunocompetent and chronic diarrhea in the immunosuppressed

-Oocysts have four sporozoites, which are released and then infect new cells in the intestinal wall

-Relatively resistant to chlorine

-No good antimicrobial for treatment: use supportive therapy with rehydration

Image courtesy of the author

FIGURE 5.7   Cryptosporidium parvum oocyst (red) in a fecal concentrate stained with modified Ziehl-Neelson

Toxoplasma gondii

-Life cycle in domestic cats (definitive host as the sexual reproduction takes place there)—cats do not get sick

-Trophozoites are called tachyzoites—the reproductive stage in the cat, released as oocysts in feces. Other animals can ingest Toxoplasma oocysts as well; these cysts will then be in the meat of these animals, and this can lead to toxoplasma infections acquired by eating rare meat.

-Dangerous for pregnant women if they have their first infection while pregnant but not if they have had an infection earlier

-Causes congenital infections in utero, especially in the third trimester

-Leads to stillbirths and fetal developmental problems

-Estimated that about 60% of 40-year-old women have been infected sometime (from antibody studies)

-Solution: pregnant and immunocompromised individuals should cook meats thoroughly and avoid direct contact with cat feces (also, hand washing is important after petting cats)

Trypanosoma species

-Blood parasites; can be transmitted by blood transfusion or by tsetse fly vectors (arthropods = insects)

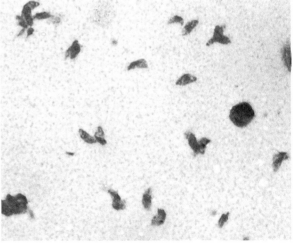

Image courtesy of the author

FIGURE 5.8   Toxoplasma gondii tachyzoites

-Three major types to know:

    a. ***T. brucei gambiense*** causes African Sleeping Sickness in Western and Central Africa

-Transmitted by a species of tsetse fly that frequents streams and is prevalent where there are large human populations

-Doesn't infect animals, just humans; milder and more chronic infection than *T. brucei rhodesiense,* although end result is the same (if left untreated)—coma and death—CNS disease

-Symptoms might not appear until months after a bite

-More than 90% of cases of trypanosomiasis are *gambiense*

    b. ***T. brucei rhodesiense*** causes African Sleeping Sickness in Eastern and Southern Africa where there are dry grasslands

-Wild animals in these areas have adapted to the parasite and are not affected,

but humans and domestic animals get acutely ill

-Fast-progressing disease; symptoms within a few days of a bite, and death within a few months—CNS disease

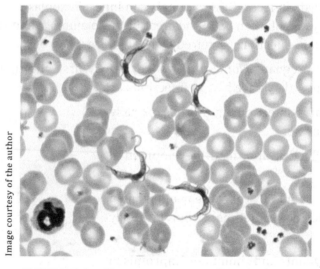

Image courtesy of the author

FIGURE 5.9   Trypomastigotes of Trypanosoma in a peripheral blood smear

c. *T. cruzi* causes Chagas disease in South America

-Bite of kissing bug or reduviid bug

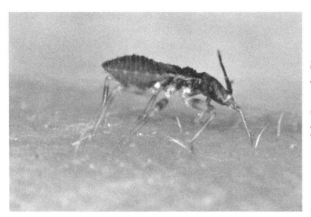

Image courtesy of the Center for Disease Control

FIGURE 5.10   *Reduviid bug*

-Chagas disease, very common in SA, cardiac complications, typical "eye of Romana," 10% mortality

-*Trypanosoma* can change their surface antigens more than 100 times and thus evade the immune system—this is why there is no good vaccine yet

-Treatment in early stages can be effective with the new drugs on the market, like eflornithine, which is more successful against *gambiense* than *rhodesiense*.

-Nifurtimox used for treatment of *T. cruzi*

Leishmania species

-About 20 different species cause disease, all transmitted by bites of flies (female sand flies)

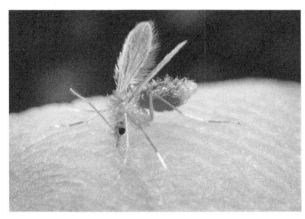

Image courtesy of the Center for Disease Control

FIGURE 5.11   *Sand fly, vector for Leishmania*

-Geographical distribution: subtropical and tropical areas of the world

-Three major species:

L. donovani in tropics causes visceral leishmaniasis (parasites invade internal organs)

–Disease is also called "kala-azar" (high mortality, malaria-like)

L. braziliensis causes mucocutaneous leishmaniasis

L. tropica causes Oriental sore or "rose of Jericho," (cutaneous leishmaniasis)

-Type of treatment depends on the species of *Leishmania* and the disease

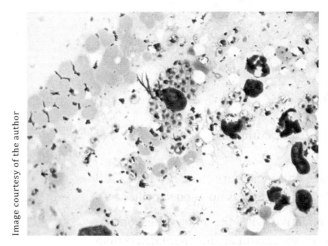

Image courtesy of the author

FIGURE 5.12   L. braziliensis amastigotes in tissue from a case of visceral leishmaniasis

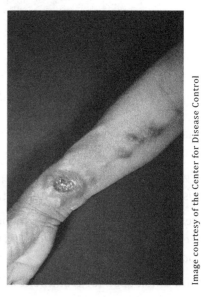

Image courtesy of the Center for Disease Control

FIGURE 5.13   Cutaneous leishmania with the original lesion spreading up the lymphatics

Babesia microti

-Tick-borne protozoal infection, *Ixodes* sp. (same tick that carries Lyme disease)

-Common in northeastern United States

-Microbes replicate in RBC; resemble plasmodium in red blood cells; end result hemolysis and anemia

-Relatively mild to moderate disease

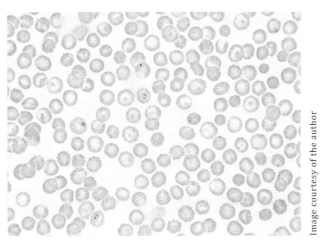

Image courtesy of the author

FIGURE 5.14   *Babesia microti in a peripheral blood smear*

Plasmodium species

-Cause of malaria; worldwide problem

-About 300 million people infected each year, causes 2 million–4 million deaths/year

-Four main types infect humans, but *P. knowlesii* (monkey malaria) is emerging as a significant zoonosis

-All transmitted by female Anopheles mosquito

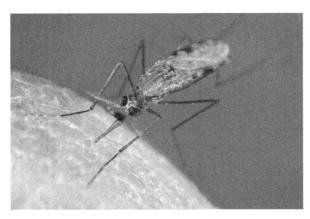

Image courtesy of the Center for Disease Control

FIGURE 5.15   *Anopheles mosquito, vector for malaria*

a. *Plasmodium falciparum*

-"Malignant malaria;" severe

-Change properties of the RBC they infect and make them "sticky"—will clump together and occlude capillaries

-Problem with drug resistance

b. *Plasmodium malariae*

-Parasite counts usually low; can cause chronic lifelong infections

-Also called "quartian" malaria—fevers are at longer intervals than the other types of malaria

c. *Plasmodium vivax*

-Has the possibility to remain latent in the liver; this should be taken into consideration when choosing the treatment drug because only one will eliminate the latent "hypnozoites"

-Mild clinical picture, low percentage parasitemia

d. *Plasmodium ovale*

-Has the possibility to remain latent in the liver for long periods

-Mild clinical picture, lower percentage parasitemia

e. *Plasmodium knowlesii*: emerging pathogen, zoonosis

-"Monkey malaria;" high incidence in southeast Asia

-Resembles *P. malariae* morphologically

-Most cases are relatively mild

-No drug resistance yet; easy to treat

-Most dangerous form is *P. falciparum* (cerebral malaria, extreme anemia, circulatory collapse) because it infects all ages of red blood cells, and the level of parasites in the blood gets very high (percentage parasitemia).

-Mosquito bites the infected humans at night, ingests gametocytes; sexual cycle of reproduction is carried out in the mosquito gut, and sporozoites migrate to the salivary glands of the mosquito. When the mosquito then bites a new host, it injects the parasites with the saliva

-Sporozoites migrate to the blood stream and liver within 30 minutes.

-In liver, sporozoites enter liver cells and undergo schizogeny (asexual reproduction, where the nucleus divides many times before the cell divides) and release thousands of merozoites, which enter the blood stream, infecting red blood cells

-Symptoms of malaria:

  Paroxyms (fever and chills): caused by the release of toxic breakdown

  products when the RBCs rupture and release more merozoites

  Anemia: lysis of red blood cells

-High mortality rate in children

-Individuals with sickle-cell trait have resistance to falciparum malaria

-Diagnosed by blood smears (thick drop and thin smear)

-No vaccine available; parasite has many life forms and can vary the antigens

-Problem with rising resistance to antimalarials (e.g., chloroquine)

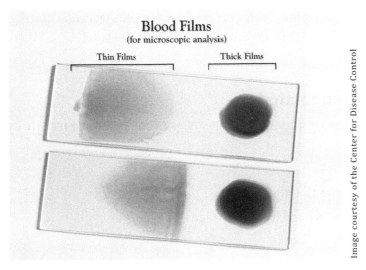

Image courtesy of the Center for Disease Control

FIGURE 5.16 *Diagnostic blood smears for morphological diagnosis of malaria*

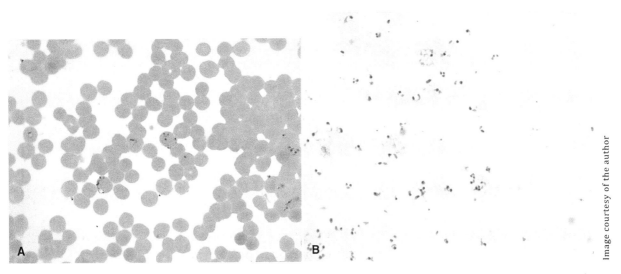

Image courtesy of the author

FIGURE 5.17a & b: *Microscopic appearance of Plasmodium falciparum in a thin (a) and a thick smear (b)*

Metazoa

Three major categories:

    A. Nematodes

    B. Trematodes

    C. Cestodes

-In general, infestation with worms does not always cause diarrhea. Diarrhea is actually more often the exception than the rule!

A. HUMAN NEMATODE (ROUNDWORM) INFECTIONS

Intestinal nematodes:

-Roundworms with complete digestive system, including mouth, intestine, and anus

-Two categories:

    a.   Eggs are the infective stage

    b.   Larvae are the infective stage

TABLE 5.2   *Nematode Infections*

Species	Acquired by	Human site
Transmitted person to person:		
Enterobius vermicularis	Ingestion of eggs	Large intestine
Ascaris lumbricoides	Ingestion of eggs	Small intestine
Hookworms	Skin penetration by infective larvae	Small intestine
Strongyloides stercoralis	Skin penetration by infective larvae; Autoinfection	Small intestine (adults) General tissue (larvae)
Trichuris trichuria	Ingestion of eggs	Large intestine
Trichinella spiralis	Ingestion of larvae	Muscle tissue
Anisakis species	Ingestion of larvae	Stomach
Dracunculus medinesis (Guinea worm)	Ingestion of larvae	Systemic
Transmitted person to person via arthropod vector:		
Brugia malayi	Mosquito + larvae	Lymphatics (adults) Blood (larvae)
Onchocerca volvulus	Simulum fly + Larvae + bacterium (Wolbachia species)	Skin (larvae,adults) Eye (larvae) Lymphatics (adults) Blood (larvae)
Loa loa	Deer fly + larvae	Tissues, eye

Enterobius vermicularis (pinworm)

-Spends whole life cycle in human; no intermediate host

-Human to human infection; eggs infective stage

-Live in large intestine; females (about 1 cm long) migrate to anus and lay eggs

-Eggs are glued to the skin around the outside of the anus—this glue is very irritating and causes intense itchiness

-Usually not serious; causes anal itching but rarely can reach appendix or uterus

-Specimen taken by laying scotch tape against outside of anal opening and rolling it on a glass slide

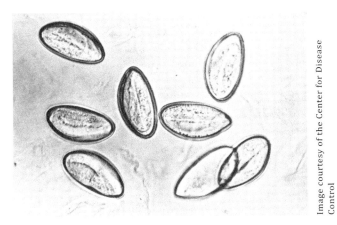

Image courtesy of the Center for Disease Control

FIGURE 5.18   *Pinworm eggs*

Ascaris lumbricoides

-Large, 30 cm when adult

-Lives in small intestines of pigs, cows, and horses

-Eggs in soil are very hardy due to thick protein coat on egg; survive a long time

-Infection by "accidental ingestion" of eggs

-Adult worms distinct sexes (dioecious)

-Diagnosis of infestation by examination of feces

   -Eggs reported as "fertilized or unfertilized"—this is important because if the eggs are fertilized, you know there may be a large infestation

-Eggs hatch in intestine of human host; larvae migrate to the lungs where they continue growth and development

-Can crawl up respiratory passages and exit by the nose or mouth (happens in children who do not have a good "swallow reflex," but adults usually just swallow them down to the stomach and intestines

-Rarely, larvae can also find their way to joints, where the adult worm may develop

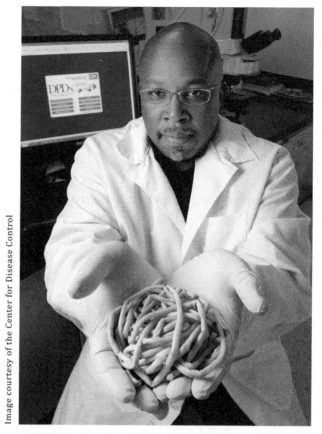

Image courtesy of the Center for Disease Control

FIGURE 5.19   *Bolus of expelled Ascaris worms after treatment*

Trichuris trichuria (also known as "whipworm")

-Relatively benign infestation of children; found in tropical and subtropical countries; associated with rat feces

-Small, slender worm

-Usually asymptomatic

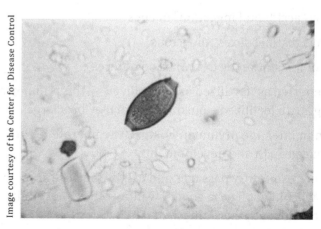

Image courtesy of the Center for Disease Control

FIGURE 5.20   *Whipworm egg from a fecal specimen*

Hookworms

-Two species:

1) *Necator americanus:* sucks ~0.03 ml blood/day (found in the Americas)

2) *Ancylostoma duodenale:* sucks 5X more blood/day (found in Africa, etc.)

-Can cause significant anemia

-Only found in warm climates (tropical and subtropical)

-Eggs in soil hatch; infective stage larvae penetrate intact skin (i.e., soles of feet between toes); migrate to lymphatic system; then end up in the circulation

-Carried to lungs, coughed up, and swallowed down to small intestine, where they attach to mucosa with their "hooks"

-Can't complete life cycle in host—eggs excreted to soil for recycling

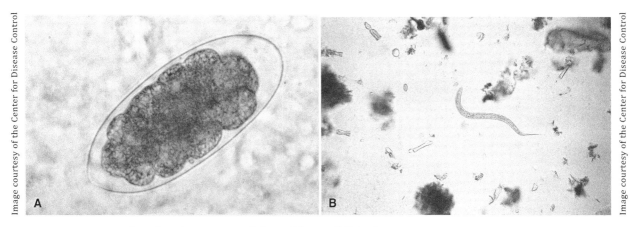

Image courtesy of the Center for Disease Control

A   B

FIGURE 5.21a & b: *Hookworm egg* **(a)** *and larva* **(b)** *in feces*

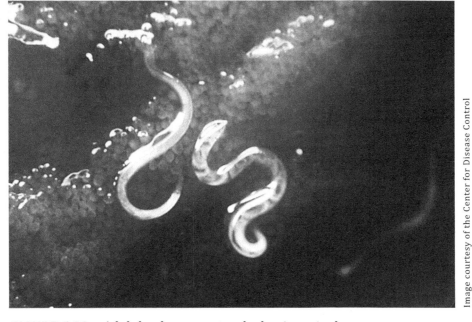

Image courtesy of the Center for Disease Control

FIGURE 5.22   *Adult hookworms attached to intestinal mucosa*

Strongyloides stercoralis

-Same method of infectivity as hookworm, but the female larvae penetrate the bowel wall and cause a generalized infection

-Eggs are not laid in intestine; larvae can be excreted, but there is no requirement for excretion to outside environment, thus "autoinfection" is common, where the larvae can reinfect while inside the body

-Usually cause abdominal pain and diarrhea; can also cause lung inflammation if the parasite is in the lung as well as skin lesions

-Chronic infections common especially in immunocompromised where, if the worm disseminates through the body, can cause septic shock and death

-Eggs are similar to hookworm but rarely seen; the larvae are similar

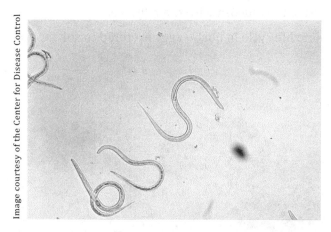

Image courtesy of the Center for Disease Control

FIGURE 5.23   *Strongyloides larvae in feces*

Trichinella spiralis

-Smallest nematode parasite of humans

-Acquired from infected undercooked meat—the larvae are in nurse cells in the striated muscle

-Nurse cells release larvae in the stomach because of the low pH; larvae then escape and enter the circulation and tissues, where they encyst and cause muscle weakness

-Life cycle can be completed in one animal

-Bears, walrus, and pigs are very common sources of infection

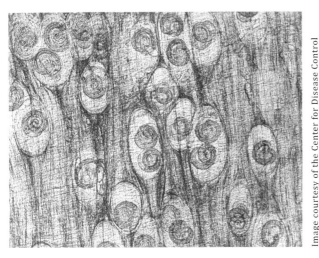

Image courtesy of the Center for Disease Control

FIGURE 5.24   *Encysted Trichinella spiralis in striated muscle*

Anisakis

-Small fish nematodes; accidentally infect humans (1–3 cm in length)

-Fishing practices (large catches, fish held for many hours in a hold before being gutted) contribute to increased rate of Anisakis in raw fish eaters

-Fairly uncommon, although increasing in prevalence with increased consumption of sushi (properly prepared fish for sushi will not have larvae in the meat)

-Can also prevent this by heating fish to 60 °C for 10 minutes, blast-freezing to −35 °C for ~16 hours, or freezing fish at −23 °C for a week

Dracunculia species (Guinea worm):

-Fecal–oral transmission, but the growing larvae penetrate the intestines and travel in the subcutaneous tissues

-Can be up to 1 m in length

-Emerge from body by causing a blister, which erupts and the worm emerges—when it senses water, it releases larvae into the water, perpetuating the cycle

-Treatment: usually removal of worm (slowly winding it out 1 inch/day so as not to break it and cause undue inflammation)

-Probably the origin of the snake winding around the staff in the medical symbol (rod of Asclepius)

-WHO has an eradication program, which has been successful, and the number of cases are drastically decreasing in Africa

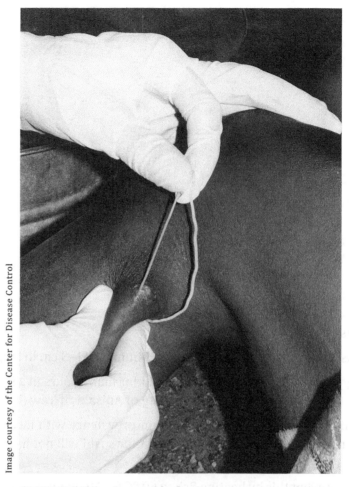

Image courtesy of the Center for Disease Control

FIGURE 5.25   *Removal of a Guinea worm*

Blood and tissue helminths (Filaria)

-Main filarial infections in humans are:

1. Lymphatic filariasis (elephantiasis)

   -Adult worms live in lymphatic tissue

2. Onchocerciasis (river blindness)

   -Adult worms live in subcutaneous tissue

   -Adult worms are infected by a bacterium (Wolbachia), which cause the intense inflammation in the eye, leading to "river blindness"

-Transmitted by bites of mosquitoes

-Microfilariae (offspring of adult worms) circulate through bloodstream or migrate through subcutaneous tissue

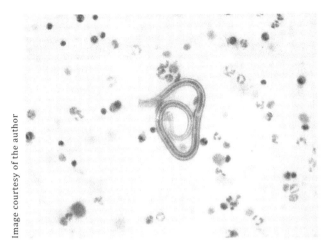

Image courtesy of the author

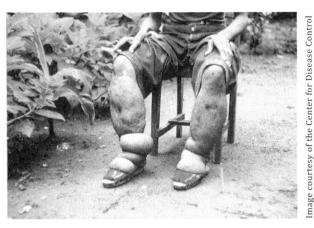

Image courtesy of the Center for Disease Control

FIGURE 5.26a *Wuchereria bancrofti in a peripheral blood specimen*

FIGURE 5.26b *Elephantiasis in a patient from the Philippines*

-Form lumps in skin—larvae seek oxygen and try to get to the surface. Diagnosis can be done by "skin snips," where a lump is incised and the fluid examined in a microscope for microscopic worms)

-High prevalence in Africa, Asia, and tropical Latin America

-Major species of filaria:

Wuchereria bancrofti

Brugia malayi

Loa loa

Human cestode (tapeworm) infections

-Cestodes do not have a full digestive system, rather a head and a body composed of segments that each contain male and female sexual organs, and obtain food by absorption through the cuticle

-Most have an "intermediate host" that they must go through in order to maintain the infectious life cycle; only a few can autoinfect humans

-Two types of infection:

Intestinal infection: mild clinical picture, produced by pork, beef, and fish or rodent tapeworms

Deep tissue infection: serious infections, pork tapeworm (cysticercosis) or dog tapeworm (echinococcus)

TABLE 5.3   Deep Tissue Infections

Species	Source	Other hosts	Body site
Taenia saginata	Larvae in beef	None	Intestine
Taenia solium (adult worm)	Larvae in pork	None	Intestine
Taenia solium (larvae)	Eggs in food, water contaminated with human feces	Pigs	Brain, eyes
Diphyllobothrium latum	Larvae in fish	Fish-eating mammals	Intestine
Hymenolypsis nana	Eggs or larvae in beetles	Rodents	Intestine
Echinococcus granulosus (hydatid disease)	Eggs passed by dogs	Sheep	Liver, lung, brain

Taenia saginata

-Beef tapeworm; life cycle requires both humans and cattle

-Infectious tissue larvae (cysticerci) are ingested by humans from infected, undercooked meat and mature into adult tapeworms in the intestine

-Adult worms can be as long as 10 m, attached to the intestinal wall by sucking discs on the head or "scolex" of the worm

-Hermaphrodites

-Mild symptoms, if any, and no complications

-Segments of the tapeworm fall off the worm and can be excreted as whole segments or as individual eggs

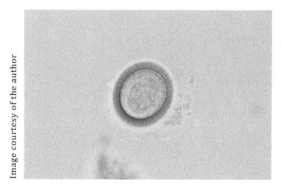

Image courtesy of the author

FIGURE 5.27a   *Taenia egg*

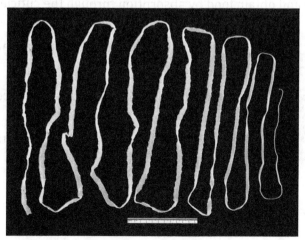

Image courtesy of the Center for Disease Control

FIGURE 5.27b   *Adult Taenia saginata*

Taenia solium

-Intermediate host is the pig, usually about 3 m, but can be longer as adult

Two types of disease:

1) Infection by egg: ingestion of eggs or segments (proglottids) with eggs; hatching of eggs in the intestine after passing through the stomach acid; larvae then escape and can migrate through the body. A preferred site for them to reside and become encysted is the brain. This can occur through autoinfection with an adult worm residing in the body.

2) Infection by larvae: similar to *T. saginata*; ingestion of larvae, which survive stomach acid and attach to the intestinal wall with the suckers/hooks on their scolexes. Ribbon-band of segments form and either drop off as a whole or as eggs, which are released and excreted in feces.

-Person-to-person transmission is possible; also autoinfection

-Larvae in central nervous system encyst and are a major cause of seizures and syncope in many underdeveloped countries

Diphyllobothrium latum

-Fish tapeworm; ingestion of larvae in undercooked contaminated fish (Scandinavia, Pacific northwest in North America)

-Can get to 10 m in length; attach to intestinal wall with grooves on the scolex

-Use vitamin B_{12} and cause B_{12} deficiency—with megaloblastic anemia

-Mild to moderate symptoms, some diarrhea, abdominal pain

-Eggs are excreted in the feces

Hymenolypsis nana

-Most common tapeworm globally, common in all tropical areas

-Small, 1-4 cm

-Do not need an "intermediate host"—can autoinfect a human

-Few symptoms unless the worm infestation is huge

-Infections by ingesting egg (fecal–oral transmission)

-Cysticeroid stage can develop in the intestine of humans in heavy infections—this can cause some tissue damage leading to symptoms of enteritis, diarrhea, cramps, etc.

Echinococcus species (dog tapeworm)

E. multilocaris and *E. granulosus* most common

-Small tapeworm found in canines (dogs, coyotes, foxes, wolves), which are the definitive hosts where the sexual reproduction takes place

-Humans are accidental hosts if the eggs that canines excrete are ingested. Eggs hatch, and the larvae travel through the bloodstream to the organs where the hydatid cyst develops

-Echinococcus forms "hydatid cysts" in liver or lungs (and other organs) of humans. These cysts are brood capsules and contain heads of tapeworms. These cannot develop into tapeworms in the human, but as they grow in size, they can cause irritation and inflammation and also tissue damage due to displacement of tissue

-If hydatid cysts are disrupted and break apart, this can cause life-threatening shock in the human

-In Alberta most cases are due to *Echinococcus granulosus,* and most have cysts in the lungs. Surgery is not indicated normally due to the risk of rupturing the cyst and releasing anaphylactic substances

Human trematodes

TABLE 5.4   *Trematodes (Flukes)*

Species	Source	Other hosts	Body site
Paragonimus westermani	Contaminated food and water	Carnivores	Lungs
Clonorchis sinensus	Contaminated water	Fish	Liver
Schistosoma mansoni, hematobium, japonicum	Contaminated water		Intestine and bladder (hematobium)

Paragonimus westermani

-Intermediate host is fresh water snail, where the metacerceria develop

-Humans ingest the metacerceria usually in seafood; these excyst in the duodenum, and the free larvae penetrate through to the lungs

-Infects human lungs and causes inflammation. Pseudotubercle formed; symptoms are cough and hemoptysis

Clonorchis sinusensis (Chinese or Oriental liver fluke)

-Very common in the Far East; small fluke

-Intermediate host is the snail; cercariae released and enter a fish, where they develop into a cyst like metacerciaral structure

-Metacercariae in undercooked or raw fish muscle are ingested by humans; cyst is acid-resistant, so larvae hatch in the small intestine and migrate to the liver

-Live on bile and produce an inflammatory reaction in the gall bladder, bile ducts, and liver. Can obstruct the bile duct

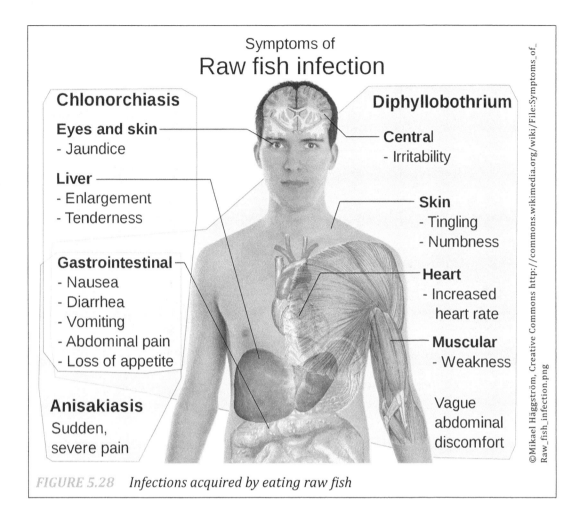

Symptoms of
Raw fish infection

Chlonorchiasis

Eyes and skin
- Jaundice

Liver
- Enlargement
- Tenderness

Gastrointestinal
- Nausea
- Diarrhea
- Vomiting
- Abdominal pain
- Loss of appetite

Anisakiasis
Sudden,
severe pain

Diphyllobothrium

Central
- Irritability

Skin
- Tingling
- Numbness

Heart
- Increased
  heart rate

Muscular
- Weakness

Vague
abdominal
discomfort

©Mikael Häggström, Creative Commons http://commons.wikimedia.org/wiki/File:Symptoms_of_Raw_fish_infection.png

FIGURE 5.28 Infections acquired by eating raw fish

Schistosoma species

-Intermediate host fresh water snail; definitive host is the human; infected by cercariae that penetrate intact skin in contaminated waters

-Very important disease worldwide; causes debilitating disease

-Adult worms not affected by host immune system: they cover themselves with a protein layer that mimics host tissues

-Eggs reside in the venous plexus of bladder or intestine, depending on species

Three main types of pathogenic *Schistosoma* in humans:

    S. haematobium: urinary schistosomiasis
    -Results in inflammation of bladder wall
    -Chronic sequalae—bladder cancer
    -Found in Africa and the Middle East

    S. japonicum: intestinal parasite, found in the Far East

    S. mansoni: intestinal parasite, found in Africa, South America, and the Caribbean

    -More than 250 million people infected

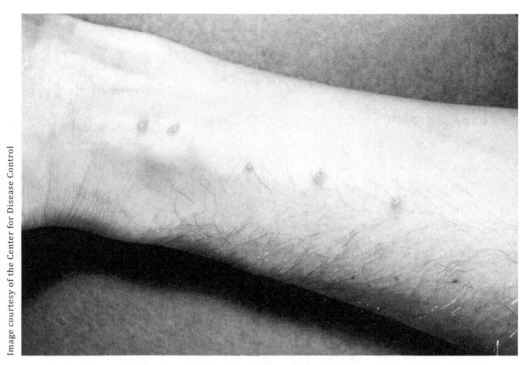

Image courtesy of the Center for Disease Control

FIGURE 5.29   Rash of "swimmer's itch"

"Swimmer's itch": caused by cercariae of nonhuman schistosome (ducks and other waterfowl)

-Do not enter the circulation; self-limiting infection in the skin, which causes intense itching

Different types of *Schistosoma* can be differentiated by the appearance of the eggs and source of specimen (urine for hematobium and feces for mansoni and japonicum).

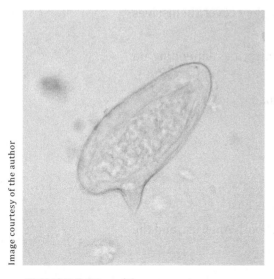

Image courtesy of the author

FIGURE 5.30   a)S. mansoni;

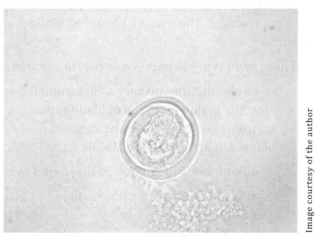

Image courtesy of the author

FIGURE 5.30   b) S. japonicum;

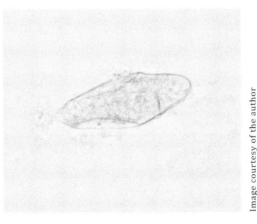

Image courtesy of the author

Figure 5.30—cont'd   c) S. hematobium

TABLE 5.5   *Nematode Zoonoses Transmitted from Animals*

Species	Acquired by	Human site
Angiostrongylus cantonensis	Ingestion of larvae in snails, crustacea	CNS (larvae)
Anisakis simplex	Ingestion of larvae in fish	Stomach, small intestine (larvae)
Capillaria philipinensis	Ingestion of larvae in fish	Small intestine (adults, larvae)
Toxocara canis	Ingestion of eggs excreted by dogs	Tissues, CNS (larvae)
*Trichinella spiralis**	Ingestion of larvae in pork, wild mammals	Small intestine (adult), muscles (larvae)

Ectoparasites

-"Ectoparasites" like scabies, mites, and lice live in or on the skin and do not enter deep tissues but can act as vectors for infection and can cause skin irritation leading to scratching and secondary bacterial infection

Scabies

-Caused by *Sarcoptes scabei var hominis* (human scabies), an arthropod, 400 um mite

-Dog mange is caused by a closely related *Sarcoptes* species; does not cause human infection

-Infectious from human to human

-Fertilized adult female burrows in the skin to lay eggs

-Presence of mites tunnelling in skin and the eggs cause an extensive allergic reaction, and the areas are excruciatingly itchy—can move up to an inch a minute

-Preferentially live on finger webs, elbows, armpits, and breasts and around the groin and buttocks

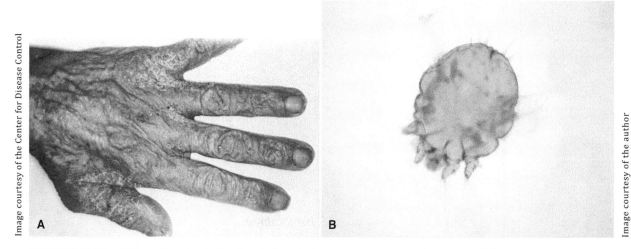

Image courtesy of the Center for Disease Control

Image courtesy of the author

FIGURE 5.31a & b: *Scabies infection (a) and the causative mite Sarcoptes (b)*

-Heavy infestations are called "Norwegian scabies"

-Secondary infections with staphylococci and streptococci common

Pubic lice or "crabs" (*Phthirus pubis*) and head lice (*Pediculus humanus*):

-Surface dwellers; do not burrow

-Feed by penetrating the skin with mouth and sucking blood

-Female pubic louse lays eggs (called nits) and glues them to hair shafts

-Eggs hatch in 5–10 days, releasing new lice

-Secondary infections when lice feces crushed into wounds

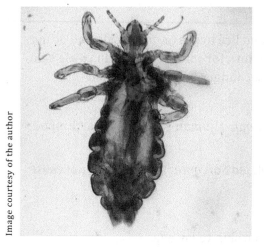

Image courtesy of the author

FIGURE 5.32a   *Head Louse*

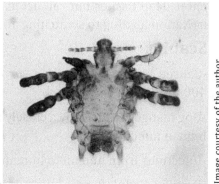

Image courtesy of the author

FIGURE 5.32b   *Pubic Louse*

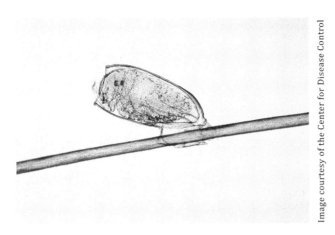

Image courtesy of the Center for Disease Control

FIGURE 5.33   *Louse nit (egg) attached to a hair*

Interested? Want to learn more?

For more reading, several texts online at the U of A library are recommended:

1.   Brooks, GF, Carroll KC, Butel JS, Morse SA, editors. Jawetz, Melnick, and Adelberg's Medical Microbiology, 24th ed. Blacklick OH-McGraw Hill; 2007

2.   Ryan KJ, Ray CG, editors. Sherris Medical Microbiology, 5th ed. New York – McGraw-Hill, 2010.

Chapter 6

Nosocomial Infection, Disinfection, and Sterilization

Learning Objectives:

1. Define common terms used to describe disinfection, sterilization, and nosocomial infection, and identify a few major causes of nosocomial infections.
2. Explain how we can control the environment in a hospital or a laboratory.
3. Define and describe the process of sterilization.
4. Identify the spore test as a method of quality control for autoclaving processes.
5. Identify chemicals that can be used to sterilize objects and surfaces.
6. Explain why alcohol-based hand sanitizers are not as effective against endospores and naked virus as hand washing.

Nosocomial Infection: infection acquired while in a hospital or institution, usually either from the environment or from other people (staff/visitors)

-Generally accepted to mean infections occurring that are **NOT** part of the primary disease the patient had (it **could** be originating from their own flora!)

Endogenous: self-infection from another part of the body

Exogenous: from another person or from an environmental source

-Many hospital infections are preventable.

-Semmelweiss (about 1850) first showed that puerperal fever with *Streptococcus pyogenes* was a hospital-acquired infection.

-**Hand washing** is the most important preventative measure.

-Infections most commonly acquired in the hospital:

a. ***Urinary tract infection** (majority of infections and most are *Escherichia coli*)

b. Surgical wound infection (often patient's own flora)

c. Lower respiratory tract infection

d. Bacteremia

   - Primary bacteremia as result of catheter or contaminated intravenous fluids

   - Secondary bacteremia to some other infection in body (e.g., urinary tract infection)

Nosocomial infections

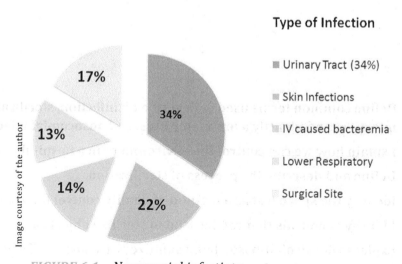

Type of Infection

- Urinary Tract (34%)
- Skin Infections
- IV caused bacteremia
- Lower Respiratory
- Surgical Site

Image courtesy of the author

FIGURE 6.1   Nosocomial infections

-Other infections occurring in the hospital setting are outbreaks of RSV, Influenza, rotovirus, or norovirus gastroenteritis, etc.

Consequences of hospital infection

-Serious illness or death

-Prolonged hospital stay

-Expensive antimicrobials may be needed

-Patient may become a carrier or source and spread the infection in the community

-Spread of multiresistant organisms

Prevention of hospital infection

HAND WASHING!

-Alcohol-based hand sanitizers: useful in conjunction with hand washing, but remember that nonenveloped viruses (e.g., norovirus) and bacteria that have endospores (e.g., *Clostridium difficile*) are not affected by alcohol!

-Exclude sources of infection from environment.

-Provide "sterile" instruments and dressings, fluids, and bed clothes.

-Interrupt the transmission of infection from source to patient.

-Prevent patient contact with staff who are carriers of pathogens (includes immunization of staff, reporting of diarrheal disease, etc.).

-Enhance the patients' ability to resist infection.

-good nutrition, preoperative antimicrobials.

Clostridium difficile: Anaerobic Gram positive bacillus, spore forming. Common cause of nosocomial infections.

Sherry, aged 46, homemaker with a previous complicated medical history—several surgeries for bladder abnormalities. Last surgery was in April 2007 and was complicated by infection, necessitating treatment with an antibiotic, clindamycin. (*Note that clindamycin is a broad spectrum antibiotic that targets many different types of bacteria.) One week after discharge, she had fever, severe abdominal cramps, and diarrhea. Stool specimens were collected and sent for analysis.

Result: positive for *C. difficile* exotoxins. Sherry was treated with metronidazole (antibiotic that targets anaerobic bacteria); diarrhea was reduced but not eliminated, and she returned for a follow-up in two weeks. *C. difficile* toxin was still present in fecal samples. She then received another treatment with metronidazole; this didn't help, so she was given oral vancomycin (active against Gram positives). Her

Continued

diarrhea then stopped, and she was able to resume her volunteer work at a nursing home.

Sherry was well for six months, then had a relapse of diarrhea, fever and abdominal pain, and she returned to her doctor, who again prescribed vancomycin. This time her pain increased, and her fever soared to 41 °C. She was admitted and diagnosed with toxic megacolon (gangrene of the colon); needed emergency surgery. After a lengthy hospital stay, she was released and remained healthy for two months. She again relapsed with diarrhea and pain, was given oral vancomycin, but was still toxin-positive after three weeks. Infectious disease was consulted and decided on a pulse regiment of antibiotics: three weeks on and two weeks off for the next two months. The diarrhea finally resolved, and she was negative for toxin. Sherry has resigned her volunteer position at the nursing home.

Clostridium difficile is present as normal flora in about 3%–5% of healthy individuals. Sherry may have had this organism from the beginning or may have acquired it from the nursing home, where this type of infection is very common. When Sherry was treated with clindamycin, the antibiotic wiped out her "good bacteria" or normal flora in her intestine, allowing the *C. difficile* to thrive and take over, producing toxin A (enterotoxin causing watery diarrhea) and toxin B (a cytotoxin that damaged and killed intestinal mucosal cells). A severe intestinal inflammation developed with a pseudomembrane covering the intestinal wall (comprised of pus, dead mucosal cells, and bacteria). Antibiotic treatment was difficult because the bacterium produces spores that are not metabolically active and cannot be inhibited by antibiotics; only actively growing bacteria are susceptible. Spores can survive months in the environment and are difficult to inactivate with disinfectants.

Syndromes with *C. difficile* range from mild diarrhea (called AAD or antibiotic associated diarrhea to AAC (antibiotic associated colitis) to PMC (pseudomembranous colitis) to toxic megacolon (life threatening gangrene). An elderly person who acquires this infection may die. An interesting detail is that young children <2 years of age NEVER get *C. difficile* (maybe a difference in the intestinal mucosa).

Factors that predispose patients to hospital (nosocomial) infection

1. Age
2. Specific immunity
3. Underlying disease
4. Other infections
5. Specific medical therapeutics (i.e., cytotoxic drugs)
6. Trauma—burns, stab wounds,
7. Surgery, catheters, peritoneal dialysis

Postoperative infections: a type of nosocomial infection

Risk factors for postoperative Infections

1. Length of preoperative stay: the longer the stay, the more chance of colonization
2. Surgical procedures done on areas with a preexisting infection
3. Length of operation: the longer the operation, the greater the risk
4. Nature of the operation: for example, GI tract surgery has a higher incidence of postoperative infection than carpal tunnel repair (GI tract surgery is called "dirty surgery")
5. Presence of foreign bodies; for example, pacemaker, prostheses, shunts
6. State of tissues: blood supply, drainage, and tissue breakdown products

Prevention of postoperative infections

1. Pre- and per (during) operative antibiotics
2. Postoperative antibiotics
3. Stringent infection control, use of isolation tents, etc.

Hazards to healthcare workers

Diseases: infectious diseases pose a risk for healthcare workers involved in the primary care of patients. Some of the more serious of these are:

HIV

Hepatitis B, Hepatitis C

TB and other respiratory pathogens (including *N. meningitidis*)

Hemorrhagic fever viruses (unlikely in Canada)

Tularemia, plague (uncommon, but possible)

Emergent viruses such as SARS (rare)

Common sources of infection to healthcare workers

1. Infected patients
2. Soiled bedding, towels, dressings, and other fomites (fomites = inanimate object)
3. Contaminated needles
4. Surgical equipment

Avoidance of infection

Hand washing: number one preventive measure

Gloves, gowns, masks, and goggles

Proper handling of needles and sharps

Disinfection of the environment

What to do if you do get accidentally contaminated?

Immediately:

1. Wash needle sticks and cuts with soap and water.
2. Flush splashes in the nose, mouth, or skin with water.
3. Irrigate eyes with clean water, saline, or sterile irrigants.
4. Report the incident to the supervisor as soon as possible.
5. Immediately seek medical attention.

    -In the case of HIV, antiretroviral therapy may be indicated quickly.

    -In the case of Hepatitis A or B, this may mean vaccination or immuno-globulin therapy.

Controlling the Environment in Healthcare Facilities

Ventilation: should be clean and free of pathogens

-Ultra clean air (passed through high efficiency filters like HEPA) used in "tents" for hip replacements during operations or in the lab for preventing personnel from infection with the organisms they are working with

-Standards for correct air flows essential during construction

-Isolation rooms with "air locks"

Positive-pressure rooms: air flows only from the patient room to the corridor, not from the corridor into the room, protecting patient from infection.

Negative-pressure rooms: air flows from the corridor into the patient room but never out of the patient room, protecting everyone from the infection the patient has.

Sterilization and disinfection

Most important consideration that determines the efficiency of sterilization is whether the object to be sterilized is free of organic matter (blood, feces, tissue).

TABLE 1: *Definitions*

Term	Definition
Antiseptic	Disinfectant used on the skin
Aseptic technique	Use of methods to exclude microorganisms
Bactericidal	Kills bacteria
Bacteriostatic	Inhibits growth of bacteria; doesn't kill
Disinfectant	Chemical used to destroy many microorganisms and viruses
Fungicide	Kills fungi
Pasteurization	Brief heat treatment used to reduce the numbers of organisms and to kill pathogenic organisms
Sanitization	Reduction of number of organisms to standard public health level
Sterilization	Destruction of all forms of microbes, including spores
Viricide	Inactivates viruses

Sterilization

-May be achieved by:

    A. Heat

    B. Irradiation (gamma or UV)

    C. Filtration

    D. Chemicals

A. HEAT: preferred method because of ease of use, low cost, and efficiency

Disadvantages: cannot be used for living tissues or materials destroyed by high temperatures (e.g., plastics, blood serum, vaccines)

-Heat resistance differs between different organisms; must consider the thermal death point for choice of appropriate sterilization programs

Types of HEAT

Dry heat: sterilizing mechanism is the oxidation of cell components by high temperature

a) Hot air sterilization

-Sterilization by heating in a hot air oven 160°–180 °C for one to two hours

b) Incineration

-Very useful for destruction of biological hazards (i.e., anthrax-contaminated animal carcasses)

c) Moist heat

1. Boiling

-Easiest method but is not totally effective in killing all forms of pathogenic bacteria and viruses

2. Autoclaving

-Best method for sterilization; uses moist heat (saturated steam) and pressure (autoclave)

-Usual autoclaving cycle is 121 °C for 15 min at 15 psi (pounds pressure per square inch. This will kill *C. botulinum* spores—the industry standard.

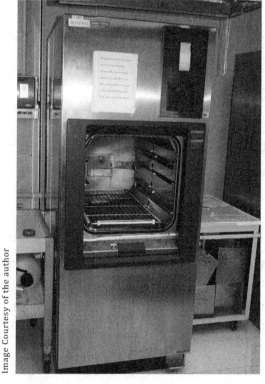

Image Courtesy of the author

FIGURE 6.2   a) Autoclave

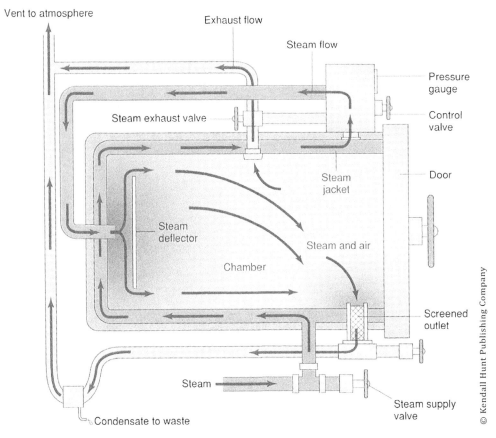

Vent to atmosphere

Exhaust flow

Steam flow

Pressure gauge

Control valve

Steam exhaust valve

Door

Steam jacket

Steam deflector

Steam and air

Chamber

Screened outlet

Steam

Steam supply valve

Condensate to waste

© Kendall Hunt Publishing Company

FIGURE 6.2—cont'd   b) Autoclave function

-Used to sterilize surgical instruments and dressings, to decontaminate medical waste, and to sterilize media and solutions for microbiology laboratory methods

-Test efficiency by using a "spore test"

Spore test: test to determine if a preparation of endospores from a bacterium will be effectively inactivated by the autoclave. Normally a nonpathogenic strain of *Bacillus* spores are used and may be sold in small vials containing some growth medium. The vial is placed in the autoclave together with the goods to be sterilized, and after the autoclaving procedure is done, the vial is put into a 37 °C water bath and observed for growth. If the endospores were NOT inactivated, they will grow into bacteria and cause the pH of the growth medium to change, which is reflected in a change of color in the medium containing a pH indicator. If the autoclaving procedure was effective, the endospores will not grow in the ampule. This test must be done often to ensure that there is proper functioning of the autoclave.

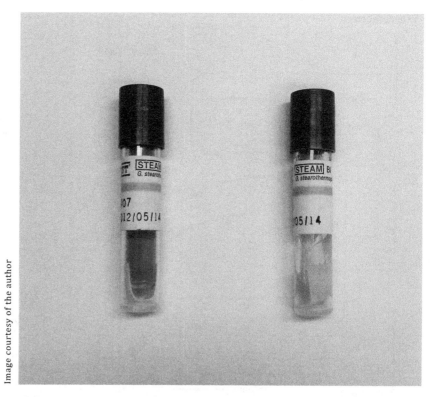

FIGURE 6.3   Spore test showing yellow color, indicating lack of sterility as compared to a sterile test

3. **Pasteurization**: mild heating to reduce numbers of bacteria and remove pathogenic bacteria

-Heating at 63 °C for 30 minutes or 72 °C for 15 seconds—usual procedure

-Often used for foodstuffs like milk and beer

B. Irradiation: two types

i. **Ionizing radiation**: gamma rays (i.e., from cobalt), X rays, high-energy electron beams

- Effect is the result of the ionization of water, forming highly reactive hydroxyl radicals, which react with cellular components and destroys them; DNA is broken down

ii. **Nonionizing radiation**: rays of longer wavelength and thus lower energy (i.e., UV light)

- Acts to inactivate DNA by causing improper bonding between the strands of DNA (thus stops replication of the microorganisms)

-Most effective wavelength is 260 nm, which is the wavelength absorbed best by DNA

-Disadvantage: rays do not penetrate very far into the material, and the UV source must be close to the surface of the object

-Microwaves do not have an efficient antimicrobial effect (however, the heat generated in the foodstuff may be sufficient to kill)

C. Filtration: passage of substance through a screen-like filter that has pores or small holes of a specified size predetermined to prevent the passage of microbes.

-Used to sterilize heat sensitive liquids (i.e., some culture media, vaccines, drugs)

-Usually used with a vacuum, which is needed to pull the substance through the membrane

-Membrane filters may be made of plastic polymers or cellulose with pore sizes as low as .01 micron (this will remove viruses)

- **HEPA** filters: high-efficiency particulate air filters with pore size of .3 microns (e.g., air filters used in operating rooms)

D. Chemicals: many different chemicals available, but very few agents will sterilize

Relative resistance of microbes to chemical agents

Prions	**Hardest to inactivate with chemicals**
Endospores	
Mycobacterium species	
Cysts of protozoa	
Trophozoites (vegetative) protozoa	
Gram negative bacteria	
Fungi	
Nonenveloped viruses	
Gram positive bacteria	
Enveloped bacteria	**Easiest to inactivate with chemicals**

Summary: List of Chemicals

1. **Phenols and phenolics**:

Phenol: antibacterial effect at concentrations >1% **but** is irritating to skin

Phenolic: chemically altered phenol; less irritating to skin

-**Mode of action**: disruption of lipids in cell plasma membranes, causing leakage and cell death

-Remain **active** in the presence of organic substances (i.e., pus, feces, saliva)

-Example of a phenolic: **Lysol™**

Bisphenol: derivative of phenol

-Hexachlorophene (PHisoHex™) (good against Gram positives)

Biguanide: derivative of phenol

-Chlorhexidine

-Active on most vegetative bacteria and fungi

-Not active on Mycobacteria (TB) or spores, protozoan cysts, "naked" viruses

2. **Halogens** (e.g., iodine and chlorine)

Iodine: available as tincture (solution in alcohol) or as an iodaphor (combination of iodine and an organic molecule from which iodine is released slowly)

-Used as a skin disinfectant

-Example: Betadine™

Chlorine: strong oxidizing agent

-Hypochlorous acid forms when chlorine gas is introduced to water

-Calcium hypochlorite: used to disinfect dairy equipment (chloride of lime)

-Sodium hypochlorite: household disinfectant and bleach

-Example: Chlorox™

3. **Alcohols**: kill bacteria and fungi but not endospores and nonenveloped viruses

-Mechanism is protein denaturation and disruption of the lipid membranes

-Used for skin "degerming"

-Not good for treating wounds because alcohol causes a coagulation of the proteins, creating an environment where the bacteria can grow

-Ethanol optimum concentration is 70% (denaturation needs water to work)

-Isopropanol = rubbing alcohol—is better than ethanol—does not evaporate as fast

4. **Heavy metals (**e.g., copper, silver have antimicrobial effects by denaturing enzymes)

5. **Surface-active agents** (surfactants)

-Soaps

-Not much value for disinfection but good for mechanical removal of lipids

6. **Quaternary ammonium compounds**

-Modification of NH_4^+

-Strongly bactericidal for Gram positive bacteria, fungicidal, viricidal for enveloped virus, amoebacidal

-Do not kill endospores or mycobacteria

-Inactivated by organic substances

-Some bacteria (e.g., *Pseudomonas* spp.) can grow in them

-Example: Cepacol™ mouthwash

7. **Aldehyde**: most effective antimicrobial chemical

-Can be considered a sterilizing agent

-Inactivate proteins

-Formaldehyde and glutaraldehyde

-Used to disinfect hospital instruments that cannot be autoclaved

-Example: Cidex™ (glutaraldehyde)

8. **Gaseous chemosterilizers**: chemicals that sterilize in a closed chamber

-Denature proteins

-Problem with toxicity (nasty to work with and dangerous)—mostly used in industry

-Example: ethylene oxide

9. **Peroxygens**: oxidizing agents

-Ozone, hydrogen peroxide, peracetic acid

-Hydrogen peroxide can be very effective if left in contact with object for an extended time (even for inactivating endospores)

-Peracetic acid most effective—used as a sterilant

Summary: Chemical Sterilizers

Only peroxygens, gaseous chemosterilizers like ethylene oxide, aldehydes, and strong solutions of halogens (e.g., chlorine) can sterilize.

Interested? Want to learn more?

For more reading, several texts online at the U of A library are recommended:

1. Brooks, GF, Carroll KC, Butel JS, Morse SA, editors. Jawetz, Melnick, and Adelberg's Medical Microbiology, 24th ed. Blacklick OH-McGraw Hill; 2007

2. Ryan KJ, Ray CG, editors. Sherris Medical Microbiology, 5th ed. New York – McGraw-Hill, 2010.

Chapter 7

Antimicrobials

Learning Objectives:

1. List some problems associated with chemotherapy for bacteria, viruses, fungi, and parasites.
2. Define mechanisms of antibiotic resistance.
3. Define spectrum of activity, broad-spectrum drugs, MIC, SIR, drug of choice, bactericidal, and bacteriostatic.
4. List five modes of activity for antimicrobials, and learn the examples given.
5. Explain why monitoring antibiotic levels should be done in some patients for some antimicrobials.
6. List the common superbugs, and identify the reason they are classed as superbugs.

Antimicrobial agents are defined as chemicals that are used to prevent or treat infection by inhibiting the growth of or by killing microbial agents. This includes antibiotics, antivirals, antifungals, and antiparasitics. Some of these drugs are toxic to the human body and thus are only used topically (on the skin or eye surface), but most of them are either parenteral (injectable) or oral drugs. Many of the drugs work by inhibiting the metabolic or replicative processes of the microorganisms, for example, by preventing cell wall synthesis like penicillins, protein synthesis like the macrolides and aminoglycosides, or disturbing DNA synthesis.

In addition to the drugs that directly affect microorganisms, there are a growing number of immunoactive substances that are being developed. A good example of this is interferon. Interferon is a natural substance produced by cells around a virus-infected cell that acts to prevent the healthy cells from being invaded by viruses.

Successful treatment of an infection with an antimicrobial must be done early in the disease process before the infection has a chance to cause irreparable tissue damage.

If there has been tissue damage, the drugs may not penetrate into the tissue; if there are too many bacteria, the drug may not be able to effectively inhibit all of them; if abscesses have formed, the antibiotics may not be able to penetrate through the walls of the abscesses to attack the bacteria within. In all cases, a prerequisite for efficient treatment is the presence of a well functioning immune system. The drugs can beat down the microbes, but the immune cells mop up the remaining microbes and control the infection.

In recent years, antimicrobial resistance has emerged, making effective treatment of some types of infections very problematic.

Historical Perspective

Natural substances with some activity against microbes have been used for centuries with significant success (e.g., the bark of the cinchona tree contained quinine, a drug that is still used to treat malaria).

The early antimicrobial substances damaged the host as much as the pathogen! An example of this was the use of arsenic (called salvarsan) to treat syphilis. Salvarsan was formulated by Paul Ehrlich, an important antimicrobial pioneer in the early 20th century. He came up with the idea that "magic bullets" were needed that would selectively harm pathogens and not harm the host.

Alexander Fleming discovered that a substance that was made by a mold, *Penicillium notatum,* could inhibit the growth of bacteria. This led to the development of penicillin, but it took many years from the discovery (1929) to the first clinical trials (1940s) because it was difficult to extract enough penicillin from the fungal cultures. It wasn't until the World War II that penicillin was in common use, and even then, it was precious and hard to obtain.

In 1935 a researcher named Gerhard Domagk discovered that sulphonamide, a synthetic substance, could inhibit bacterial growth. For many years the only antibiotics available were sulfa drugs and penicillin; then in the 1960s, many more antibiotics were synthesized and discovered.

An antibiotic is defined as a substance produced by microorganisms that, in small amounts, can inhibit the growth of another microorganism. Many of the antibiotics we use today are derived from the bacterium *Strepto-myces* living in soil, *Bacillus* species and *Penicillium* and *Cephalosporium* molds. Antibiosis is a term used to describe inhibition of growth, and this is where the name "antibiotic" came from.

"Antibiotic" has come to mean all antibacterial substances, even those totally chemically synthesized.

What do we want in a good antibiotic?

1. Toxic to microbes, harmless to human cells

2. Effective at low concentrations

3. Able to penetrate through tissues

These three things are not always attainable, so often we have to balance the pros and cons and choose the best antibiotic for the job. In general though, we can think back to the differences between prokaryotes and eukaryotes to choose targets for antimicrobials that will avoid toxic effects on the human body (eukaryotes) as much as possible.

Antibiotics like penicillin are nontoxic to eukaryotic cells because they disturb the synthesis of peptidoglycan in bacterial cell walls, a substance not found in eukaryotic cells. Prokaryotes have 70S ribosomes, and the drugs that inhibit protein synthesis act on the 70S ribosomes. Here we have a bit of a problem because the human mitochondria contain a 70S ribosome, even if the cells themselves use an 80S ribosome for protein synthesis. The drugs that affect protein synthesis have to be used carefully because they can have some toxic effects on human cells. Prokaryotes must synthesize folic acid to make DNA and RNA; human cells do not. Thus, if you can target the folic acid synthesis in bacteria, you have a drug that will have minimal harmful side effects on human cells. Sulfa is such a drug.

Five Major Classes of Antibiotics

1. Drugs that result in inhibition of cell wall synthesis (e.g., penicillin, ampicillin, cephalosporin, vancomycin)

2. Drugs that result in inhibition of protein synthesis (e.g., aminoglycosides, macrolides, tetracyclines)

3. Drugs that cause injury to the plasma membrane of cells (e.g., polymixin B (a topical agent because it is harmful to human cells))

4. Drugs that inhibit nucleic acid synthesis (e.g., quinolones, rifamycin, imidazoles)

5. Drugs that inhibit the synthesis of essential metabolites (e.g., sulfa and trimethoprim)

Broad Spectrum Antibiotics and Narrow Spectrum Antibiotics

-Antibiotics that inhibit many different types of bacteria (Gram positives and Gram negatives) are called "broad spectrum." A good example is tetracycline, which has activity against both Gram positive and Gram negative bacteria.

-Antibiotics that are more specific in their action, inhibiting fewer types of organisms, are "narrow spectrum." Penicillin is an example of a narrow spectrum drug, mostly effective on certain types of Gram positives.

*In general we want to use narrow spectrum drugs as much as possible because they will not usually wipe out our normal flora that we need to prevent pathogens from infecting us. There are circumstances where broad spectrum drugs must be used, so they are not always a "bad choice:"

1. Serious infections where we do not know the identity of the infection bacteria and it is imperative to get some effect on the pathogen as soon as possible

2. Multibacterial infections where several types of bacteria are working together to cause an infection

Advantages of "broad spectrum" antibiotics: ability to inhibit or kill many different species of bacteria before knowing what the culture results are. Broad spectrums can be given as a first treatment option then discontinued, and narrow spectrum drugs can be continued.

Clostridium difficile AAD (antibiotic-associated diarrhea) or AAC (antibiotic-associated colitis) or PMC (pseudomembranous colitis):

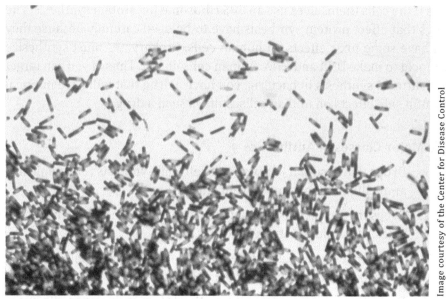

Image courtesy of the Center for Disease Control

FIGURE 7.1   C. difficile Gram's stain

-Normal gut flora (primarily *Bacteroides* species) can easily be abolished by treatment with broad spectrum antibiotics like clindamycin and tetracycline. *C. difficile* is usually resistant to these drugs and, in addition, exists as a spore form that is impermeable to all antibiotics. If this organism is present in the gut, it can then start growing uninhibitedly and produces the exotoxins that cause the inflammatory diarrhea.

-Produce exotoxins A and B: A is an enterotoxin that causes fluid accumulation and watery diarrhea, B is a cytotoxin that damages the mucosal surface of the intestinal lining, leading to ulceration and inflammation. The pseudomembrane is composed of dead epithelial cells, pus, and bacteria; it covers the surface and prevents normal functioning.

-Complications include toxic megacolon (gangrene of the intestines) and surgical emergency.

-It is often acquired nosocomially from the hospital environment.

-Prevention measures include hand washing (not alcohol-based hand sanitizers).

-Treatment includes antibiotics active against Gram positive anaerobes (metronidazole and vancomycin), fecal implants to restore normal flora, and possible probiotics?

*Children younger than 2 years do not get *C. difficile* diarrhea (different type of mucosa?).

Disadvantages of "broad spectrum" antibiotics: usually have an effect on reducing or eliminating the normal flora in the body to the level that allows other microbial species to take over and cause an opportunistic infection.

*example: *Clostridium difficile* diarrheal disease

*example: *Candida albicans* genital yeast infection

Inhibition of the normal flora (lactobacilli) by broad spectrum antibiotics can "pave the way" and allow overgrowth of yeast (which are not susceptible to antibiotics). Lactobacilli normally metabolize glycogen and produce acid, keeping the genital tract at an acid pH. When the lactobacilli are decreased in number by broad spectrum antibiotics, the pH rises to neutral and allows *Candida albicans* to thrive.

-It is often manifested as vaginal yeast infections in women when treated with broad spectrum antibiotics such as tetracycline or ampicillin. It can also be found in women who have used douching for feminine hygiene.

-*C. albicans* is always present in the intestine as "normal flora" and to some degree in the female genitalia.

Continued

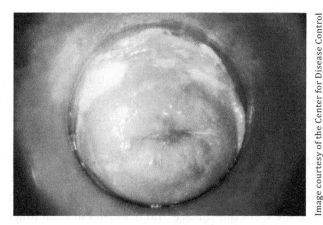

Image courtesy of the Center for Disease Control

FIGURE 7.2   Candida albicans infection of the cervix

Bacteriostatic Versus Bactericidal Antibiotics

-As you learn more about antimicrobials you will find they are sometimes described as "bacteriostatic" or "bacteriocidal" depending on whether they just stop bacteria from replicating or they kill the bacteria. The choice of bacteriostatic over bactericidal will depend on many aspects of the patient's clinical condition, and both are useful, particularly if the patient has a functioning immune system. Some antibiotics can be both bacteriostatic and bactericidal depending on the amount of drug given.

"Drug of Choice"

This is the drug that is deemed to be the most effective with the least side effects for a specific infection. An example is penicillin for strep throat caused by *Streptococcus pyogenes.*

Bacterial Resistance to Drugs

A bacterium that is "resistant" to an antibiotic will not be inhibited by clinically achievable concentrations of the drug. This is can pose real problems for effective treatment of some infections.

-There are several ways that bacteria can become resistant to antibiotics:

1. They can destroy the drug (e.g., production of an enzyme-like beta-lactamase that breaks the drug down).
2. They can prevent penetration of drugs through the cell wall/membrane.
3. They can alter the target site that the drug would normally bind to.
4. They can use an efflux mechanism to eject the drug out of the cytoplasm as soon as it gets into the cell. This efflux mechanism is commonly found in bacteria like Pseudomonas, which has pumps for ejecting quinolones and tetracyclines from the bacterial cells.

-Options 1–3 of the preceding list are mechanisms acquired by the uptake of foreign DNA, allowing one bacterium to "donate" DNA coding for a resistance mechanism to another bacterium.

Three Mechanisms for Foreign DNA Uptake

Conjugation: transfer of a plasmid from a donor cell to a recipient cell through the sex pilus. Plasmids are circular pieces of DNA that often contain genes for antibiotic resistance or virulence factors. When the plasmid codes for antibiotic resistance, it is called an "R" factor. Conjugation can happen between two closely related but different bacterial genus (e.g., *Staphylococcus* and *Enterococcus*, or *E. coli* and *Shigella*)

Transduction: transfer of genes from one bacterium by a bacteriophage (bacterial virus), which picks up genes from one bacterium and then deposits them in another bacterium

Transformation: uptake of free-floating DNA (genes) from the extracellular environment. Usually, these genes will be from other bacteria that have broken down after death of the cell

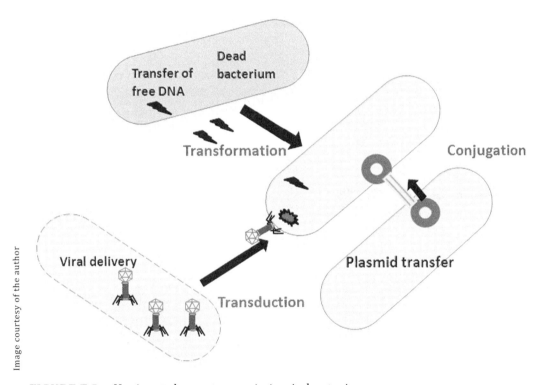

FIGURE 7.3 Horizontal gene transmission in bacteria

What happened with *Staphylococcus aureus,* and what is MRSA?

Staphylococcus aureus, a common pathogen in skin and soft tissue infections, has evolved and developed significant resistance to antibiotics during the past 50 years. In the early days of penicillin, all *S. aureus* were very susceptible to the drug, and penicillin was hailed as the "wonder drug." More than 99% of *S. aureus* strains could be treated with ordinary penicillin. This was great, until the bacteria mutated and became able to produce an enzyme called beta-lactamase (or penicillinase), which broke down the penicillin molecule into a molecule that had no antimicrobial properties (penicillinoic acid) by splitting the beta-lactam ring present in all molecules of penicillin. Now more than 99% of the *S. aureus* strains causing infection produce beta-lactamase and are resistant to penicillin.

We responded by producing semisynthetic penicillin derivatives (methicillin was the first), which had chemical structures placed strategically to protect the beta-lactam ring from binding to the enzyme. This allowed *S. aureus* to be treated and killed using these new beta-lactams much as the old beta-lactam, penicillin, did.

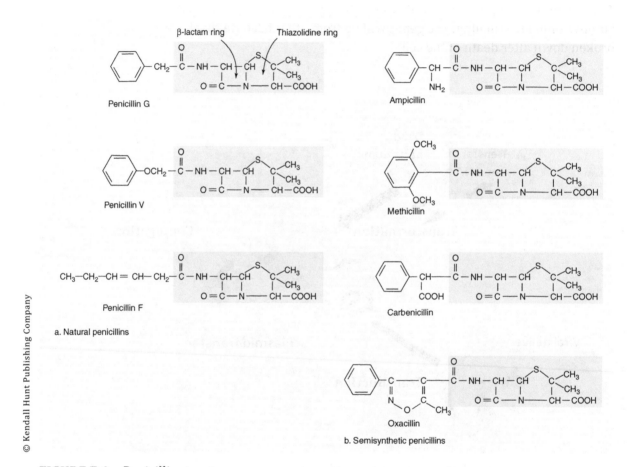

FIGURE 7.4   *Penicillin structures*

The *S. aureus* then responded to the environmental pressure of the methicillin by mutating and altering the target site within the cell wall where the methicillin could bind and prevent the synthesis of peptidoglycan. These bacteria are known as methicillin-resistant *Staphylococcus aureus* (MRSA), and the gene that codes for that target site alteration is called the Mec gene. The target site alteration is the change from the PBP2 (penicillin binding protein 2) in the cell wall to PBP2a, which has a very low affinity for the penicillin derivatives.

MRSA is now a significant problem in hospitals today. Many of the strains are not only resistant to the newer penicillin derivatives but also to other antibiotics and thus are a problem to treat. We do have another drug, not related to penicillin, that can be used for treatment of these MRSA strains, vancomycin, but responsible antibiotic stewardship is really necessary to prevent the MRSA strains from also acquiring vancomycin resistance via conjugation from another type of Gram positive bacterium *Enterococcus*. The enterococci have acquired a mutation (Van A, B, and C) which make them resistant to the action of vancomycin (VRE or vancomycin-resistant enterococci), and the fear is that the enterococci may transfer these genes to *S. aureus* by conjugation). If and when this happens, we will be left without any good treatment option for *S. aureus*. So far one or two strains have emerged, but the patients were identified and placed in isolation quickly so that the bacteria were not allowed to spread.

MRSA started as a nosocomial infection in the hospital setting, where there was a positive antibiotic pressure, and has evolved so that there are now strains of MRSA circulating in the community outside of the hospital. These can be subtyped and tracked epidemiologically.

How can we reduce the possibility that antibiotics become resistant?

-Use sparingly, only when necessary to prevent environmental buildup.

-Use combinations of drugs to reduce ability of bacteria to survive after one mutation.

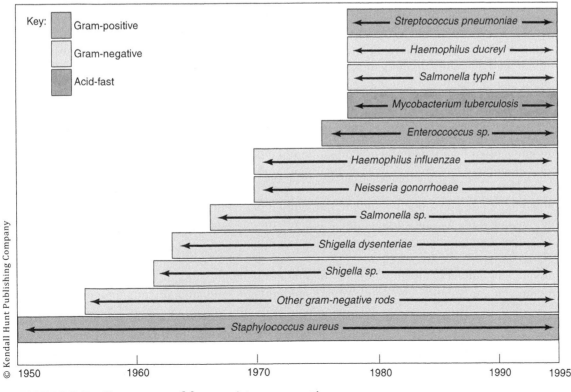

FIGURE 7.5   Emergence of drug resistance over time

Can all antibiotics be used to treat all categories of patients?

No. Think about people with allergies, pregnant women (who cannot use tetracyclines or quinolones because they damage the babies' teeth, bone, and cartilage formation), children, and individuals with liver or kidney damage (many drugs are "detoxified" in the liver and excreted through the kidney).

Side effects of antibiotics

Almost all drugs do have some side effects, but these can be more or less serious. Some are reversible, and some are permanent even after drugs are stopped:

> Gastrointestinal upsets
>
> Rash, allergy
>
> Liver damage (hepatotoxicity)
>
> Kidney damage (nephrotoxicity)
>
> Nerve damage (e.g., ototoxicity with aminoglycosides causing deafness)
>
> Teeth and bone formation in children (e.g., tetracyclines)
>
> Cartilage formation in children

Monitoring of Serum Antibiotic Levels

The serum (blood) concentration of some antibiotics should be monitored to make sure they are high enough to be effective on the bacteria but not so high that they will cause damage to organs. There are certain antibiotics that are more dangerous than others—the aminoglycosides (e.g., gentamicin, amikacin, streptomycin, tobramycin, etc.) are one group that should be monitored. These antibiotics inhibit protein synthesis at the ribosomal level and therefore will have some effect on eukaryotic cells as well as prokaryotic cells.

Monitoring is usually done by taking the blood of the patient before, one hour after and 12–16 hours after an antibiotic injection or infusion. This information will:

a. Allow us to attain effective levels of drug (over the MIC point)

b. Prevent undue toxic side effects due to too high dosing

c. Ascertain dosing intervals—want to keep the antibiotic above the MIC but below levels known to cause harmful effects

Antimicrobials: how are they administered?

Different drugs will be available in different formulations, depending on the drug. Some drugs will be available as oral tablets, others only as injection drugs to be given intramuscularly, and some for intravenous use. As a rule, if a patient has a life-threatening infection, intravenous drug will always be given to start with because this is the fastest way of attaining an effective blood and tissue concentration of the drugs.

Synergism: use of two drugs in combination may be greater than the combined effect of either drug separately:

* **example**: treatment of bacterial endocarditis: Use penicillin to damage the bacterial cell walls, and allow the aminoglycoside to enter the cell and inhibit protein synthesis.

Antagonism: combination of two drugs together is detrimental to the effect of one of the drugs

* **example**: combination of penicillin and tetracycline: Tetracycline interferes with bacterial growth, which is needed for the action of penicillin, which interferes with the synthesis of new peptidoglycan

Antimicrobials for Nonbacterial Infections:=

A. ANTIFUNGAL DRUGS

-General problem with toxicity because although the major mechanism of action is on fungal-specific structures, the drugs have other components that can harm other eukaryotic cells

-Fungal structure usually targeted is ergosterol in fungal cell membranes (humans have cholesterol). These drugs have a higher affinity for ergosterol than other sterol molecules, so preferentially act on ergosterol (but some effect on cholesterol)

-Common antifungal drugs:

Polyenes: amphotericin B used often for systemic fungal disease

Some toxicity for kidneys

-Inhibit ergosterol synthesis

Azoles: clotrimazole and miconazole commonly used topically

fluconazole and itraconazole internal use for systemic infections

-Inhibit ergosterol synthesis

Griseofulvin: active against superficial mycoses and dermatophytes

-Binds to keratin and blocks microtubule assembly, interfering with mitosis in fungi

B. ANTIVIRAL DRUGS

-Target various aspects of viral replication

1. Nucleoside and nucleotide analogues:

-Usually some limited toxicity for human cells

-Closely resemble molecules used for DNA/RNA replication, substituted for the "real" molecules resulting in nonfunctional nucleic acids

-Example: acyclovir and its derivatives: used for treating Herpes infections

-AZT (zidovudine) used for treatment of HIV, blocks synthesis of DNA from RNA by the enzyme reverse transcriptase

2.   Drugs that inhibit other enzymes

-Often analogs of amino acids, the building blocks of proteins

-Virus will try to use its proteases to break down proteins for production of new viral particles and these drugs competitively interfere with protease activity

-Often used in combination with other antivirals

-Example: neuraminidase inhibitors for treatment of early stages of Influenza A (Relenza (zanamivir) and oseltamivir (Tamiflu))

3.   Interferon

-Cytokines, produced by virally infected cells, inhibit further spread of infection

C. ANTIPARASITIC DRUGS

1.   Antiprotozoan drugs

-*Quinine and derivatives to treat malaria; problem: resistance to drugs (e.g. mefloquine for treating quinine resistant malaria)

-Imidazoles: drugs that target the anaerobic metabolism of both bacteria and protozoa (e.g. metronidazole (Flagyl™))

2.   Antihelminthic drugs

-Various mechanisms of activity

-Niclosamide: inhibits ATP production under aerobic conditions

-Used for tapeworms

-Praziquantel: alters permeability of plasma membranes of worms, exposes surface antigens on worms, rendering them susceptible to the immune system

-Used for Schistosoma, tapeworms

-Mebendazole: disrupts microtubules in cytoplasm, reduces worm mobility

-Used for Ascaris, pinworms, whipworms

-Pyantel pamoate: paralyzes worms and allows them to be eliminated naturally

-Used for roundworms

Superbugs

-Microbes that are resistant to antimicrobials and are hard to treat

1.   MRSA (methicillin-resistant *Staphylococcus aureus*)

-Mutation involving the gene Mec A; PBP2 mutated to PBP2a

2. **VRE (vancomycin-resistant *Enterococcus* species)**

-Several gene mutations, genes Van A, Van B, Van C

3. **ESBL (extended spectrum beta-lactamase)**

-Gram negative bacteria (Enterobacticeae family)

-Many different genes involved

-Increasing problem in ICU (intensive care units), extended care facilities

-ESBL-producing bacteria can inactivate even the new really good beta-lactamase antibiotics like meropenem

-NDM-1 is a variant (New Delhi metalloproteinase) that makes bacteria extremely resistant to beta-lactam antibiotics

4. *Pseudomonas aeruginosa*

-Gram negative bacterium (nonfermenter of glucose)

-"Opportunistic pathogen," normal inhabitant of soil and water

-Can live in very harsh conditions (e.g., liquid soap, Cepacol mouthwash)

-Need very few nutrients (can live in water in flower vases)

-Can infect many body sites

-Very common in burns and lungs of cystic fibrosis patients

-Endotoxin; also produces exotoxins

5. *Streptococcus pneumoniae*

-Gram positive diplococci; cause of upper and lower respiratory tract infections, meningitis

-Most common cause of community-acquired pneumonia

-Common pathogen in all ages of patients, children to elderly

-Emerging resistance to penicillin due to genetic mutations in PBP (penicillin-binding protein)

6. *Mycobacterium tuberculosis* (MDR-TB, XDR-TB)

-*M. tuberculosis* is always treated with a combination of drugs:

    First line: isoniazid, rifampin, pyrazinamide, ethambutol

    Second line: fluoroquinolones, aminoglycosides like amikacin, cycloserine, etc.

-Normally only first-line drugs used; patient becomes noninfectious in about two weeks

MDR-TB: multidrug-resistant TB: organism is resistant to isoniazid and rifampin by definition

XDR-TB: extensively drug-resistant TB: resistant to isoniazid and rifampicin and also any member of the quinolone family and at least one of the injectable drugs (like aminoglycosides)

-Second-line drugs are more toxic with more side effects than first line drugs

-Treatment might be necessary for up to two years

Susceptibility Testing for Antimicrobials (Mostly Antibiotics)

DEFINITIONS

MIC = minimum inhibitory concentration: the minimum amount of drug that will inhibit the growth of the bacteria (not kill!)

MBC = minimum bactericidal concentration: the minimum amount of drug that will kill the bacteria

Kirby-Bauer test: routine test used in the bacteriology laboratory to measure the extent of drug susceptibility exhibited by specific strains of bacteria. Filter paper discs are impregnated with different amounts of antibiotics and tested with the bacterial isolated from an infection to see how well the drug inhibits growth.

E-test: method of determining MIC for individual antibiotics

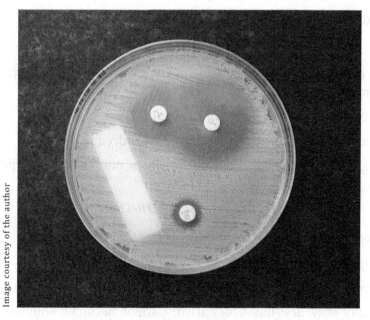

Image courtesy of the author

FIGURE 7.6   Kirby-Bauer susceptibility test

SIR: susceptible, intermediate, and resistant:

-Specific pathogens are classified as being S, I, or R to specific drugs that could be used for treatment. This information is used to choose the appropriate antibiotic for treating the infection. Only S is usually used, although a drug that is I for the bacterium could be used if the drug is used for a urinary tract infection and the kidney is known to concentrate the drug in the urine.

E-test: gives the MIC value of the drug tested for the specific bacterial isolate

-Plastic strips are impregnated with a gradient of the antibiotic—lowest concentration at the bottom of the strip, highest at the top—a culture plate is streaked with bacteria, the e-test strip is placed on the surface, and the plate is incubated at 37 °C and allowed to grow. The MIC can then be read off of the strip—the intersection of the area of no-growth with the area of growth around the antibiotic containing strip

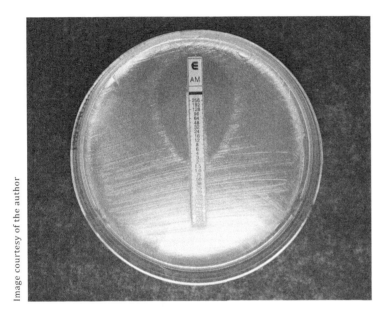

Image courtesy of the author

FIGURE 7.7   E-test for determining MIC of a bacterial isolate

Interested? Want to learn more?

For more reading, several texts online at the U of A library are recommended:

1.   Brooks, GF, Carroll KC, Butel JS, Morse SA, editors. Jawetz, Melnick, and Adelberg's Medical Microbiology, 24th ed. Blacklick OH-McGraw Hill; 2007.

2.   Ryan KJ, Ray CG, editors. Sherris Medical Microbiology, 5th ed. New York – McGraw-Hill, 2010.

3.   Mandell GL, Bennett JE, Dolin R, editors. Mandell, Douglas and Bennett's Principles and Practices of Infectious Diseases, 7th ed. Churchill Livingstone Elsevier, Philadelphia, 2010.

Chapter 8

The Innate Immune Response

Learning Objectives:

1. List the major components of the innate first line of defense.
2. List and define the cell types involved in the second line of defense.
3. Describe the mechanisms in diapedesis, chemotaxis, and phagocytosis.
4. Explain how opsonization increases the efficiency of the immune system.
5. Differentiate between MHC I and MHC II.

The Immune System

The body's defence system functions to:

- Keep microorganisms out
- Remove microorganisms that get in
- Combat microorganisms that remain inside
- Fight cancer

IMPORTANT CRITERION for Proper Immune Functioning

- Immune system must be able to distinguish between **self** (host) and **nonself** (pathogen or something that doesn't belong).

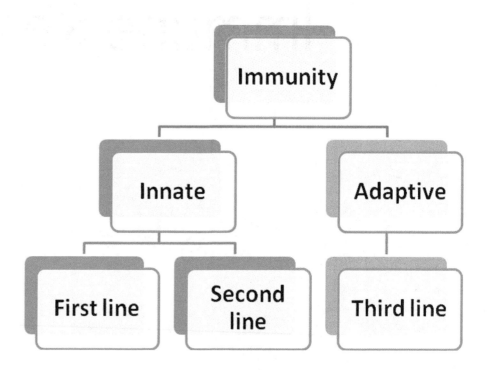

Functions of the Two Branches of Immunity

The two branches of the immune system do not function separately in a void. There is a lot of "cross talk" or "collaboration" between innate and adaptive immunity—they help each other perform optimally, and there are many redundancies to make up for possible deficits.

A. NONSPECIFIC (INNATE, NATURAL)

-Already in place at birth, no "priming required"

-First and second lines of defense

-Prevent colonization, replication, and spread of infectious agents

-Physical barriers are always the first hindrance to infection

-When physical barriers are breached, the second line of defense comes into play

-Phagocytes (cells that engulf organisms), inflammatory responses, and complement proteins become activated and help activate the immune functioning

-Antimicrobial substances are produced, like acute phase proteins

*example: C-reactive protein (CRP) in the liver

lysozyme, an enzyme that breaks down bacterial cell walls and is found in body secretions like tears

-Nonspecific functions occur rapidly and are essential for survival of the species

-Give the host time to develop the slower developing, more specific responses in the third line of defense

B. SPECIFIC (ADAPTIVE, ACQUIRED)

-Third line of defense

-Takes time to develop

-Specific "memory" of infection with a specific organism

-If the host is challenged later with the same organism, there is a more rapid, more efficient response on second exposure because the cells are already primed and ready to go!

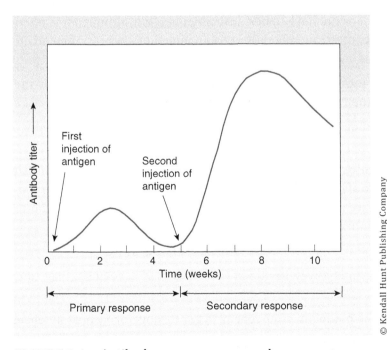

FIGURE 8.1   Antibody response on second exposure to a pathogen

-Three elements of the third line of defense:

1. B cells (or B-lymphocytes)

2. T cells (or T lymphocytes)

3. Antibodies (produced by plasma cells, which in turn are derived from B lymphocytes

TABLE 8.1   *Nonspecific and Specific Resistance*

Nonspecific Resistance: innate—we are born with these defenses

First line	Second line
1. Skin	1. Phagocytes and NK cells
2. Mucous membranes	2. Inflammation
3. Normal flora	3. Complement
	4. Antimicrobial substances

Specific Resistance: develops later; more specialized and has memory function

Third line of defense
1. Specialized lymphocytes:
-B cells and T cells
2. Antibodies

You probably know more about the immune system than you think...

When you get a cut or a sliver, you experience heat, redness, swelling, and pain in the area—**this is an inflammatory response**. An inflammatory response does not have to be caused by infection, although it is often associated with infection. When there is an infection, there is often an elevated white blood cell (WBC) count.

You need more WBC during an infection because these cells mediate the immune response to the infecting organism.

-When you get a sore throat, you may have swollen lymph nodes in the neck.

Lymph nodes are where the cells of the immune system multiply to prepare to fight off the infection. This is why you get an enlarged gland when you are infected—the lymph node physically grows to accommodate all of the immune cells.

The Host–Pathogen Relationship: A Constant Battle

-Pathogen finds a way to attack the host; host develops a way to defend itself.

BUT the pathogen often learns to get through or by host defenses.

-Different types of immune responses can occur that are tailored for the many different types of pathogens the host can encounter.

Lymph node

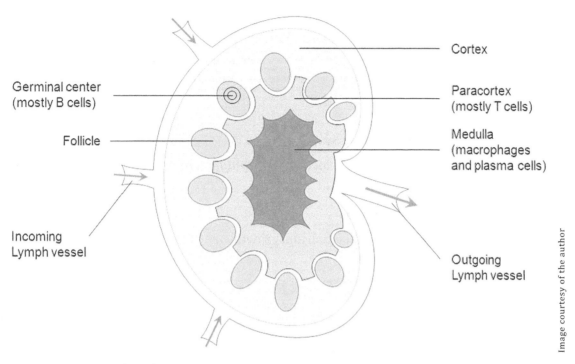

Cortex

Germinal center
(mostly B cells)

Paracortex
(mostly T cells)

Follicle

Medulla
(macrophages
and plasma cells)

Incoming
Lymph vessel

Outgoing
Lymph vessel

Image courtesy of the author

FIGURE 8.2   Lymph node anatomy

-Successful pathogens have evolved mechanisms to avoid host defense mechanisms.

Different pathogens use different strategies to overcome host defenses.

Viruses

-Invade host cells and take over cellular machinery for their own use

-Live inside of host cells and try to hide from immune system

-Some may down regulate markers on the host cell that signal infection within the cell

Bacteria

-Usually live outside of host cells

-Many have specific mechanisms like capsules, enzymes, and exotoxins to avoid or destroy host defenses (and cells)

Parasites

-Can be very large (some worms are as long as 10 m in length)

-Some cloak themselves with a layer that makes them invisible to the immune system. This coating consists of host-derived molecules. The immune cells will then see the parasite as "self."

Fungi

-Different strategies, depending on the fungus

-Some yeast can produce a capsule for evading phagocytosis

-Some molds are large and not easily accessible for phagocytosis

-Some molds can change their morphology in the body and become yeast, which may be able to replicate and survive in macrophages (dimorphic)

How the Immune System Reacts

The innate defences focus on *stopping* microorganisms before they get in!

-Block adherence

-Block invasion

-Inhibit colonization and growth

Components of the Cellular Immune Response

Composition of Blood

Plasma: fluid portion of blood, with clotting proteins intact and nonactivated

Erythrocytes: red blood cells; carry oxygen to tissues

Platelets: involved in clotting and plugging capillaries, production of immune-reactive chemicals like serotonin

Leukocytes: white blood cells; granulocytes and mononuclear cells

Serum: liquid part of the blood, with blood clotting factors removed

Plasma: liquid part of the blood, with blood clotting factors intact (chemicals used to prevent blood clotting)

Hematopoiesis in Humans

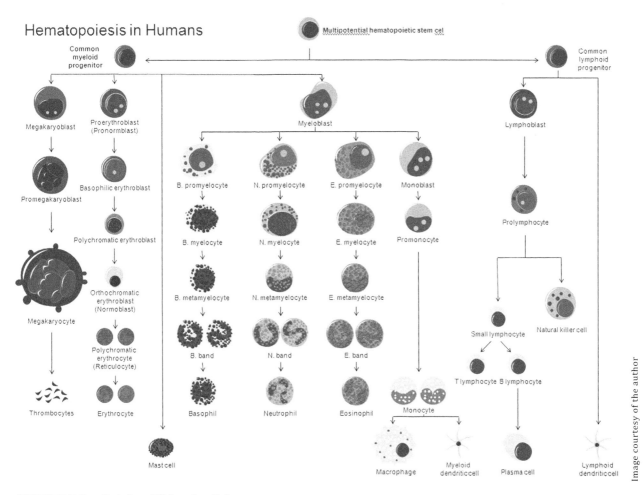

FIGURE 8.3   *Origin of "blood cells"*

Image courtesy of the author

Leukocytes

A. GRANULOCYTES

- Three types of white blood cells that have granules, or pouches, of chemicals and enzymes in the cytoplasm

- These are neutrophils, basophils, and eosinophils

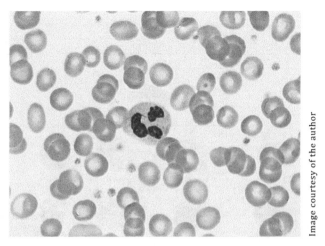

FIGURE 8.4   Neutrophil in a peripheral blood smear

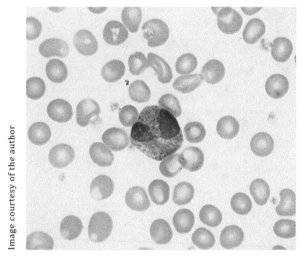

FIGURE 8.5   Eosinophil in a peripheral blood smear

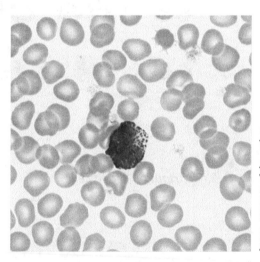

FIGURE 8.6   Basophil in a peripheral blood smear

B. MONONUCLEAR CELLS

-Includes monocytes (become macrophages when activated in tissues), natural killer (NK cells), and lymphocytes

- Natural killer cells (NK) cells (look like small lymphocytes)

Where do all of the different kinds of leukocytes come from?

-All blood cells originate as stem cells in the bone marrow.

-T-lymphocytes and B-lymphocytes function in the adaptive system

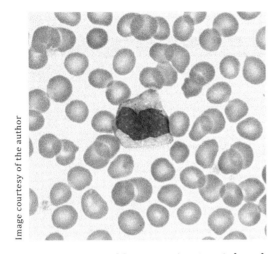

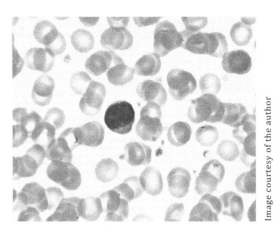

Image courtesy of the author

Image courtesy of the author

FIGURE 8.7   *Monocyte in a peripheral blood smear*

FIGURE 8.8   *Lymphocyte*

-Different cell types develop as a result of chemical signals called **cytokines**, which are produced by activated white blood cells.

-Each cell type has a specific function, and each cytokine will have specific functions.

Immunity is mediated by cells in blood and lymphatic fluid

-Blood is circulated through a pressurized system, pumped by the heart through arteries and veins.

-Blood is circulated through a pressurized system; lymph is not.

-Blood is pumped by the heart through the arteries and veins; lymph is the drainage from capillaries. This lymph is called interstitial fluid when it enters tissues.

-Lymph is an ultra-filtrate of blood and does contain some white blood cells, which are also found in the lymph nodes.

-Lymphatic system is comprised of channels that are connected to lymph nodes.

-Lymph nodes contain high concentrations of B-lymphocytes and T-lymphocytes, so they are a good site for "antigen presentation."

-Lymph nodes also act as filters for microorganisms and foreign material.

-Filtered lymphatic fluid is returned to blood circulation for recycling.

****

TABLE 8.2   *Example of Major Cytokines*

Cytokine	Cell Source	Effects
Interleukin-1	Macrophages, B cells	Activation of lymphocytes, stimulation of macrophages
Interleukin-2	T cells	T-cell growth factor
Interleukin-3	T cells	Colony-stimulating factor
Interleukin-4	T cells	B-cell growth factor
Interleukin-5	T cells	B-cell growth factor
Interleukin-6	T cells, B cells, macrophages	B-cell growth factor
Interleukin-7	Bone-marrow stromal cells	Stimulates growth and differentiation of B cells
Interleukin-8	Macrophages, skin cells	Chemotaxis of neutrophils
Interleukin-9	T cells	Induces proliferation of some T helper cells in the absence of antigen, promotes growth of mast cells
Interleukin-10	T cells	Inhibition of cytokine synthesis
Interleukin-11	Bone-marrow cells	Stimulates B cell development
Interleukin-12	Monocytes	Induction of T_H1 cells
Interleukin-13	T cells	Blocks IL-12 production; regulator of inflammatory response
Interleukin-14	T cells	Induces proliferation of activated B cells
Tumor necrosis factors α and β	Macrophages, lymphocytes, T cells	Activation of macrophages, granulocytes, and cytotoxic cells
Interferon-α/β	Macrophages, lymphocytes	MHC class I induction, antiviral effect
Interferon-γ	T cells, natural killer cells	MHC induction, macrophage activation, endothelial cell adhesion
Monocyte colony stimulating factor	Monocytes	Stimulates division and differentiation of monocytes
Granulocyte colony stimulating factor	Macrophages	Stimulates division and differentiation of macrophages
Migration inhibition factor	T cells	Inhibits migration of cells

©Kendall Hunt 16.03

First Line of Defense (External Barriers)

-Skin, mucous membranes, antimicrobial secretions, and normal flora work together to maintain integrity of the body.

-Keratin

-Cells in superficial layers of skin slough off and take microorganisms with them.

-High or low pH in secretions/organs inhibit antimicrobial growth.

A. SKIN: TWO LAYERS WITH TIGHT JUNCTIONS

Dermis: tightly woven connective tissue

Epidermis: epithelial cells in layers

-Layers flatten out toward the outside—keratin embeds the outer layers.

-Tight junctions between cells form an impermeable barrier.

-Keratin is a protective protein in the upper epidermidis for waterproofing the skin.

-Sweat glands, blood vessels, nerves, and hair follicles are in the deeper dermis layer.

Intact skin is an effective barrier against infection

-Skin provides a very inhospitable environment for microbial growth.

-Skin is a very dry environment; most microorganisms require a moist environment.

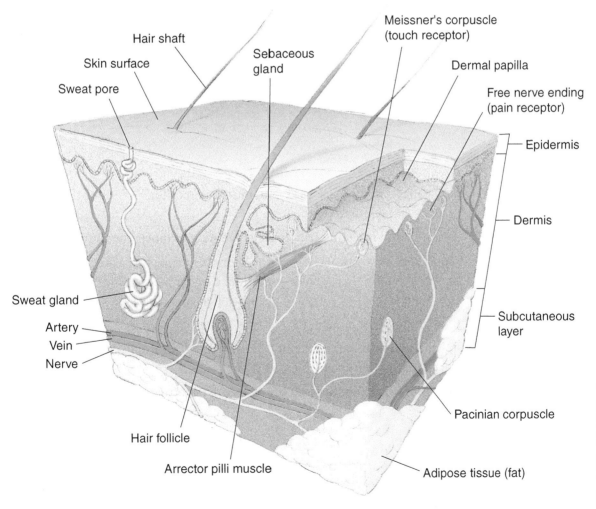

FIGURE 8.9 *Skin structure*

-Sweat contains high concentration of salt; salt inhibits growth of most microorganisms.

-Sebaceous glands in the skin secrete sebum, a fatty acid (oily protective barrier), which is antibacterial and antifungal and lowers skin pH,

Dendritic cells (e.g., Langerhans cells): antigen-presenting cells that live in tissues and process and present antigen to helper T cells in the lymph tissues (bringing in the "adaptive system). These cells survey the tissues looking for "antigen" or foreign substances and can be microorganisms.

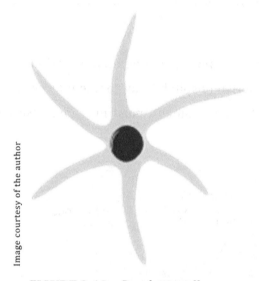

Image courtesy of the author

FIGURE 8.10   Dendritic cell

B. MUCOUS MEMBRANES (INTERNAL "SKIN")

-Cells of the mucosa are bathed in mucus and other secretions that help to flush away the microorganisms.

-Peristalsis in intestine (rhythmic movement to move intestinal contents)

-Ciliated cells in respiratory tract (hair-like projections on the surface of the cells that, with a wave-like motion, carry mucus and microbes up and out of the system—this is sometimes called the "ciliary elevator")

-Body fluids flush organisms out (e.g., urine)

-Mucous membranes that line the GI and respiratory and genitourinary tracts are thin permeable barriers.

Antimicrobial Substances Associated with Mucous Membranes

-Inhibit or kill microorganisms

Lysozyme: degrades peptidoglycan, breaks down cell wall (e.g., tears, saliva)

-G+ bacteria primarily but also has some effect on Gram negatives under certain conditions when the outer layer of the cell wall is disrupted

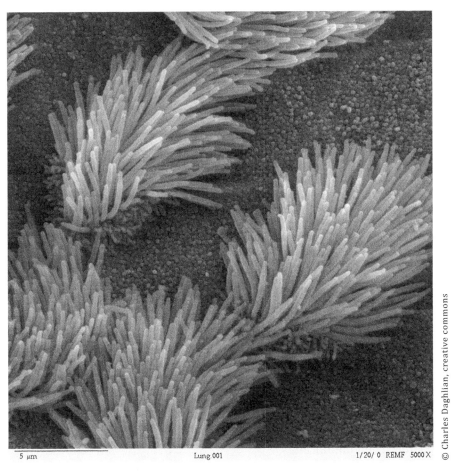

© Charles Daghlian, creative commons

5 μm   Lung.001   1/20/ 0 REMF 5000 X

FIGURE 8.11   SEM (scanning electron micrograph) of bronchial epithelium with cilia

Peroxidase: enzymes (break down H_2O_2) and produce oxidizing compounds that can affect bacteria (e.g., catalase)

Lactoferrin: iron-binding protein often in secretions (deprives proliferating bacteria of iron, so restricts growth)

Transferrin: iron-binding protein in the blood

-Both lactoferrin and transferrin bind to and remove free iron, preventing microbes from using it for growth.

Defensins: short antimicrobial peptides found on mucous membranes and in phagocytic cells. Function to form pores in target; results in microbial cell destruction.

Summary: Defense Mechanisms of Mucous Membranes

Goblet cells: secrete mucus— traps microbes

Mechanical removal: coughing, sneezing to expel organisms

Ciliary escalator: ciliated epithelial cells in trachea and nasopharynx

- Cilia push bacterial cells back up and out of the respiratory tract; protect lungs from colonization

- Bacteria trapped by mucous can be coughed out, or swallowed and killed by stomach acid

Secretions: "flushing" to prevent infection

Tears: flush the surface of the eye and remove potential pathogens

Saliva: prevents microbial colonization in mouth; flush out spaces between teeth

Crevicular fluid: fluid that flows into gingival crevice (between teeth)—similar composition to blood serum

- Contains immune cells and molecules

Urine: flush epithelial surface in urethra

Innate Defense Mechanisms in the Gastrointestinal System

-Stomach contains gastric juice.

- Highly acidic (pH 1–2)

- Most microorganisms cannot survive.

-Paneth cells in the intestines make proteins called defensins, which damage bacterial cell membranes.

-Movement of food provides some defense against infection in the small intestine.

-Following exposure, the pathogens must adhere to a body surface in order to infect.

-This makes sense because even though bacterial cells are small, they can't "transport" from one place to another (you can't enter a room without opening a door).

-Food moves quickly through the small intestine; bacteria is carried along with the food.

-It is difficult for bacteria to "grab on" to the intestinal walls to mediate adherence.

-No adherence = no invasion

c. Normal microbiota (or "normal flora")

-**Microbial antagonism**: active opposition between two microbes

-Competition for nutrients, oxygen, iron, etc.

-Physical presence using available binding sites

-Production of substances like bacteriocins that kill other bacteria

****

Second Line of Defense

-Consists of: phagocytic WBC: neutrophils and macrophages

Inflammation

    Complement

    NK cells

    Antimicrobial substances

A. PHAGOCYTIC WBC (WHITE BLOOD CELLS)

-Ingest and destroy foreign material (e.g., organisms)

-Attract more immune cells to the area

-Prevent further spread of infection

-Trigger initiation of adaptive immune response

Phagocytosis: "phago" = eat; "cyt" = cell; "osis" = condition of

-Ingestion of microorganisms by a cell

-Means to counter infection

Phagocytes: cells that perform phagocytosis

-White blood cells (WBC): neutrophils and macrophages, dendritic cells and Langerhans cells in tissues

    How?

-Phagocytosis

-Inflammation and fever

-Antimicrobial proteins

-Complement

-Direct extracellular killing by NK cells and eosinophils

How do neutrophils recognize pathogens?

-Bacteria: all proteins start with formylmethionine group, our proteins do not, so neutrophils sniff out those proteins and realize it is an invader.

    Neutrophil: polymorphonuclear leukocyte (PMNL)

- Originate in bone marrow
- Short-lived cell because it does not have mitochondria
- Prominent in acute infections
- Defense against pyogenic bacteria (e.g., strep, staph)
- Contain granules: small pouches of enzymes

    examples: myeloperoxidase: responsible for green color of pus

    lysozyme (breaks down peptidoglycan)

    proteases and acid hydrolases (break down protein structures)

Deficiencies in neutrophil function

- Result in increased bacterial infections (by pyogenic or pus produc-ing organisms)

- Often recurrent skin, pulmonary, and GI infections

How do macrophages recognize pathogens?

-One important way: through **pattern recognition receptors**, which act as the "eyes" for the cell to look for microbes.

-**Toll-like receptors (TLRs)** are **pattern recognition receptors** and bind specific structures on microorganisms. When this binding occurs, the mac-rophages become activated and can actively produce cytokines, and able to more efficiently phagocytose organisms.

- TLR recognize molecules that are unique to microbes and are never found in multicellular organisms.

  *example: peptidoglycan in bacterial cell wall binds to TLR-2

  lipopolysaccharide (LPS) on Gram negative bacteria binds to TLR-4

  flagellin binds to TLR-5

Note that there are TLR internally in macrophages that recognize viral ele-ments like single-stranded RNA.

Phagocytosis of a microbe

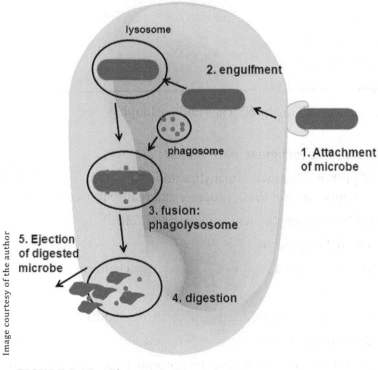

FIGURE 8.12   Phagocytosis

Macrophage/Dendritic Cells

-Mature from monocytes and proliferate in lymph nodes

-Microorganisms pass through tissue with macrophages, are recognized, and are ingested (phagocytosed)

-Also dispose of worn out blood cells to clear the debris

-Activated macrophages secrete cytokines

-Responsible for "antigen presentation" to lymphocytes

Both neutrophils and macrophages "phagocytose" microorganisms

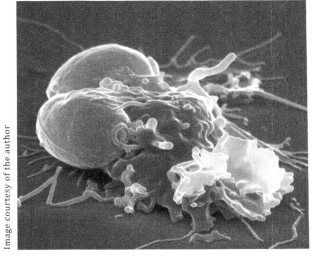

Image courtesy of the author

FIGURE 8.13a   *Leukocyte (neutrophil) attaching to a yeast cell (SEM)*

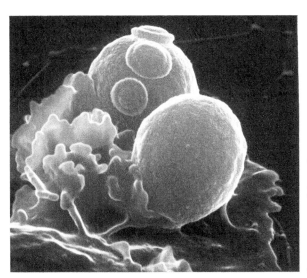

Image courtesy of the author

FIGURE 8.13b.   *Pseudopods ruffle and enclose the yeast cell (SEM)*

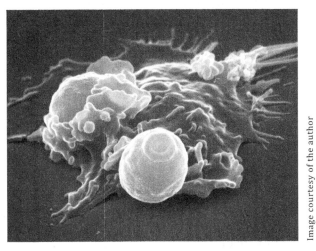

Image courtesy of the author

FIGURE 8.13c   *Leukocyte (neutrophil) engulfing a yeast cell (SEM)*

Important Chronologic Events in Phagocytosis

1. Chemotaxis

-Directed movement of the cell to the antigen in response to cytokine, complement by-products, or microbial chemical molecules

2. Attachment (also called adherence)

-Plasma membrane of phagocyte extends projections (pseudopods) to enfold the microorganism (hug of death)

-Adherence can be inhibited by some virulence factors (e.g., *S. pneumoniae* capsule)

3. Ingestion

- Pseudopods meet and fuse, and pull the foreign invader into the cell.

- Phagosome forms (membrane around the vacuole with the micro-organism).

4. Fusion of phagosome with lysosome

Lysosomes: vesicles that contain digestive enzymes, bactericidal substances, lysozyme, lipases, and proteases and have a low pH

Phagolysosome = fused lysosome and phagosome

5. Digestion

-Enzymes in phagolysosome break down particulate matter

-Most types of bacteria can be destroyed by lysosomal contents

6. Release of products

-If a neutrophil has digested an organism, it just releases all debris to the extracellular environment

-If a macrophage has digested the organism, MHC II will bind some of the peptides from the microorganism and transport it to the cell surface where it is anchored in the cell membrane—this is **antigen presentation** (some debris will also be expelled).

Bacterial Resistance to Phagocytosis

S. pyogenes: M protein in cell wall prevents adherence

Coxiella burnetii: replicates at low pH in the phagolysosome

Listeria monocytogenes, *Shigella flexneri*: contain enzyme to lyse phagolysosome and free bacteria to multiply in the cytoplasm, avoiding the chemicals contained in the vacuole

Some microbes are able to grow in phagocytes:

Chlamydia

Rickettsia

Mycobacterium tuberculosis

Leishmania

Plasmodia

HIV, other viruses

B. INFLAMMATION

-Intimately tied to activation of the immune system and cells

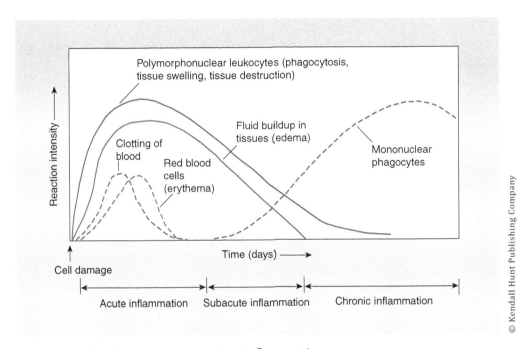

FIGURE 8.14 Events accompanying inflammation

Four cardinal signs of inflammation: **SHRP** (swelling, heat, redness, and pain)

-Release of chemical mediators, which affect vascular permeability and fluid movement in tissues

Basophils are part of the innate immune system and are important for inflammation

-Basophils are similar to **mast cells** in the tissues and function to release inflammatory mediators like histamine

-Also important in allergy

Two Types of Inflammation

1. Acute inflammation: immediate, nonspecific; **neutrophils** main cell type involved

-**Chemotaxis**: neutrophils migrate in response to a chemical gradient of:

   a. Complement products (e.g., C5a)

   b. Formyl peptides in bacterial proteins

   c. Chemotactic cytokines

-**Opsonization**: neutrophils/macrophages are phagocytic and have Fc receptors that will bind to the Fc region on antibody molecules. They also have C3b receptors. Coating the cells with C3b **or** antibody **or** C-reactive protein makes the process more efficient.

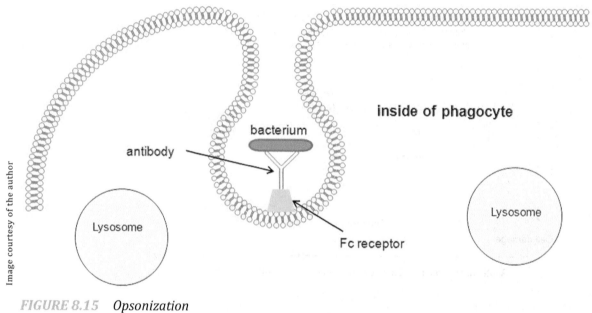

FIGURE 8.15   *Opsonization*

-**Neutrophil killing**: neutrophils can kill by the formation of superoxide radicals or by enzymatic digestion

2. Chronic inflammation: takes longer to evolve, more likely specific; lymphocytes and **macrophages** (mononuclear cells) most important

-More likely to result in permanent damage to tissue structures due to fibrosis and scarring.

-**Mononuclear phagocytes**: dominant players in chronic inflammation. Monocytes become macrophages when activated (or histiocytes-resident tissue macrophages)

-Mononuclear phagocytes also respond to chemotactic factors but move more slowly. They are all phagocytic and prefer opsonized microbes. They use some of the same killing mechanisms as neutrophils use in acute inflammation.

Mononuclear phagocytes differ from neutrophils in the following ways:

- Long life span in tissue

- Produce cytokines (e.g., TNF and IL-1, which produces fever)

- Present antigen in MHC II (e.g., CD4 or T helper cells)

Lymphocytes: B and T cells both participate in inflammation

Eosinophils: granulocytes, similar to neutrophils, have oxidative killing mechanisms like neutrophils have. Often seen in tissues in allergic diseases and in worm infections

Granulomatous inflammation: granuloma = localized collection of mononuclear phagocytes. Sometimes giant cells where many macrophages have fused together.

-Seen in:

    Foreign body granuloma

    Tuberculosis

    Fungal infection

    A few other diseases like sarcoidosis and Crohn's disease

Chronic inflammation and tissue repair: new blood vessel growth and fibrosis results in scarring.

C. THE COMPLEMENT SYSTEM

-Set of plasma proteins that are involved in phagocytosis and lysis of bacteria

-Very complex pathway; at least 20 proteins involved; sequential activation of proteins in a stepwise manner

-Attack extracellular pathogens

-May or may not involve antibodies as activators

-Important in:

    -Lysis of foreign cells with the membrane attack complex formed when the last members of the complement pathway form pores in the target cell membrane

    -Development of inflammation

    -Activated complement components (e.g., C3b important **opsonin** for phagocytosis)

    -C3a and C5a important in mast cell degranulation

    -C5a important in attracting leukocytes (chemoattractant)

Three pathways of complement activation

    1. **Classical pathway**

-Binding of antigen and antibody to C1 activates the classical pathway (C1 cleaves C2 into C2a and C2b; also C4 to C4a and C4b, then C2a and C4a combine to activate C3, splitting it to C3a and C3b).

-C3b is important for opsonisation of microbes, and it continues activating the pathway, splitting C5 to C5a and C5b, etc.

-The end result of all complement activation pathways is the formation of **MAC (membrane attack complex)**.

2.   Alternate pathway

-No antibodies are involved.

-C3 combines with factors B, D, and P on the surface of a microbe and is split to C3a and C3b—the pathway then starts from this point and ends in formation of **MAC (membrane attack complex)**.

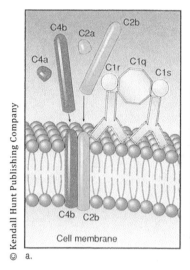 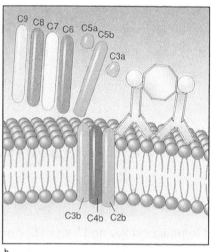 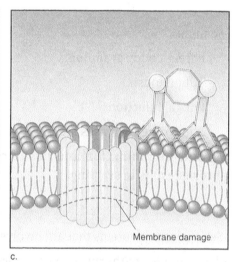

FIGURE 8.16   Complement activation by the classical pathway (antibody mediated)

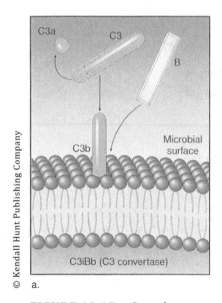 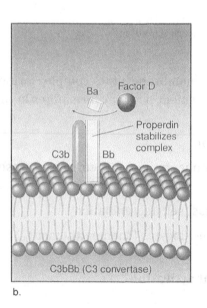 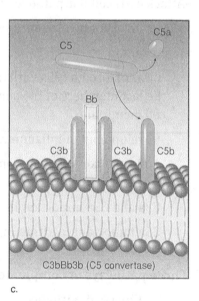

FIGURE 18.17   Complement activation by the alternate pathway

3. Lectin pathway

-No antibodies are involved.

-When macrophages phagocytose, they release cytokines that stimulate the liver to produce lectins, which are proteins that bind to carbohydrates.

-When a lectin binds to a microbe, it can then split C2 and C4, and the split produces C2a, and C4b combine to activate C3 to C3a and C3b.

-The end result is formation of **MAC (membrane attack complex)**.

> ***example***: mannose-binding lectin (MBL), which binds to mannose found on cells of some bacteria and viruses.

When a pathogen becomes coated with complement proteins (opsonisation), one of two things can happen:

1. Phagocytosis and digestion in the macrophage

2. Direct killing: C5b, C6, C7 + C8, and C9 form a complex protein that acts as a pore in the microbial cell membranes and results in lysis of the organism **(MAC) or membrane attack complex**:

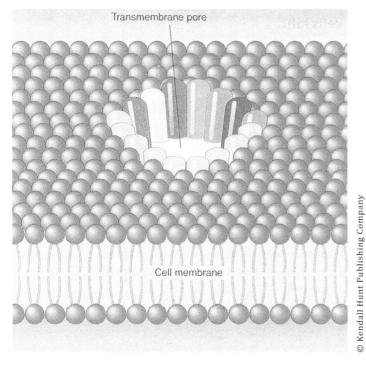

Transmembrane pore

Cell membrane

© Kendall Hunt Publishing Company

FIGURE 18.18   Membrane attack complex formed from complement on the surface of a microbe

Complement deficiency (genetic lack of one of the later comple-ment components, like C5, C6, C7, C8 or C9): increased susceptibility to bacterial infections like *Neisseria meningitidis* and *N. gonorrhoeae.*

D. NK CELLS AND EOSINOPHILS: EXTRACELLULAR KILLING

Natural killer cells: first line of defense against intracellular pathogens like virus and intracellular bacteria. No memory—look like a small lymphocyte though!

-Kill "targets" directly. NK cells check out the MHC I that is on all nucleated cells in the body to see if there is a self-peptide or a microbial peptide bound in the molecule.

Also checks to see if there is a MHC I on the surface of a cell (some cancers do not have MHC I).

Targets for NK cell killing:

Tumor cells

Viral/intracellular bacteria infected cells

How do NK cells kill?

-They release "cytolytic granules" containing perforin and granzyme.

-Target cell undergoes apoptosis (tidy self-destruction).

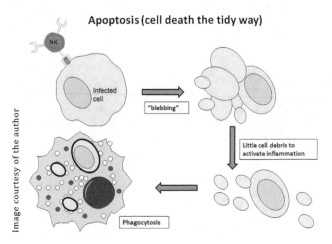

Image courtesy of the author

FIGURE 8.19   *Apoptosis by NK cells*

Eosinophils: granulocytes specialized for killing parasites

-Parasites are too big for phagocytosis, so lots of eosinophils can attach to a worm (with or without help of an antibody) and release chemicals to damage the worm cuticle—high number of eosinophils in circulation lead one to suspect a parasitic infection or an allergy.

E. ANTIMICROBIAL SUBSTANCES

Acute phase proteins: proteins produced in liver during infection

-High levels are usually indicative of a bacterial infection or inflammation.

-CRP (C-reactive protein) can act to opsonize bacteria for easier phagocytosis.

Proteolytic and hydrolytic enzymes (mainly in immune cells granules): digest and kill microorganisms

Interferon: produced by tissues in response to viral infections (purpose is to protect surrounding cells from viral infection)

****

MHC (major histocompatibility complex)

-Also called HLA (human leukocyte antigen); found on the outside membrane of body cells (this is what we "type" when transplanting organs)

-Comes in two kinds: MHC I and MHC II

MHC I

-Found on almost all nucleated body cells

-Marker for "self" because can bind to self-produced peptides

-Viral peptides or intracellular living bacterial peptides can be bound in MHC I, indicating an infection in the cell

-Presents endogenous antigen

-Many viruses decrease MHC I production when they infect cells; some (like CMV) actually direct the host cell to make a "fake" MHC I to fool the NK cells

-Some cancer cells do not have MHC I on their surface, so this is a problem and NK cells will then kill that target cell

> **NK cells check out the MHC I to find out if there is a problem, and if there is, they will kill the cell with cytolytic granules that force apoptosis.**

If only self-peptides are found in the MHC I, the NK cell will ignore that host cell.

MHC II

-Found only on **APC** (antigen-presenting cells) (APC present antigen to lymphocytes):

APC: macrophages, dendritic cells, and B-lymphocytes

-Function is to bind peptides from a phagocytosed pathogen and expose them on the surface of the macrophage or other APC

-The MHC II interacts with the T-helper lymphocytes in the adaptive immune system. If there is a peptide bound in the MHC II, then the T helper cells will activate and induce both B-lymphocytes and T-cytotoxic lymphocytes to become activated and produce immune responses to kill the original pathogen

-Presents exogenous antigen originating from outside the cell

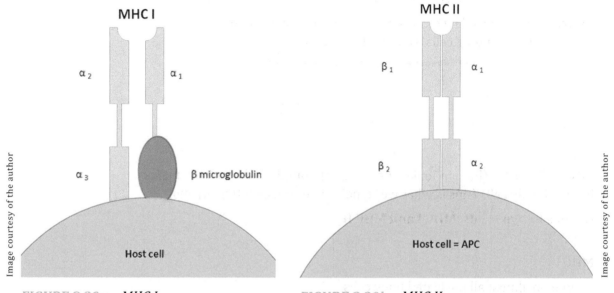

Image courtesy of the author

FIGURE 8.20a MHC I

Image courtesy of the author

FIGURE 8.20b MHC II

Interested? Want to learn more?

For more reading, several texts online at the U of A library are recommended:

1. Brooks, GF, Carroll KC, Butel JS, Morse SA, editors. Jawetz, Melnick, and Adelberg's Medical Microbiology, 24th ed. Blacklick OH-McGraw Hill; 2007.

2. Ryan KJ, Ray CG, editors. Sherris Medical Microbiology, 5th ed. New York – McGraw-Hill, 2010.

3. Mandell GL, Bennett JE, Dolin R, editors. Mandell, Douglas and Bennett's Principles and Practices of Infectious Diseases, 7th ed. Churchill Livingstone Elsevier, Philadelphia, 2010.

And...

-For great YouTube videos of immune functioning, see videos by Khan Academy.

Chapter 9

The Adaptive (or Acquired) Immune System Specific Defenses of the Host

Learning Objectives:

1. Describe the components of the adaptive immune system and their functions.
2. List the five types of antibody and their functions in health and disease.
3. Differentiate between the functions of MHC 1 and MHC II.
4. Differentiate between necrosis and apoptosis.
5. Explain how a defect in T-helper cells can cause immunodeficiency.

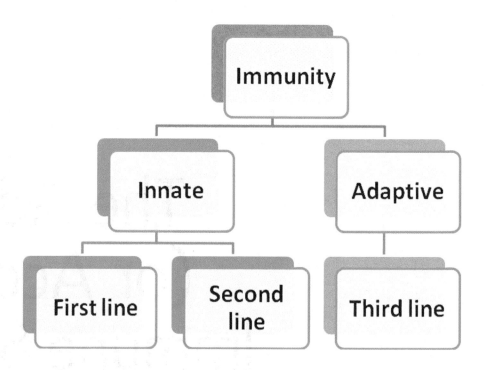

Third line of defense

- **SPECIFIC** immunity
- Adaptive, acquired
- Takes time to develop (~5–7 days)
- Mediated by **B-lymphocytes and T lymphocytes**
    - B cells: antibody-production factories
    - T_C cells: T cytotoxic cells responsible for cell-mediated immunity
    - T_H cells: T helper cells: interact with antigen-presenting cells and mediate the activation of B and Tc cells

Definitions

Antigen: substance (usually foreign) that is capable of provoking an immune response

- Bacteria, protozoa, virus, helminths, pollen, insect venom, transplanted tissue, etc.
- **Epitope**: site on antigen that the antibody recognizes

Antibody: protein produced by the immune system in response to a *specific* antigen

- Function to destroy or inactivate the antigen that triggered its formation
- Produced by **B cells** in response to "antigenic stimulation"
- Also initiate complement pathway

Four Fundamental Properties of Acquired or Adaptive Immunity

1. **LEARNING**
    - Distinguish between self and foreign

2. **SPECIFICITY**
   - Can recognize very tiny region of pathogen
3. **DIVERSITY**
   - Must have broad coverage; many pathogens exist
4. **MEMORY**
   - "Remembers" antigen for future reference

Sequence of Events in a Bacterial Infection

1. Antigen in tissues is recognized by neutrophils (innate system), which move to the site in order to phagocytose the antigen
2. At the same time, tissue macrophages are also detecting the presence of antigen and arrive at the infection site shortly after the neutrophils.
3. Tissue macrophages bind the antigen, process it, and transport it to the lymph node where there are many T-lymphocytes (both B and T).
4. Antigen is presented on the MHC (protein on the outside of the macrophage that binds peptides from protein antigens) of the tissue macrophages to the T and B cells in the lymph node.
5. The T and B cells in the lymph nodes scan the antigen bound in the MHC and, when the right match is found, become activated to effector cells and memory cells, which will remain in the body in case the same antigen is reintroduced in the future (basis of immunity).

The adaptive (acquired) immune response has two branches:

1. B cell-mediated (antibody-mediated)
2. T cell-mediated (cell-mediated)

TABLE 9.1   *Comparison of B Lymphocytes and T Lymphocytes*

Type	Site of Maturation	Type of Immunity	Half-life	Mobility	Function
B Lymphocytes	Bone marrow or lymphoid tissue	Humoral	Short (days to weeks)	Relatively localized	Differentiate into antibody-secreting plasma cells
T Lymphocytes	Thymus	Cell-mediated	Long (months to years)		Widely distributed Are involved in delayed hypersensitivity T helper (TH) cells: activate B lymphocytes, produce cytokines, and are involved In cell-mediated immunity Cytotoxic T (TC) cells: destroy cells with antigen on their surfaces

Humoral Response: B-Lymphocytes (B Cells)

-Most effective against **EXTRACELLULAR** antigens:

– Bacteria

– Toxins

– Free virus

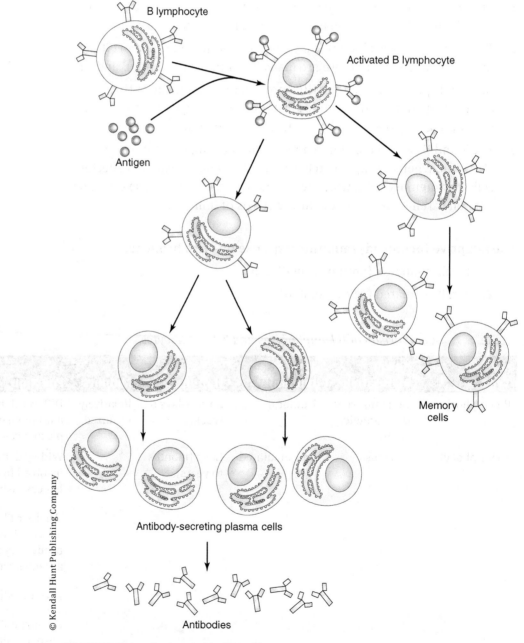

FIGURE 9.1   *Activation of B cells*

-T helper cells are required for B cell response

-B cells originate AND mature in **B**one marrow

-Can act as antigen-presenting cells (APC)

-Antigen binding to the unique antigen-binding receptor on a B cell causes it to divide rapidly and to produce antibody specific for only that antigen

-**Plasma cell**: effector B cell that is capable of antibody production

B Cell and Antibody Facts

-Each B cell can ONLY make one **specificity** of antibody (meaning the antibodies, regardless of class, will bind only to one and the same antigen.

-Another name for antibody is IMMUNOGLOBULIN (Ig).

-Antibodies in the body can be found either:

1. Stuck to the surface of a B cell (e.g. B cell receptor—BCR)
2. Secreted—circulating in the blood and lymph or patrolling mucosal surfaces

Antibodies have two main functions structurally separated:

1. Bind specifically to pathogens
    a. By the variable region
    b. Antibody repertoire is large enough that virtually any structure can be recognized
2. Recruitment of other cells to destroy the pathogen
    a. Constant region (also known as Fc region)
    b. Minimal variability

Memory

Memory B cells produced during the first exposure to an antigen facilitate quick response to "familiar" antigens when reexposed to infection a second time. This is the basis for the success of vaccines.

Antibodies and the Fetus (Neonate)

-Infants are born with the mothers IgG (only antibody that crosses over the placenta) and do not produce their own IgG until about 6 to 12 months of age.

-Neonates can only produce IgM (ability starts during last trimester in utero).

-Neonates receive IgA from mother's breast milk.

Antibodies bind to a specific site on the surface of a pathogen

-A single pathogen may contain numerous epitopes.

-Different antibodies can recognize different epitopes on the same pathogen.

-Remember, an **EPITOPE**: is the portion of an antigen that is bound by an antibody

-Antibodies usually recognize external epitopes on pathogens.

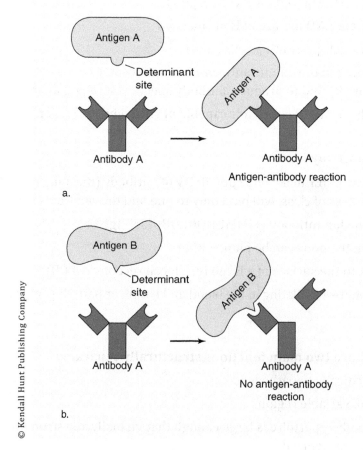

FIGURE 9.2   *Antigen–antibody binding*

Antibody Structure

1. Variable region (Fab or the arms of the antibody): antigen-binding sites

2. Constant region (Fc or the stem of the antibody): binds receptors on immune cells

- Some white blood cells (WBC) like macrophages have receptors that can bind to the Fc region of antibodies, and these receptors are called "Fc receptors."

Biological Activities of Antibodies

1. Opsonization

- Opsonization means "prepare to eat"

- Coating antigen with antibody can enhance phagocytosis

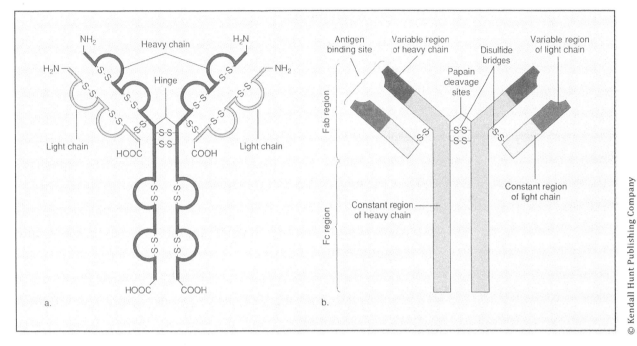

FIGURE 9.3 Antibody structure

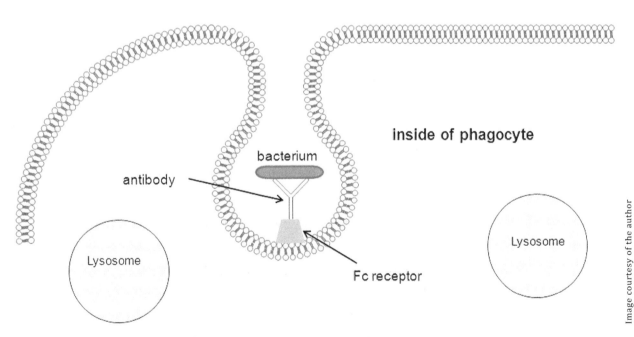

FIGURE 9.4 Opsonization

2. **Activation of complement**
   - Antibody binding to antigen (e.g., bacteria) can act as the activating step for the complement system.
   - Activation leads to:
     * Lysis of the bacterial cell
     * Opsonization
     * Inflammation

Refer to Complement activation from Chapter 8

3. **Agglutination**
   - Antibodies have more than one binding site and can bind two antigens per molecule.
   - Antibodies can "clump" antigens together by joining them.
   - Used in laboratory testing; also, the larger aggregates are more easily ingested by phagocytes.

4. **Neutralization**
   - Antibodies can bind surface of pathogen to block adhesion of pathogen to the host cell—if the pathogen can't adhere to the cells of the body, it can't infect.
   - Antibodies can bind toxins to block their activity.

Antibody Isotypes: Five Types or "Classes"

-Each isotype has a specific biological activity.

-A single B cell is capable of expressing each isotype at different times in immune response (called "class switching").

-Antigen specificity of antibodies from a single B cell is the SAME regardless of isotype.

Each immunoglobulin isotype has a specific biological activity

IgM
   * 5%–10% of total serum immunoglobulins
   * First Ig produced in primary response to antigen
   * Membrane-bound form attaches and acts as the surface BCR (B cell receptor)
   * Pentameric form = serum IgM (five molecules joined with a J chain)
   * Can bind numerous Ag simultaneously
   * Highly efficient because of the multiple binding sites
   * Good at activating complement

TABLE 9.1   Classes of Immunoglobulins

Classes	Structure	Molecular Weight (Daltons)	% of Total Antibody	Serum Level (mg/ml)	Number of Antigen-Binding Sites	Heavy Chains	Light Chains	Major Characteristics
IgG		150,000	80	3	2	γ	κ or λ	Major circulating antibody *infants born with mother's IgG
IgM	J chain	900,000 (pentameter)	10	1.5	10	μ	κ or λ	First antibody to be specifically produced during immune response *neonates can only produce IgM
IgA	J chain	160,000 (monometer) 385,000 (dimer)	5–15	1.5–4	2 4	α	κ or λ	Often the first antibody to contact invading microorganisms; major secretory antibody; exists as monomer in serum and as dimer in secretions *in breastmilk
IgE		190,000	0.002–0.05	0.0001–0.0003	2	ε	κ or λ	Involved in Type I hypersensitive reactions
IgD		185,000	1	0.03	2	δ	κ or λ	Present on surfaces of lymphocytes

IgD

-0.2% of serum immunoglobulins

-Membrane-bound Ig on mature B cells (along with IgM)

-Biological effector function unknown

IgG

- 80% of serum immunoglobulins

- Capable of crossing placenta; important in protection of fetus

- Activates complement

- Binds Fc receptors on phagocytic cells—mediates opsonization
  long-lived antibody

IgA

-10%–15% of serum immunoglobulins

-Predominant Ig in external secretions

    Breast milk

    Saliva

    Tears

    Mucous

-Prevents attachment of pathogens to mucosa—inhibits colonization

-Protects newborns during first months of life

IgE

-Very low serum concentration normally

-Mediates hypersensitivity reactions

    Hay fever

    Asthma

    Hives

    Anaphylactic shock

-Binds Fc receptors on mast cells and basophils

    IgE in allergy:

- IgE specific for an allergen binds Fab receptors on mast cells or basophils and crosslinks the molecules, causing an activation signal to be generated, which tells the mast cell to degranulate and release histamine and other chemicals.

*Remember:

    – **Not all antibodies are protective against disease.**

    – **Some antibodies that arise during an infection are only useful for using as markers for infection (lab tests).**

T-Lymphocytes: Cell-Mediated Immunity

-Effective against **intracellular antigens** and otherwise **altered self-cells**

    – Virus, tumors, transplants

-CTL (cytotoxic lymphocytes) directly kill altered self-cells by apoptosis (this requires cell to cell contact).

-T helper cells are required for CTL response because they activate the cytotoxic cells after exposure to the antigen.

-Immune cells respond to SPECIFIC pathogens.

   Two kinds of T cells:

    Helper T cell (T_H cell) (CD4): send signals to activate other parts of immune response

    Cytotoxic T cell (T_C cell; CTL, CD8): directly kill altered self-cells

    Virally infected cells (intracellular pathogens), tumor cells

-T cells bind antigen through the T cell receptor (TCR) in conjunction with MHC

-TCR only recognizes antigen that is bound in the MHC of the T helper cells

    MHC = <u>M</u>ajor <u>H</u>istocompatibility <u>C</u>omplex (note that in humans this is often called HLA or human leukocyte antigen)

-Compare with B cells that recognize free extracellular antigen

MHC = major histocompatibility complex

-**SELF** marker on surface of cells

-Specific to each individual

    – The only people with the same MHC are identical twins

-First discovered to have a role in graft rejection

MHC Diversity

-On the SAME cell, a single individual can express:

    6 different   MHC I

    8 different   MHC II

-Wide diversity of antigens that can be recognized

MHC present (bind to and display) protein breakdown products made within the cell (peptides or pieces of the proteins)

-Peptides may be self or foreign:

    Self: everything is OK

    Foreign: may be "danger"

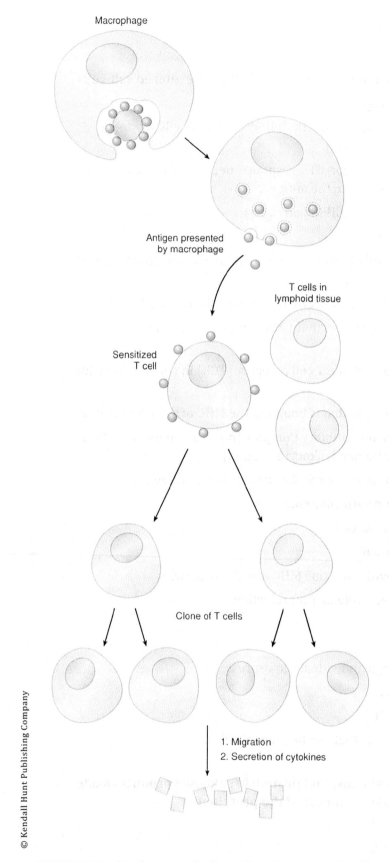

Macrophage

Antigen presented
by macrophage

T cells in
lymphoid tissue

Sensitized
T cell

Clone of T cells

1. Migration
2. Secretion of cytokines

FIGURE 9.5   *Mechanism of cell-mediated immunity T cells*

Two classes (or types) of MHC:

MHC I: present on all nucleated body cells

MHC II: present on macrophages, dendritic cells, and B cells

- "APC or antigen-presenting cells"

MHC molecules are like highway warning signs

Under normal conditions (absence of infection):

- MHC I and II present "self-peptides"—T cells know there is no danger.
- When there is an infection, MHC can let the T cells know that they have to act and protect the system.

The two types of T cells react with different MHC types

Tc = CTL = cytotoxic lymphocytes

- Directly kill infected cells
- Recognize antigen presented on MHC class I

T_H = T helper cell

- Important for initiation of the adaptive immune response
- Recognize antigen presented on MHC class II

Where do the peptides come from?

-Peptides for MHC I and MHC II are obtained by degradation of (microbial) proteins in the host cells.

-Normal self-peptides are derived from normal proteins produced by host cells; these are normally degraded in the body.

MHC class I presents endogenous peptides (peptides that are manufactured in that cell)

-Cell is infected by virus or is an altered self-cell or cancer cell.

-Viral proteins are made by the host cell's machinery.

1. Viral proteins are degraded and loaded onto MHC I in the endoplasmic reticulum of the host cell.
2. MHC I with viral peptide is transported to host cell surface.
3. Killer T cell (T_c cell) can recognize MHC I complexed to a peptide, bind, and then release chemicals to kill that cell by apoptosis.

MHC class II presents peptides from extracellular antigens

1. Phagocytic cell takes up bacteria or toxin.
2. Bacteria is inside of phagocytic compartment.
3. Lysosome fuses with phagosome.
4. Bacteria are digested.
5. Peptides from bacterial digestion are loaded on MHC II.
6. MHCII/peptide is transported to cell surface.

7. MHCII/peptide complex can be recognized by T_H cells.

8. Foreign peptide on MHC II indicates that an APC has encountered and phagocytosed an antigen.

9. Antigen is usually bacteria or toxin.

When there is no infection...

-Peptides from normal self-proteins are processed and presented on MHC I and MHC II.

-Self-peptides **DO NOT** activate the immune response (exception: autoimmunity).

TCR/MHC I binding recognition results in DEATH to the infected self-cell

-Foreign peptide on MHC I indicates an intracellular infection (usually viral or may be a tumor cell).

-Because the cell being recognized is infected, it is of no benefit to the body and must be destroyed.

TCR/MHC II binding results in APC activation

-MHC II binding does not result in direct killing because the APCs are not infected—they are just signaling danger.

-Consequences of TCR/MHC II binding: B cells make antibodies, and macrophages become more efficient phagocytes.

TABLE 9.3   Some Autoimmune Diseases in Humans

Disease	Organ or Tissue	Mechanism of Damage
Grave's disease	Thyroid	Autoantibodies bind thyroid-stimulating hormone receptor, resulting in overstimulation of thyroid
Juvenile diabetes (insulin-dependent diabetes mellitus)	Pancreas	T-cell destruction of pancreatic cells
Myasthenia gravis	Muscle	Autoantibodies bind acetylcholine receptors on muscle, preventing muscle contraction
Pernicious anemia	Stomach	Cell-mediated immunity and autoantibodies bind to parietal cells, resulting in vitamin B_{12} deficiency and defective red cell maturation
Rheumatoid arthritis	Joints	Immune complexes deposited in joints, resulting in inflammation and cartilage destruction
Sympathetic ophthalmia	Eye	Autoantibodies bind to eye antigens after eye trauma, resulting in inflammation, photophobia, and blurred vision
Systemic lupus erthematosus	Widespread (small blood vessels, kidney glomeruli)	Autoantibodies bind to self-antigens, especially those in the cell nuclei, resulting in deposition of immune complexes in tissue

T helper cells (CD4) are central to the adaptive immune response

-HIV virus lives in CD4 cells and destroys them, leaving the host susceptible to opportunistic infections.

-CD4 cell number is greatly reduced in HIV infection, and the life span is shortened (inability to mount immune responses to foreign antigens).

Normal: 1000 CD4 cells/mm^3

AIDS: $\leq$ 200 CD4 cells/mm^3

Cell Death

Necrosis: whole cell is destroyed at once, releasing immune-stimulatory debris; leads to induction of inflammatory pathway

Apoptosis: programmed cell death, various parts of the cell are enclosed in cell membrane "bubbles"

- Prevents release of potentially damaging cellular elements into host tissues

- No inflammation ensues

Cancer

-In cancer, apoptosis is inhibited, and proliferation of cells is unimpeded (e.g., Burkitt's lymphoma caused by EBV).

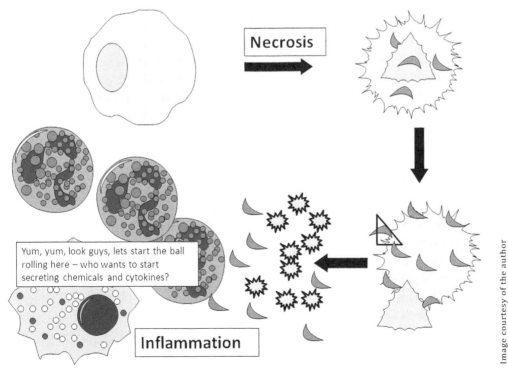

FIGURE 9.6 *Necrotic cell death leads to inflammation*

Apoptosis (cell death the tidy way)

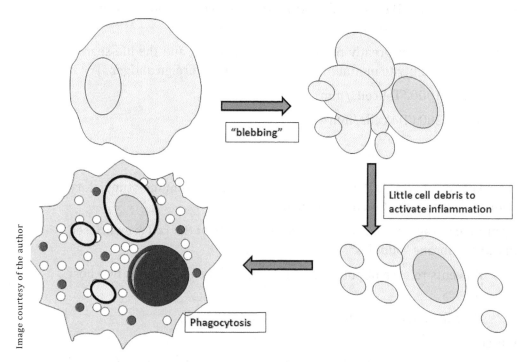

Image courtesy of the author

FIGURE 9.7   Apoptotic cell death does not lead to inflammation

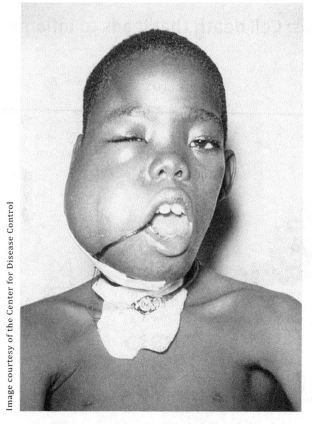

Image courtesy of the Center for Disease Control

FIGURE 9.8   Burkitt's lymphoma, the most common childhood cancer in Africa

-EBV blocks apoptosis (example of how a virus can cause cancer).

This is a mechanism of pathogenicity for EBV, which prevents the cell from dying and immortalizes cells).

Interested? Want to learn more?

For more reading, several texts online at the U of A library are recommended:

1.   Brooks, GF, Carroll KC, Butel JS, Morse SA, editors. Jawetz, Melnick, and Adelberg's Medical Microbiology, 24th ed. Blacklick OH-McGraw Hill; 2007.

2.   Ryan KJ, Ray CG, editors. Sherris Medical Microbiology, 5th ed. New York – McGraw-Hill, 2010.

3.   Mandell GL, Bennett JE, Dolin R, editors. Mandell, Douglas and Bennett's Principles and Practices of Infectious Diseases, 7th ed. Churchill Livingstone Elsevier, Philadelphia, 2010.

And...

-For great YouTube videos of immune functioning, see videos by Khan Academy.

Chapter 10

Hypersensitivity and Vaccines

Learning Objectives:

1. Describe the four types of hypersensitivity, and give an example of each.
2. Describe the different types of vaccine formulations, and give an example of each.
3. Differentiate among the four types of immune responses.
4. Identify reasons for the use of passive administration of immunoglobulins in protective passive immunity.

Hypersensitivity = Allergy

-When the immune system isn't doing us a favor and goes awry

FOUR MAJOR TYPES

Type I: immediate IgE mediated

- Localized (e.g., hives)
- General anaphylaxis leading to **SHOCK**

Type II: cytotoxic (cell-bound antigens)

- Transfusion reactions, HDN (hemolytic disease of the newborn or Rh disease)

Type III: immune complex-mediated (soluble antigens)

- Serum sickness, Arthus reaction, lupus erythematosis...

Type IV: delayed cell-mediated

- Contact hypersensitivity (e.g., latex "allergies," nickel "allergies," poison ivy, tuberculin test)

How Common Is Allergy?

Many of us have some type of allergy, and most are mild; however, a minority of people have life-threatening allergies. There is a genetic association for Type I allergy. According to the American Academy of Allergy Asthma & Immunology (www.aaaai.org/media/statistics/allergy-statistics.asp), more than half of all U.S. citizens test positive to one or more allergens. The same is likely true for Canadians.

We don't know why the body has developed these reactions to foreign particles we call allergens (or antigens). The "hygiene hypothesis" is a theory that has been proposed to explain the increased numbers of allergies in populations that are relatively free from pollution and exposure to known allergens. In this theory, individuals who have grown up in a very "clean" environment suffer more from allergies than those who have grown up with a lot of antigen exposure. This might be true, although we really don't know for sure. There is speculation that because we have such clean environments and do not normally get infested with worms, our immune system becomes somehow dysfunctional! It does seem that people who live in developing nations and who often have worm infestations have fewer problems with Type I allergies, but this is just an observation, not evidence-based medicine.

TABLE 10.1   *Comparison of Different Types of Hypersensitivity*

Characteristics	Type I	Type II	Type III	Type IV
Antibody type	IgE	IgG, IgM	IgG, IgM	None
Antigen source	Exogenous	Cell-bound	Soluble	Tissues and organs
Time to reaction	15–30 min	Min–hrs	3–8 hrs	48–72 hrs
Appearance on skin	"Wheal and flare," hives	Lysis and necrosis	Erythema, edema, necrosis	Erythema, induration
Factors involved	Basophils and eosinophils	Antibody and complement	Antibody	T cells
Examples	Allergic asthma, hay fever, peanut allergy, latex allergy, shellfish allergy	Erythroblastosis fetalis (HDN), transfusion reactions	SLE, postinfectious glomerulonephritis, serum sickness, Arthus reaction, farmer's lung, reactive arthritis	Tuberculin test, poison ivy, latex allergy, nickel allergy granuloma

TYPE I ALLERGIC REACTIONS

These allergic reactions are due to an **IgE** response to allergens. Type I allergic reactions are called anaphylactic reactions and can be of two general types:

-Local (may be hay fever, allergic asthma, or skin lesions like hives)

Note that not all asthma is a Type I allergic reaction.

-Systemic (life-threatening conditions leading to shock and death)

TABLE 10.2   *Common Allergens*

Method of Contact	Allergen
Ingested	Peanuts, fish, milk, wheat, shellfish, eggs, tree nuts
Inhaled	Pollen, dust mites, pet dander, perfumes
Injected	Drugs, insect venom
Direct contact	Latex, poison ivy and oak, nickel

A Type I reaction does not happen the first time a person is exposed to the allergen; they must be **sensitized** first. Allergens or antigens are usually a protein or a polysaccharide. Sensitization means that the allergen will have been presented to the immune system and immune reactions have been initiated. As we learned in Chapter 9, B cells will produce antibodies to that antigen or allergen.

In allergic individuals, IgE antibodies are the most abundant type of immunoglobulin class produced. During the first exposure, mast cells in tissues and basophils in the circulation will bind IgE antibodies by the Fc portion of the antibody molecule via a high-affinity receptor expressed on their surface.

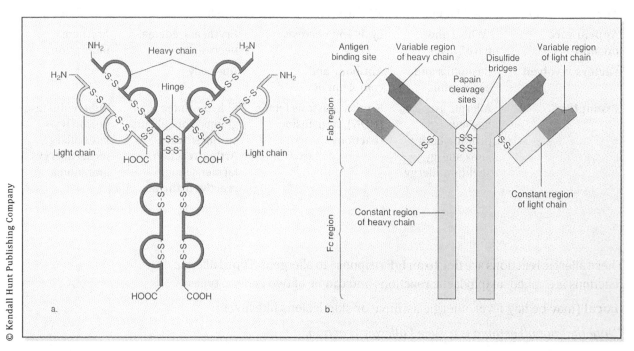

FIGURE 10.1   *Antibody structure*

The binding power is so strong that the binding is close to irreversible. If the individual is exposed to the same allergen a second time, the antigen will bind the Fab (antigen-specific) arms of the IgE that is bound to the mast cells and basophils. Allergens bind and cross-link or connect the IgE molecules on the cells. This cross-linking results in a signal being transmitted to the mast cell/basophil, inducing them to release their granule content into the tissues.

Mast cell granules contain several inflammatory mediators:

- Histamine

- Serine protease, serotonin, prostaglandin D2, leukotriene C4, platelet activating factor, and cytokines like eosinophil chemotactic factor

Histamine is one of the most important mediators causing anaphylaxis. Histamine binds to cells possessing a receptor for the chemical, like smooth muscle cells and endothelial cells lining the blood vessels. It causes bronchoconstriction in the lungs, narrowing the airways, and a separation of the endothelial cells in blood vessels, which allows cells and fluid to leak into tissues, causing edema and hives. Uterine cramps, involuntary urination, and defecation are additional symptoms due to smooth muscle contraction.

If mast cells throughout the body release histamine, the effect is systemic. Blood pressure may drop dramatically due to fluid leaving the blood vessels, and death from shock can result in as short of a time as 1–30 minutes. Antihistamines must be given promptly because this is an immediate reaction. It is common practice for people who know they have a serious allergy to carry an EpiPen™, which they use to inject epinephrine (also known as adrenalin) to counteract the histamine.

Ninety percent of all food-associated allergies are caused by shellfish, peanuts, milk, egg, tree nuts, fish, soy, and wheat. Some allergies disappear as the individual ages (e.g., milk allergies) but others are for a lifetime (e.g., peanut and shellfish allergies).

Type I

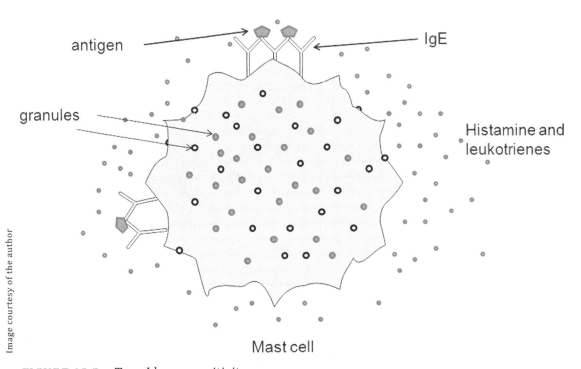

FIGURE 10.2   *Type I hypersensitivity*

Immunotherapy for Type I Hypersensitivity

-Immunotherapy is sometimes used to try to "desensitize" allergic individuals to their allergens. This is done by injecting very small amounts of the allergen over a period of months, gradually increasing the dose. This is done to stimulate the production of IgG antibodies, which are thought to be able to neutralize the allergens before they can cross-link the IgE molecules on the mast cells.

-A new therapy employing anti-IgE antibodies is being developed, which is aimed to prevent the binding of IgE to the high affinity receptors on the mast cells.

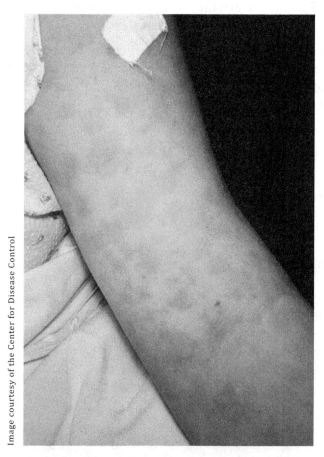

Image courtesy of the Center for Disease Control

FIGURE 10.3   Hives—an allergic skin rash

TYPE II HYPERSENSITIVITY REACTIONS

Type II reactions, also known as cytotoxic reactions, are dependent on the interaction of cell-bound antigens and complement **IgG** or **IgM** antibodies. Two well-known examples are hemolytic disease of the newborn (HDN) and transfusion reactions where someone has been transfused with the wrong blood type. In this type of immune-mediated reaction, the antigen is bound to a cell (insoluble), and in the case of both HDN and transfusion reactions, the cell is an erythrocyte (RBC).

Hemolytic Disease of the Newborn and Rhesus Antibodies

Approximately 85% of us have an antigen known as Rhesus factor on our red blood cells (Rh+). Individuals who lack this antigen are called Rh-. A potentially dangerous situation can occur when an Rh- woman and an Rh+ man produce offspring. If the fetus is Rh+, the baby's antigen-carrying red blood cells will mix with the mother's blood at parturition. The mother's immune system sees the Rh+ antigen as an invader, and an immune response is produced, resulting in IgG antibodies to Rh+ cells being produced.

The first baby is in no danger, but if the couple has another baby and this second baby is also Rh+, the mother's antibodies can pass through the placenta and bind to the baby's red blood cells. Add circulating complement to the mix, and there will be lysis of the red blood cells, which could be life-threatening for the baby. The term "blue baby" refers to babies born with hemolysis and not enough oxygen being transported to cells and tissues. This condition is also known as erythroblastosis fetalis due to the high percentage of immature, nucleated red blood cells in the baby's circulation in an attempt to provide more oxygen-carrying capacity to the unborn baby.

Before the baby is born, the mother's circulation will filter out most of the toxic by-products of red blood cell hemolysis, but after birth the baby will not only have anemia but also will develop severe jaundice due to high levels of bilirubin, a breakdown product of hemoglobin. Bilirubin is toxic to brain tissues. The infant may have to have a blood exchange transfusion to survive.

Prevention of Erythroblastosis Fetalis or HDN

If the mother is given RhoGAM®, a commercially available suspension of anti-Rh antibodies before birth of the first child, these antibodies will react with the baby's Rh+ red blood cells, destroying them before they can elicit an immune response in the mother. Pregnant women are tested to find out if they are Rh− during routine prenatal workups and monitored to determine if the baby she is carrying could be Rh+.

ABO Transfusion Reactions

The principle for transfusion reactions is the same as for HDN.

Wrongly matched ABO blood group transfusions are another example of this type of hypersensitivity. People with blood group A have A antigens on their RBC and anti-B antibodies circulating in the serum. If a blood group A person gets transfused with group B blood, which contains anti-A antibodies, hemolysis will result.

Type II Hypersensitivity: ABO Transfusion Reaction

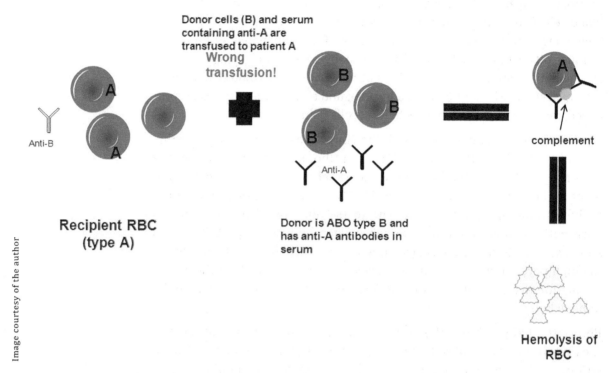

FIGURE 10.4   Type II hypersensitivity; an example—ABO mismatch

TYPE III HYPERSENSITIVITY REACTIONS

In Type II hypersensitivity, the antigen was cell-bound, but in Type III reactions, it is soluble. In this type of hypersensitivity, immune complexes (antigen + antibody complexes) containing **IgG (and sometimes IgM)** that are soluble and have been circulating in the blood attach to tissues in some organs, like the skin, kidneys, lungs, joints, and blood vessels, notably to the basement membranes. This only happens if there is slightly more antigen than antibody available. If there is more antibody than antigen, the antibodies, which are usually IgG, fix or activate complement, and this results in phagocytes removing the immune complex from circulation.

The deposited immune complexes on the basement membranes can activate complement and cause some inflammation. Complement split products like C5a attract neutrophils to the site, which release the contents of their granules, causing tissue damage and more inflammation. The result could be permanent damage to organs.

Some well-known examples are:

Serum sickness: Horse serum used to be used to administer antitoxin (like antitetanus and antidiphtheria) to people exposed to these organisms. The foreign antigens in the horse serum caused the production of antigens and immune complex. In a proportion of people, a disease called serum sickness developed, where the patient usually got severe skin reactions, fever, and generalized inflammatory disease. We use primarily human serum now for such treatments and avoid this Type III hypersensitivity reaction. However, certain drugs can also cause "serum sickness." Most cases are mild and disappear when the drug is stopped, but severe reactions resulting in death have occurred.

Arthus reaction: a local reaction that occurs after a skin injection of antigen/antibody that is a localized inflammation of the blood vessels. These reactions are sometimes reported after a vaccination, especially with tetanus or diphtheria toxoid. This type of reactivity was used in the "Schick test," which was used to determine the susceptibility of an individual to diphtheria. A positive Schick test meant that you did not have immunity to the organism's toxin and so were a candidate for revaccination.

SLE: **Systemic lupus erythematosis**: in this autoimmune disease, antibodies are formed to nuclear cell antigens (host antigens). The resulting antibody–antigen complexes can cause a Type III hypersensitivity, resulting in heart failure or kidney failure.

Reactive arthritis: the antigens can be various bacterial antigens.

Poststreptococcal glomerulonephritis: antigens here are *S. pyogenes* cell wall antigens, and the immune complex deposits in the kidney, causing nephritis.

Farmer's lung: pneumonitis caused by inhaled dust, spores, etc. Note that if the antibody produced is IgE, then the reaction will be a Type I hypersensitivity reaction.

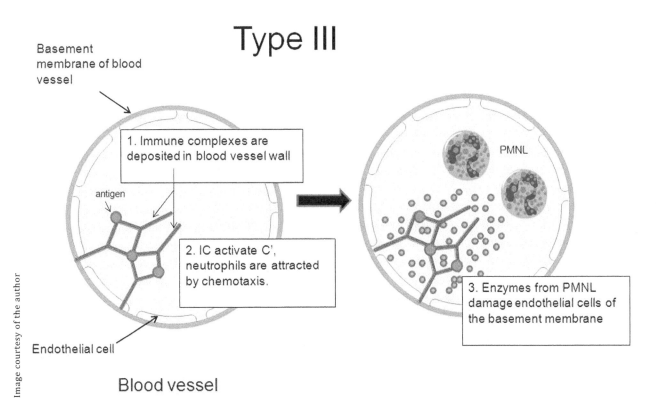

FIGURE 10.5   Type III hypersensitivity reaction

TYPE IV HYPERSENSITIVITY

Type IV hypersensitivity or "delayed-type hypersensitivity" really only describes normal T cell responses to an antigen that one has been previously exposed to. Sometimes this may cause a rash or tissue damage due to the activities of inflammatory cells. The most well-known Type IV hypersensitivity reaction is the tuberculin reaction.

With this type of reaction, when the antigen is reintroduced into the system, T memory cells originally generated during the first antigen exposure will be induced to proliferate, and T cells and macrophages will migrate to the site of irritation and gather near the offending antigen, try to "kill" it, and release cytokines, which damage tissue. This type of hypersensitivity is characterized by the formation of granulomas when infectious organisms like *M. tuberculosis* and *Aspergillus* species (a fungus) are the antigen. The reaction is "delayed" because it takes 24–72 hours for antigen-presenting cells to bind to an antigen, present to specific T helper cells, activate those cells, and secrete cytokines.

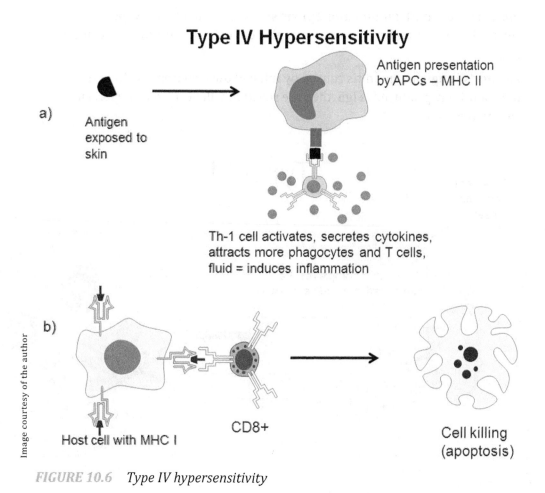

FIGURE 10.6   *Type IV hypersensitivity*

This reaction is often referred to as "**contact hypersensitivity**" or "**delayed type hypersensitivity**" and is often due to materials such as plant poisons, latex, etc. We are all familiar with the effect of poison ivy, which causes a disturbing rash called dermatitis. Nickel allergies also belong here, as do allergies to many other substances, even one type of penicillin allergy. In many of these exposures to small antigens, nothing would happen if the antigen did not react with a large skin protein, making the whole complex of antigen plus skin protein a much more interesting target for lymphocytes and macrophages. This small antigen component is called a **hapten**. In the preceding image, a) refers to the first exposure to the antigen, which primes the cell-mediated immune system and produces memory T cells, which react quickly on second exposure to the antigen.

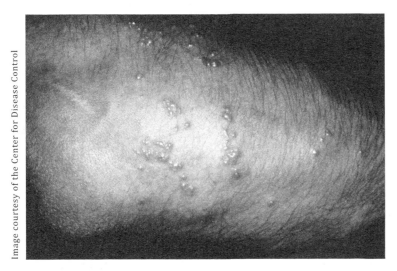

Image courtesy of the Center for Disease Control

FIGURE 10.7   Poison ivy: a Type IV hypersensitivity reaction

Although Type IV hypersensitivity reactions do cause tissue and cell damage, we can also use it to test for exposure to *Mycobacterium tuberculosis* by the "Tuberculin test" (also "Mantoux test"). Individuals who have been previously exposed to the tuberculosis antigen will test "positive" with these tests.

Tuberculin test: A small amount of PPD (purified protein derivative) from a strain of *M. tuberculosis* is injected subcutaneously and observed after two days. If the individual has been exposed to *Mycobacteria* species, the delayed hypersensitivity reaction will occur, and T-lymphocytes and macrophages will be attracted to the local injection site, causing a round raised area of inflammation. The diameter of the reaction is usually measured to assess positivity/negativity. A "Mantoux test" is the same as a tuberculin test but quantitative in that different dilutions of PPD are used to measure how large the response is. Although this skin test is used to determine if a person has been infected with latent or active tuberculosis, it is not specific to *M. tuberculosis*; other species can cause a positive result. Also, a drawback with the test is that if the person being tested has a problem with cell-mediated immunity (e.g., HIV), the test could be falsely nonreactive.

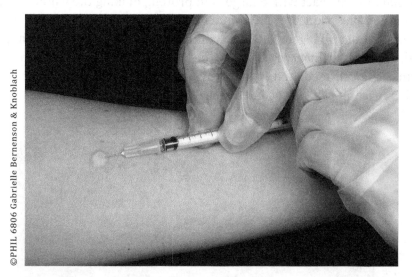

©PHIL 6806 Gabrielle Bernenson & Knoblach

FIGURE 10.8   Tuberculin testing

QuantiFERON-TB Gold Test

-New blood test for tuberculosis

-Can be used to help confirm or rule out a latent or active infection

-Does not require the patient to return to the clinic for inspection of the results

-QFT-G test is done on a blood sample collected from the patient and tests for activated T-lymphocytes by measuring the amount of cytokines released by T cells after they have been stimulated by PPD (purified protein derivative)

-Advantage: discrimination of latent from active cases of TB

-Disadvantage: labor-intensive, only done in large centers

Vaccines

The word "vaccine" comes from "vaccinia" or cowpox and started to be used when Edward Jenner performed his famous experiments with vaccinia to elicit immunity to smallpox (a closely related virus). Improved sanitation and vaccination are the two factors that have been instrumental in decreasing death due to infectious diseases globally. Vaccination reduces the number of individuals who get a disease but does not totally eliminate the chance of getting the disease. You can get the disease even if vaccinated (depending on several factors, including infectious dose and the state of your immune system), but the disease will usually be much milder than it would have been had you not been vaccinated.

It is advantageous to attain "herd immunity" in a population of vaccinated individuals. **Herd immunity** is a term used in epidemiology used to describe the situation that occurs when a sufficient percentage of the population is immune to an infectious agent, preventing the easy spread of the agent through the susceptible population.

There are four accepted types of immunity and vaccines that can be categorized into which type of immunity they induce:

1) Naturally acquired active immunity

   ◦ Infection with an infectious agent

2) Naturally acquired passive immunity

   ◦ Antibodies transferred from mother to child while in utero or by breast-feeding

3) Artificially acquired active immunity

   ◦ Attenuated vaccines, whole cell killed vaccines, and subunit vaccines

4) Artificially acquired passive immunity

   ◦ Immunoglobulin (antibodies) transferred to individual prevent infection in the short-term (last about 1–2 months), either prophylactically or post-exposure (e.g., TIG (tetanus immunoglobulin), VZIG (varicella zoster immunoglobulin), RIG (rabies immunoglobulin)). Specific antibodies of the IgG and IgM class have been identified and separated from pooled human blood for use in passive protection from disease.

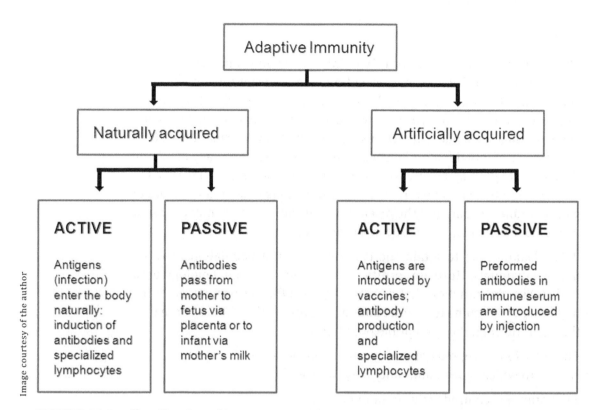

FIGURE 10.9   *Classification of immune responses*

TYPES OF VACCINES

A. Attenuated vaccines

Formulation: a live strain of a microorganism that has been handled in a manner that allows it to retain its characteristic antigens but to **not** have disease-producing ability in immunocompetent individuals

Immunity-induced: most long-lasting; involves both humoral (antibody) and cell-mediated immune system, leads to B and T memory cell development. Mimics a real infection; antigen can replicate to simulate natural immunity. Immunity often thought to be life-long but may need boosters later in life

Restrictions for use: many immunocompromised individuals will not be able to get this type of vaccine because they might become sick from the weak pathogen; this infection could be lethal

Examples: MMR (measles, mumps, and rubella), BCG (tuberculosis), Sabin (oral polio)

B. Killed whole cell vaccines

Formulation: whole microbes are killed, usually using chemicals and suspended in a solution

Immunity induced is less long-lasting and needs boosters because no living microbes are replicating and providing an ongoing antigen stimulation; not life-long

Restrictions for use: none, aside from possible allergies not related to the vaccine itself but the preservative or some other element (e.g., Influenza is grown in eggs before being killed for the vaccine)

Examples: Rabies, Salk (injection polio)

C. Subunit vaccines

Formulation: antigenic components of the microorganism are either extracted from a culture of the microorganism or genetically engineered in another organism. The best and most potent components are proteins.

Immunity-induced: less long-lasting than attenuated; less unwanted side effects than killed whole cell vaccines because of the purity of the antigens; boosters will be needed later in life

Restrictions for use: allergies to components of the vaccine

Examples: *Bordetella pertussis* (whooping cough), Hepatitis B (HBsAg is manufactured in yeast cells with genetic engineering), Gardasil (HPV vaccine, only capsids in vaccine, no DNA), Influenza A, *Streptococcus pneumoniae* (capsule), *Haemophilus influenzae* (capsule)

> **Polysaccharide vaccines**: Vaccines to *H. influenzae* and *S. pneumoniae* are based on the carbohydrate antigens in the capsule of these bacteria. Opsonizing antibodies are produced after successful vaccination, which allow the immune system phagocyte to engulf and destroy these organisms.

> **Conjugate vaccines**: Small children and some immunocompromised cannot respond adequately to antigens that are nonprotein (e.g., *H. influenzae* and *S. pneumoniae* vaccines that are based on the polysaccharide capsule antigens). They need a protein for immunization, which is a T cell-dependent antigen. Polysaccharides are T cell independent. In order to get an immune response produced in these children, the polysaccharide from a vaccine is coupled chemically with a protein. The protein used is often tetanus toxoid. This new antigen complex is now T cell-dependent, and even children <2 years can produce antibodies to the polysaccharide and the protein part of this vaccine.

D. Toxoids

Formulation: bacterial exotoxins that are chemically treated to preserve antigenicity but lack ability to function as the original toxin

Immunity-induced: humoral antibody only; need boosters every ~10 years

Restrictions for use: allergies to components

Examples: tetanus toxoid, diphtheria toxoid

E. DNA/RNA vaccines

These vaccines are currently being developed and are based on the premise that if you introduce genes from pathogens into a human cell, that cell will synthesize microbial proteins along with its normal proteins, providing a sustained antigenic stimulus. Unfortunately, it is taking time to get this research off the bench and into the marketplace—problems arise with lack of sustained effect.

Adjuvants: Adjuvants are chemical additives to vaccines that make the antigens more potent and effective. Usually aluminum salts are used for this or squalene (a natural compound). It is thought that they enhance immunogenicity by being costimulatory.

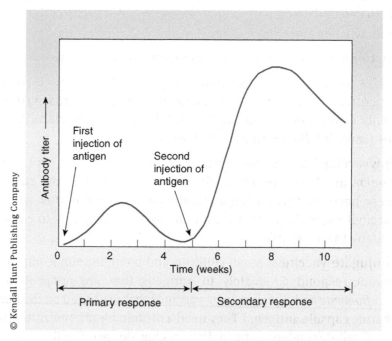

FIGURE 10.10   *Optimal (theoretical) antibody response after an immunization*

Passive Immunity with Immunoglobulins

-Not a "vaccine" but prophylactic protection against infection

-Suspension of antibodies to the specific infectious agent that have been harvested from donors

-Usually used when the individual has been exposed to an infectious agent that they are not immune to

-Examples: VZIG: varicella zoster immunoglobulin is a suspension of antibodies to the varicella zoster virus that can be given to a person who is exposed to chickenpox. The antibodies will mop up the virus and prevent infection.

-Similar immunoglobulins are available for other infectious diseases, like rabies and Hepatitis A and B.

-Protection is short lived, usually 1–2 months

Food for Thought: Vaccines and Autism

In 1998, a medical researcher named Andrew Wakefield published a research paper in the British Medical Journal claiming that the MMR vaccine caused autism in children. Other researchers tried to confirm these findings but could not. It was eventually found that the report was fraudulent, or at least data was interpreted wrongly, and autism has never been proved to be associated with vaccines. In addition, Wakefield's practice was investigated, and it was discovered that he had performed many invasive and unethical procedures on the autistic children he had studied. Wakefield lost his license to practice medicine and is now living in the United States and continuing his work against vaccines with notable celebrities like Jenny McCarthy.

What do you think? Is this a case where people always need to find a cause for abnormalities in their children?

The sad result of this whole affair is that once something is printed, people will believe even implausible conclusions. Many parents have stopped vaccinating their children with MMR, and this has resulted in a drastic increase of infections worldwide. Measles is once again a health issue, affecting 1/5 of children in the United Kingdom.

Interested? Want to learn more?

For more reading, several texts online at the U of A library are recommended:

1. Brooks, GF, Carroll KC, Butel JS, Morse SA, editors. Jawetz, Melnick, and Adelberg's Medical Microbiology, 24th ed. Blacklick OH-McGraw Hill; 2007.

2. Ryan KJ, Ray CG, editors. Sherris Medical Microbiology, 5th ed. New York – McGraw-Hill, 2010.

3. Mandell GL, Bennett JE, Dolin R, editors. Mandell, Douglas and Bennett's Principles and Practices of Infectious Diseases, 7th ed. Churchill Livingstone Elsevier, Philadelphia, 2010.

Chapter 11

Mechanisms of Pathogenicity

Learning Objectives:

1. Define primary and opportunistic pathogen.
2. Describe superantigens and the mechanism of action.
3. Identify the portal of entry for common organisms.
4. Define virulence factors, and explain how tropism determines whether an infection will occur.
5. List some of the effects that viruses exert on host cells to cause disease.

Definitions:

Pathogen: a microorganism that can cause a disease process

> **Primary pathogens**: always cause disease even in healthy immuno-competent people (e.g., *Bacillus anthracis*)

> **Opportunistic pathogens**: microorganisms that may cause disease if given the right circumstances (e.g., *Pseudomonas aeruginosa* in burn patients)

Pathogenicity: ability to cause disease by evading or overcoming host defenses

Virulence: the extent to which the microorganism is pathogenic

Virulence factors: the specific mechanisms by which a microorganism causes disease

> ***examples**: *Streptococcus pneumoniae* is a pathogen, but only if it has a capsule (the capsule is the virulence factor).

> > *Bacillus anthracis* produces exotoxins that damage tissue (the exotoxins are the virulence factor).

Tropism: the specific cell or receptor on the cell that a pathogen will preferentially infect or bind to

> ***example**: Influenza virus binds to sialic acid residues on host cells in order to penetrate the cell. Cells with sialic acid receptors are found in the respiratory tract; hence the tropism of Influenza A is for respiratory epithelium.

Measures of pathogenicity: a way for us to express the ability of a microbe to cause infection or death; gives an indication of how dangerous or easily infectious the organism is

> LD_{50} = lethal dose (used for toxin)

> - Concentration of toxin where 50% of hosts (usually experimental animals) will die if administered the toxin

> ID_{50} = number of organisms required to cause disease in 50% of inoculated or infected hosts under defined conditions (also called ED or effective dose)

> ***example**: *Vibrio cholerae* has an ID_{50} of 10^8 cells in normally acid stomachs because it is "sensitive" to acid pH (and you need a lot of bacteria before any will survive through the stomach). If the host has taken antacid and raised the pH of the stomach, reducing the acid, then the number of bacteria needed to cause a clinical infection will be much less, $\sim 10^{4\text{-}6}$ cells.

- This does not indicate how serious an infection is, only how many organisms are required to cause an infection.

Process of Infection

Adherence: organisms must be able to attach to host cells and tissues to cause an infection. This is the first step toward establishment of infection.

-Adherence is facilitated by structures on the pathogens called **ligands** or **adhesins** that attach like Lego blocks to **receptors** on the host cell.

Receptor mediated adherence

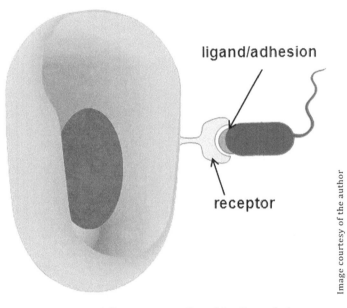

ligand/adhesion

receptor

Image courtesy of the author

FIGURE 11.1   Adherence mediated by ligands/ adhesions on organisms

-Most adhesins are glycoproteins or lipoproteins.

-Most receptors on host cells are sugars (e.g., mannose).

Structures Possessed by Bacteria for Attachment to Host Cells

1. Pili (or fimbriae), which have ligands for attachment, usually on the tips

2. Other structures include the glycocalyx, M-protein in cell walls of *S. pyogenes*, etc.

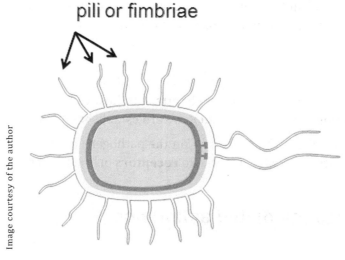

pili or fimbriae

FIGURE 11.2   Pili or fimbriae

FACTORS THAT HELP THE BACTERIA EVADE OR PENETRATE HOST DEFENSES (VIRULENCE FACTORS)

1. **Capsule**
2. **Cell wall components**
3. **Enzymes**
4. **Toxins**
5. **Superantigens**
6. **Invasins**
7. **Pathogenicity islands, Type III secretion system**
8. **Antigenic variation**
9. **Intracellular/extracellular growth**

1. **Capsule**

-Also called glycocalyx or slime layer if loosely organized

-Early in an infection, prevent the phagocyte from recognizing and ingesting the bacterium (until antibodies have been formed that help the phagocytes attach to the microbe)

-Many bacteria can produce a capsule in the right environmental conditions

     *examples: *Streptococcus pneumoniae*

                  Streptococcus pyogenes

                  Streptococcus mutans

                  Haemophilus influenzae

                  Neisseria meningitidis

                  Escherichia coli

                  Bacillus anthracis

                  Pseudomonas aeruginosa

                  Yersinia pestis

Image courtesy of the author

Klebsiella species

etc.

In a special "capsule stain," capsules around bacilli show up as clear fields around the bacteria which do not stain with the reagents.

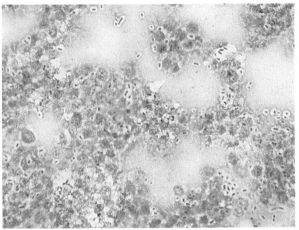

FIGURE 11.3 *Stain of* Klebsiella pneumoniae *showing the lack of staining around the bacterium, signifying the presence of a capsule*

-Some yeasts also have capsules (e.g., *Cryptococcus neoformans*)

2. **Cell wall components**

   a) **Fc receptors**

Fc receptors

-antibodies produced to the capsule enable phagocytes to ingest the organism

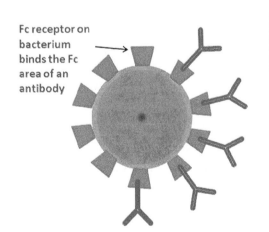

Fc receptor on bacterium binds the Fc area of an antibody

Bacterium protected from phagocytosis as the Fc portion of the molecule is not available for binding to the phagocyte.

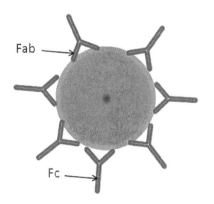

Fab

Fc

Fc region of antibody binds to phagocytes and so facilitates uptake of bacteria (phagocytosis)

FIGURE 11.4 *Fc receptors*

Some bacteria have Fc receptors in their cell walls (e.g., Protein A of *Staphylococcus aureus*). These Fc receptors will bind to the Fc (stem) of antibody molecules, exposing the Fab arms of the antibody to the environment. Phagocytes also have Fc receptors and cannot bind to Fab, so the bacterium is protected from engulfment. (If the bacterium does not have Fc receptors, the antibodies will bind to it by their Fab arms, exposing the Fc "tail" to the phagocyte, which will attach to and engulf the bacterium.)

b) **M protein**

-Heat and acid-resistant protein in the cell wall of *Streptococcus pyogenes,* which allows the bacteria to attach to epithelial cells and discourages the attachment of phagocytes

c) **Mycolic acids**

-Waxy acids in the cell wall of *Mycobacterium tuberculosis* that help protect the bacterium from digestion in the phagolysosome of a macrophage

d) **Teichoic acids**

-Help staphylococci and streptococci attach to host cells, probably due to a difference in the charge on the molecule

3. **Exoenzymes**: proteins produced in and released from microorganisms

-Many of these are important virulence factors for the organism

TABLE 11.1   *Microbial Enzymes Associated with Virulence*

Enzyme	Mode of Action	Examples of Bacteria Producing the Enzyme
Coagulase	Clots plasma	*Staphylococcus aureus*
Collagenase	Degrades collagen in muscle tissue	*Clostridium perfringens, Pseudomonas aeruginosa*
Deoxyribonuclease (DNase)	Degrades DNA in pus	*Staphylococcus aureus, Streptococcus pyogenes*
Hemolysin	Lyses red blood cells and other cells	*Staphylococcus aureus, Streptococcus pyogenes*
Hyaluronidase	Degrades the ground substance of connective tissue	*Clostridium perfringens, Staphylococcus aureus, Streptococcus pyogenes*
Lecithinase	Splits lecithin in plasma membranes	*Clostridium perfringens*
Leukocidin	Destroys white blood cells	*Staphylococcus aureus*
Staphylokinase, streptokinase	Converts plasminogen to plasmin, dissolving blood clots	*Staphylococcus aureus, Streptococcus pyogenes*

© Table 15.4 Kendall hund

4. **Toxins**

-Often primary virulence factors

-Two major types: endotoxin and exotoxin

TABLE 11.2   *Endotoxin effects in infection*

Consequence	Mechanism
Fever	Release of endogenous pyrogens (from polymorphonuclear leukocytes) that affect the hypothalamus
Inflammation	Activation of polymorphonuclear leukocytes by the presence of toxin
Increased phagocytosis	Activation of alternative complement pathway (see Chapter 16)
Rash	Hemorrhage and coagulation in capillaries of the skin
Septic shock	Increased capillary permeability with disseminated intravascular coagulation and blood stasis

© Table 15.7 Kendall hund

a) **Endotoxin**

LPS (lipopolysaccharide), lipid A only in Gram-negative cells; released when the bacterial cell dies

b) **Exotoxin**

proteins produced inside of the Gram-negative OR Gram-positive bacteria and released by the cell, either actively or when the cell breaks down

-Many exotoxins are of the A–B type, where the A part of the toxin molecule is the active or enzymatic portion and the B part is for binding to the target cell. There are two major methods by which they can enter a host cell: The active portion can be injected through the cell membrane,

A-B Toxins: 2 mechanisms

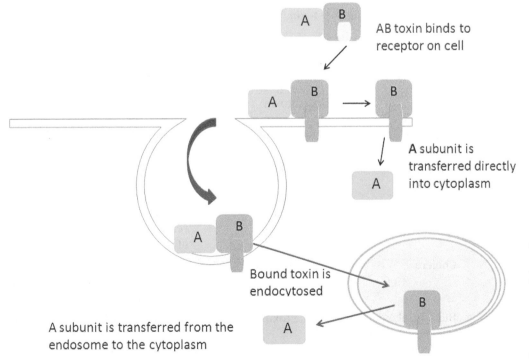

AB toxin binds to receptor on cell

A subunit is transferred directly into cytoplasm

Bound toxin is endocytosed

A subunit is transferred from the endosome to the cytoplasm

Image courtesy of the author

FIGURE 11.5   *A–B Exotoxins*

TABLE 11.3   *Example of Exotoxins*

Bacterium	Disease	Toxin	Mode of Action
Bordetella pertussis	Whooping cough	Pertussis toxin	Necrosis
Clostridium botulinum	Botulism	Neurotoxin	Blocking the release of acetylcholine, resulting in flaccid paralysis
Clostridium perfringens	Gas gangrene, food poisoning	α-toxin	Lecithinase
		β-toxin	Necrosis
		ε-toxin	Necrosis
		ι-toxin	Necrosis
		θ-toxin	Hemolysis
Clostridium tetani	Tetanus	Neurotoxin	Blocking the release of inhibitory transmitter, resulting in spastic paralysis
Corynebacterium diphtheriae	Diphtheria	Diphtheria toxin	Inhibition of the elongation step in eukaryotic protein synthesis
Escherichia coli (enterotoxigenic strains)	Gastroenteritis	Heat-stable toxin (ST)	Activation of guanylate cyclase, resulting in fluid and electrolyte loss from intestinal cells
		Heat-labile toxin (LT)	Activation of adenylate cyclase, resulting in fluid and electrolyte loss from intestinal cells
Shigella dysenteriae	Bacillary dysentery	Neurotoxin	Inhibition of protein synthesis
Staphylococcus aureus	Pyogenic infections (for example, impetigo)	α-toxin	Hemolysis
		β-toxin	Hemolysis
		γ-toxin	Hemolysis
		δ-toxin	Hemolysis
		Enterotoxin	Unknown
		Leukocidin	Degranulation of leukocytes
Streptococcus pyogenes	Pyogenic infections (for example, impetigo), scarlet fever	Streptolysin O	Hemolysis
		Streptolysin S	Hemolysis
		Erythrogenic toxin	Localized erythematous reactions (abnormal redness of the skin)
Vibrio cholerae	Cholera	Choleragen	Activation of adenylate cyclase, resulting in fluid and electrolyte loss from intestinal cells
Yersinia pestis	Bubonic plague, pneumonic plague, septicemic plague	Plague toxin	Necrosis (possible)

or the A–B toxin can be internalized in the cell in an endosome and the A portion is then extruded into the cytoplasm.

-Genes for exotoxin production are carried on bacteriophages or on plasmids.

-Exotoxins have three different types based on their function:

Exotoxins and endotoxins are very different in their modes of action and their effects on body processes.

  i. Cytotoxins (kill cells)

  ii. Neurotoxins (inhibit nerve cell function)

  iii. Enterotoxins (affect intestinal cells functioning)

-Exotoxins often damage cells, inhibit protein synthesis, and cause cell death.

-Antibodies to exotoxins are called antitoxins. If these antitoxins are treated chemically, they can be made into toxoids for vaccination purposes (e.g., tetanus toxoid).

TABLE 11.4   Comparisons of Endotoxins and Exotoxins

Characteristic	Endotoxin	Exotoxin
Bacterial source	Gram-negative bacteria	Primarily gram-positive bacteria, some gram-negative bacteria
Location in bacterium	Lipopolysaccharide	Product of bacterial cell, released extracellularly
Chemical structure	Toxic activity resides in lipid portion of lipopolysaccharide	Protein
Heat stability	Stable; can withstand 121°C for 1 hr	Unstable; usually destroyed by heating at 60°C to 80°C (except enterotoxins)
Toxicity	Low	High
Toxoid production	No	Yes (except enterotoxins)
Representative symptoms	Fever, inflammation, increased phagocytosis, rash, septic shock	Neurological complications, cell necrosis, loss of fluid and electrolytes from intestines
Representative diseases	Septic abortion	Diphtheria, botulism, tetanus, cholera

© Table 15.5 Kendall hund

5. Superantigens

-Also called Type 1 exotoxins

-Protein antigens that stimulate a very large immune response

-Normally <1% of T cells are activated by an infection, but if there is a superantigen as an activator, as many as 20% of all T cells are activated, and they release massive amounts of cytokines that enter the circulation. This has a profound systemic response, resulting in nausea, fever, diarrhea, and eventually shock and death.

  example: *Staphylococcus aureus* TSST-1 toxin, which causes toxic shock syndrome

Superantigen

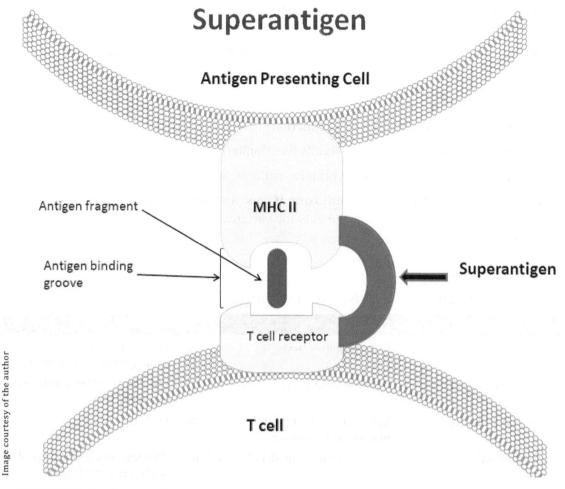

FIGURE 11.6   Superantigen

6. Invasins

-Surface proteins on some bacteria that activate actin (cytoskeleton of eukaryotic cells), usually for the purpose of making the invasion of the bacteria into the cell easier

-Invasins cause a rearrangement of the actin and in some cases form a pedestal upon which the bacteria sit and sink down into the cell. *Salmonella* species and enteropathogenic *E. coli* have these invasins

-Other bacteria use their invasins to move from one host cell to another horizontally through a tissue to avoid exiting from one cell before entering the next, thus exposing themselves to phagocytes (e.g., *Shigella* species and *Listeria monocytogenes*)

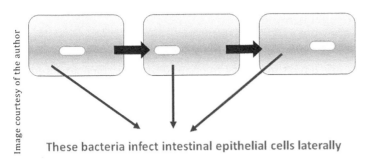

These bacteria infect intestinal epithelial cells laterally

FIGURE 11.7   Invasins allow horizontal infection in a tissue

7. Pathogenicity islands and the Type III secretion apparatus

-Some bacteria, especially the Gram negatives, have genes encoded on their chromosome or on a plasmid that code for pathogenic characteristics (e.g., coding for exotoxins or a Type III secretion apparatus)

-A pathogenicity island is a segment of the bacterial chromosome/plasmid that usually has multiple genes for virulence factors. Often, the sequence of the pathogenicity island (PAI) is very different from that of the rest of the genome, which gives rise to a theory that the island came from another organism at one time

-Type III secretion systems are molecular structures that resemble a hypodermic needle and are used by the bacteria to inject proteins, which might be toxins, into a host cell. These Type III secretion systems are encoded in the pathogenicity island

Type III Secretion System

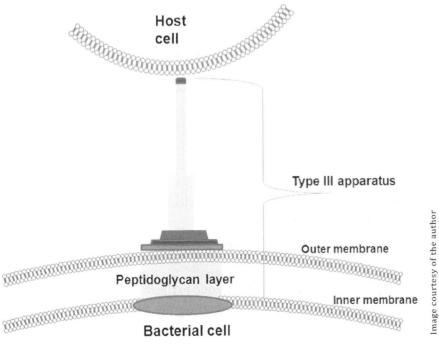

FIGURE 11.8   Type III secretion system

8. Antigenic variation

-"Fooling the immune system"

-Some pathogens have the ability to change their surface antigens to evade the immune system

> *example: *Neisseria gonorrhoeae* can change its surface antigens so that when the B cells have produced antibodies for neutralization of the bacteria, the epitopes that the antibodies are specific to have changed and the immune system faces a "new pathogen," which allows the bacteria to escape the phagocytes

-*Trypanosoma* species are also known to use antigenic variation

9. Intracellular growth

-Obligate intracellular bacteria can only grow inside of a host cell and often within a protected vacuole. This protects them from the immune system

> *example: *Chlamydia* species, *Rickettsia* species

-Facultative intracellular bacteria can multiply and live outside of host cells but can also survive and replicate inside of host cells.

> *example: *Mycobacterium tuberculosis*

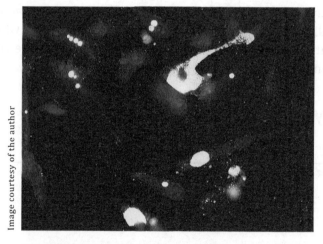

Image courtesy of the author

FIGURE 11.9 Chlamydia pneumoniae *stained with FITC, growing in human lung cells*

Virus and Pathogenicity

-Pathogenicity is different in bacteria and viruses due to the differences in structure, composition, and growth.

-Viruses invade host cells and reside intracellularly, where they are protected from the external immune system.

-Most pathogenesis caused by viruses is due to the induction of inflammation and activation of the immune system, but there are a few exceptions.

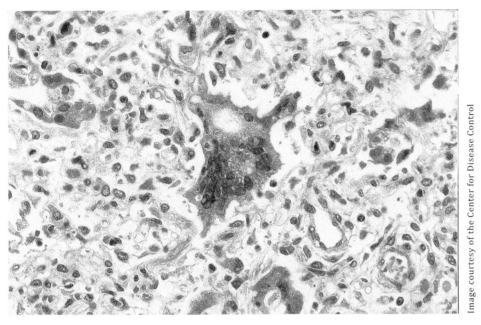

Image courtesy of the Center for Disease Control

FIGURE 11.10   Measles virus in lung tissue: syncytium formation, a CPE

CYTOPATHIC EFFECTS (CPE)

-Kill or damage the host cell as a result of viral replication

-CPE are characteristic for different types of virus.

-Formation of giant cells or syncytia are a type of CPE.

-Infected cells fuse their membranes with other cells, creating a giant cell with many nuclei that functions only as a huge virus producing factory.

-The giant cell cannot make its own proteins and eventually dies, causing inflammation and later a hole in the tissue.

   ***example**: RSV (respiratory syncytial virus), measles virus (rubeola)

VIRAL PATHOGENICITY

1.   Inhibition of macromolecular synthesis in the host cell, for example, may stop mitosis

2.   May cause the host cell to release enzymes, resulting in cell death (apoptosis)

3.   May cause a down regulation of MHC I; viral antigens will not be displayed on the cell surface, and the cytotoxic lymphocytes will not recognize that the cell is infected

4.   Syncytium formation

5.   Deregulation of cell function (e.g., effect on proteins, hormones produced)

6. Induce chromosomal changes in cells (e.g., oncoviruses)

7. Some can abolish contact inhibition responses by down regulating p53 and rb107, allowing uninhibited cell growth and tumor formation

Interested? Want to learn more?

For more reading, several texts online at the U of A library are recommended:

1. Brooks, GF, Carroll KC, Butel JS, Morse SA, editors. Jawetz, Melnick, and Adelberg's Medical Microbiology, 24th ed. Blacklick OH-McGraw Hill; 2007.

2. Ryan KJ, Ray CG, editors. Sherris Medical Microbiology, 5th ed. New York – McGraw-Hill, 2010.

3. Mandell GL, Bennett JE,Dolin R, editors. Mandell, Douglas and Bennett's Principles and Practices of Infectious Diseases, 7th ed. Churchill Livingstone Elsevier, Philadelphia, 2010.

4. Todar's Online Textbook of Bacteriology.

http://www.textbookofbacteriology.net/

Chapter 12

Normal Flora and Epidemiology

Learning Objectives:

1. Differentiate between normal flora (normal microbiota) and transient flora.
2. Define terms used to describe disease and the course of disease.
3. Identify the mechanisms by which diseases are transmitted.
4. Define the common epidemiological terms relating to burden of disease.
5. Differentiate between acute and chronic disease.

Normal Flora = Normal Microbiota

-Animals and humans are free of microbes in utero (assuming a healthy pregnancy) and only acquire normal flora bacteria at and after birth.

-Newborns' first contact with bacteria is usually lactobacilli from the mother's vaginal canal.

-With breastfeeding and exposure to the environment, foods, and other people, other types of organisms are able to colonize their skin and intestinal tracts.

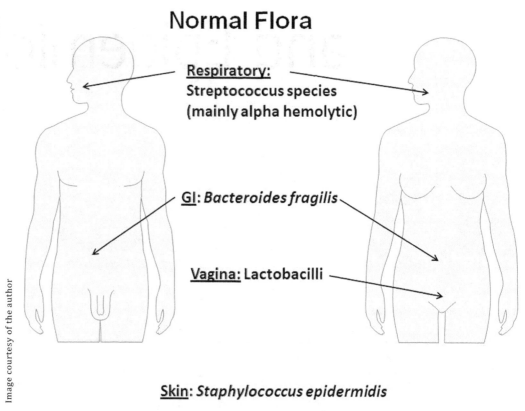

Normal Flora

Respiratory:
Streptococcus species
(mainly alpha hemolytic)

GI: *Bacteroides fragilis*

Vagina: Lactobacilli

Skin: *Staphylococcus epidermidis*

Image courtesy of the author

FIGURE 12.1   *Dominating normal flora of the body*

Transient Flora = Transient Microbiota

-Microorganisms that may be present on body surfaces temporarily (days, weeks, months) eventually disappear.

-They are removed by hand washing (**normal** flora is **NOT** removed by hand washing!).

-They can be either pathogenic (disease-producing) or nonpathogenic.

-They do not necessarily cause disease unless special conditions prevail (e.g., bacteria can enter a cut).

FUNCTION OF NORMAL FLORA

Microbial Antagonism

-Normal flora prevent the overgrowth of harmful microorganisms.

-It involves competition for nutrients, cellular receptors, production of substances that affect pH and available oxygen, and production of substances that can kill or inhibit growth of other bacteria.

-If the balance is upset, disease can result.

   *examples:

   - *Escherichia coli* in the large intestine:

      E. coli has the capacity to produce bacteriocins (proteins that inhibit the growth of other bacteria of the same or closely related species, such as pathogenic *Salmonella* or *Shigella* species.

   - *Clostridium difficile* disease

Zoonosis: disease transmitted to humans from an animal (usually the human is an accidental host)

   - Animal may be a healthy carrier of the organism or may be clinically diseased (e.g., rabies, tularemia, plague, *Chlamydia psittaci* pneumonia, West Nile virus).

Disease Stages (Any Infection)

-We all know that the most common types of infections have an incubation period, a period where we get some symptoms that eventually worsen, and then a stage of full-blown disease, at which point the immune system kicks in and starts working to eradicate the organism. This is followed by a period in the illness when we return to health (See Figure 12.2).

-After infection, we can spread the disease to others even if we haven't yet acquired symptoms, and after an infection, we can excrete the organism for long periods of time (months) even after we are clinically cured. This is a major problem for preventing spread of disease in a population.

-With the exception of primary pathogens, infection can always exist in an asymptomatic form in some people. Their immune system will recognize the pathogen and "seroconvert," meaning that they go from having no antibodies to the organism in their blood to producing significant measurable amounts of specific antibodies to that organism. This is also a challenge for epidemiologists because these asymptomatic carriers can spread disease even if the numbers of organisms may not be as high as in symptomatic individuals. The figure "iceberg of infection" (Figure 12.3) emphasizes the fact that usually only a small number of people infected with an organism get the classically recognizable disease and the vast majority are undetected in a population unless the population is monitored with blood specimens.

Disease Stages

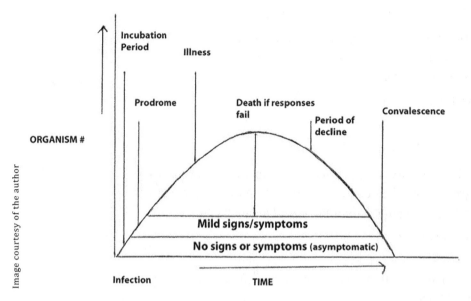

FIGURE 12.2   Stages of disease

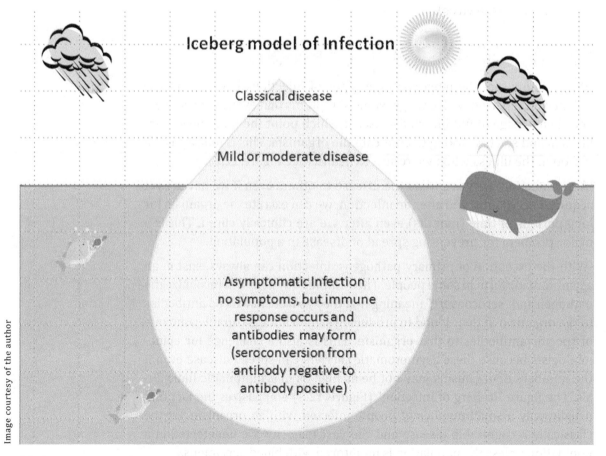

FIGURE 12.3   Iceberg model of infection in a population

Transmission of Disease

Horizontal transmission: transmission from one person to another through contact, vectors (insects), or vehicles (air, water, food)

> *example: sexually transmitted infections, respiratory infections like Influenza A, spread by coughing and sneezing or direct contact

Vertical transmission: transfer of a pathogen from a pregnant mother to her fetus

> *example: *Streptococcus agalactiae* (Group B strep or GBS) from the vaginal tract to the respiratory tract of the baby during birth

Transmission of infectious agents according to the Canadian Hospital Infection Control Association (CHICA)

-Three major categories of transmission: contact, vehicle, and vectors

-Diseases can be classified according to the most dangerous (for the population) method of transmission

> *example: Tuberculosis (*M. tuberculosis*) is classified as airborne transmission even if it can be transmitted by direct contact, indirect contact, or droplet.

1. **Contact transmission**

   a) **Direct contact**: person-to-person (e.g., kissing, touching, sexual contact)

   b) **Indirect contact**: agent transferred from the reservoir to the susceptible host by a nonliving inanimate object (fomite) (e.g., towels, drinking glasses, etc.)

   c) **Droplet transmission**: microbes are spread in mucus droplets that travel up to 1 m in air, then drop to the ground. These droplets are >5 nm in size and can be produced by sneezing and coughing

2. **Vehicle transmission**

-Transmission of infectious agents by a medium that may be air (airborne), water, food, blood, IV fluids, etc.

> *example: *Mycobacterium tuberculosis* by the airborne route—microorganisms are riding on very small mucus droplet nuclei <5 nm in diameter, and they float indefinitely in the air, making this type of transmission the most dangerous and feared.

***Do not confuse droplet and airborne transmission**—very different infection control practices must be used to control the spread of diseases with the two types of spreading.

3. **Vector transmission** (arthropods like ticks, mosquitoes)

   a) **Mechanical transmission**: passive transport of the organism on the body of the vector (e.g., spread of *Shigella* bacteria on the legs of a house fly)

   b) **Biological transmission**: part of the life cycle of the infectious organism is in the arthropod vector (e.g., malaria—the *Plasmodium* species must undergo part of its life cycle in the body of the Anopheles mosquito in order for it to be infectious).

Epidemiology

-The study of when and where diseases occur

-Purpose: to control disease transmission

Pandemic: occurrence of a disease on more than one continent or worldwide (e.g., Influenza A H1N1)

Epidemic: many people infected in a geographical area (e.g., yellow fever in the Panama Canal, turn of the 1900s)

Endemic: disease is always in the population at a low level (e.g., common cold)

Outbreak: cluster of cases of a disease in a geographical area (e.g., norovirus outbreaks in nursing homes)

Notifiable diseases: diseases that physicians and laboratories are required by law to report to Public Health. Health Canada has a list of such diseases, and the province usually adds a few diseases according to the local spectrum of infections.

Examples of a few notifiable diseases in Alberta that are deemed to be dangerous for the population:

   Gonorrhoea, syphilis, chlamydia

   Tuberculosis

   Pertussis (whooping cough)

   Malaria

   Hepatitis A, B, C

   Invasive meningococcal and streptococcal disease

   Trichinosis

   HIV

Incidence: number of new diseases occurring within a specified time period (e.g., 457 cases of Influenza A were reported in the town of XX between Jan. 1 and Mar. 30, 2010)

Prevalence: number of diseases in the population at a given point in time (e.g., 15% of school-aged children have Influenza A in town XX)

Morbidity: incidence of specific diseases

Mortality: number of deaths from diseases

Food for Thought

Smallpox is an example of the only disease yet eradicated because of the application of epidemiology by the World Health Organization (1977). This disease was responsible for hundreds of millions of deaths in past years.

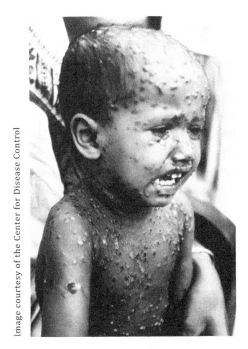

Image courtesy of the Center for Disease Control

FIGURE 12.4   Smallpox victim

Caused by a DNA virus, the orthopoxvirus, also called variola virus: enveloped, large (~300 nm). Last case was in Somalia in 1977. Two viral strains still exist, one in the United States at CDC in a freezer and the other in Russia in a freezer. Should they be kept or destroyed?

Vaccination campaigns, tracking cases, and isolating cases are responsible for totally eradicating this disease. How was this possible? Every case of disease was symptomatic; there were no asymptomatic cases, so they were easy to identify, and there is no animal reservoir. Vaccination campaigns were run successfully using a closely related virus, vaccinia, because there is good cross-immunity between the two viruses. Vaccinia is safe as a vaccine.

Disease begins as a respiratory tract infection with inhalation of droplets or contact with viral particles on objects. Virus infects tissues and spreads through the bloodstream to tissues where the lesions erupt.

Continued

First recorded case of bioterrorism in North America perpetrated against the first nations when people were given blankets contaminated with smallpox virus from British and American soldiers. Lesions are always in the same stage of development, which is the way you differentiate them from chickenpox lesions.

Lesions often become secondarily infected with *Staphylococcus aureus* and other skin bacteria, and sepsis can result, leading to death. Smallpox didn't kill very many people, but the complications did!

Why can't we eradicate other diseases as effectively as smallpox?

Other Terminology Used to Describe Types of Disease

Acute disease: characterized by an acute inflammatory response where the dominant responding cell type is the neutrophil

-Often accompanied by pus production (e.g., a boil caused by *S. aureus*)

Chronic disease: characterized by a slowly progressing chronic inflammatory response where the predominant responding immune cells are the mononuclear cells like macrophages and lymphocytes

- Often accompanied by the development of granulomas containing macrophages and lymphocytes (e.g., tuberculosis, fungal diseases)

Subacute disease: intermediate between acute and chronic; usually a disease process that takes a long time to develop fully (e.g., BSE in cattle or vCJD in humans)

Latent disease: causative organism may lie dormant for long periods of time before starting to replicate and causing disease (e.g., Herpes simplex virus or Varicella virus)

Terminology Used to Describe the Extent of Disease

Local infection: infection limited to one site

Systemic infection: disseminated or generalized spread of infection through the body via the blood, lymph, and sometimes through the tissues

Focal infection: after the spread of a systemic infection through the body, the organisms remain in specific areas (e.g., the liver for hepatitis)

Primary infection: acute initial infection

Secondary infection: appears as a complication of primary infection; may be caused by another organism taking advantage of the damage done by the primary infection

Terminology Used for Different Infectious Causes in Blood

Bacteremia: bacteria in the blood (nonreplicating)

Septicemia: replicating bacteria in the blood

Toxemia: toxins in the blood

Viremia: virus in the blood

Fungemia: fungi in the blood

Parasitemia: parasites in the blood

Interested? Want to learn more?

For more reading, several texts online at the U of A library are recommended:

1. Brooks, GF, Carroll KC, Butel JS, Morse SA, editors. Jawetz, Melnick, and Adelberg's Medical Microbiology, 24th ed. Blacklick OH-McGraw Hill; 2007.

2. Ryan KJ, Ray CG, editors. Sherris Medical Microbiology, 5th ed. New York – McGraw-Hill, 2010.

3. Mandell GL, Bennett JE,Dolin R, editors. Mandell, Douglas and Bennett's Principles and Practices of Infectious Diseases, 7th ed. Churchill Livingstone Elsevier, Philadelphia, 2010.

4. CHICA (Community and Hospital Infection Control Association)

http://www.chica.org/educ_overview.php

Chapter 13

Skin and Wound Infections

Learning Objectives:

1. Explain why the skin is a good barrier to infection.
2. Identify the normal flora of skin.
3. Describe common causes of bacterial, viral, fungal, and parasitic skin infections.
4. Identify commonly occurring infections when skin is breached.
5. Describe problems arising from the use of artificial devices.
6. Define the different levels of infection affecting the skin (cellulitis, gangrene, etc.).

Skin Infections

Skin Infections

The skin is the largest organ in the body and comprises both the external skin and the mucosal membranes that line the body orifices. It is a physical and chemical barrier to infection as discussed in the innate immunity section. Moist areas of the skin, for example, armpits and groin, have a higher density of microbial flora than dry areas like forearms and legs.

The normal skin flora usually has a higher than normal resistance to drying and salt. Most normal flora that live on the skin can be called "halophiles." An example is *Staphylococcus* species. Normal mucosal membrane flora tolerate acidic environments (e.g., alpha-hemolytic streptococci).

Skin infections can result from external sources or internal sources (e.g., a systemic infection causing lesions on the skin from the "inside").

Normal Flora of the Skin

-Both aerobic and some anaerobic bacteria grow on and in the skin.

-Major species include:

Staphylococcus epidermidis*dominates

Other *Micrococcus* species

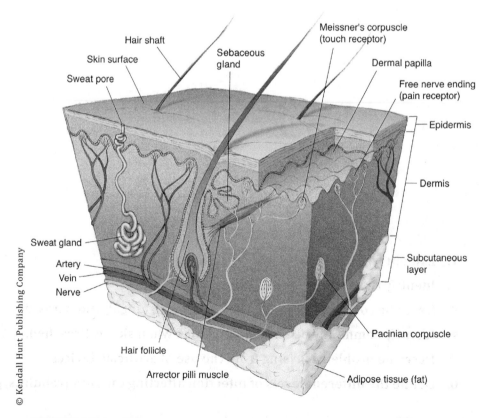

FIGURE 13.1   *Skin anatomy*

Diphtheroids: *Corynebacterium* sp.: aerobes, on surface

Propionibacterium sp.: anaerobes, live under the surface in follicles and glands

Some yeasts (e.g., *Malassezia furfur*)

Types of Skin Lesions

1. **Macules**: reddened flat or slightly raised areas on the skin
2. **Vesicles**: small, fluid-filled, blister-like lesions (<1 cm-diameter)
3. **Bullae**: large, fluid-filled, blister-like lesions (>1 cm-diameter)
4. **Papules/pustules**: papule is a fluid-filled type of a vesicle that is located deeper in the skin but causes a raised lesion on the skin surface; when the papule is filled with pus, it is called a pustule

Mucous Membranes

-Line body cavities ("body as a tube"—continuous mucous membrane-lined conduit from the oral cavity to the anal opening).

-They can be considered as "internal skin."

-Sheets of epithelial cells attached to a basement membrane, folded to provide large surface area (estimated to be about the size of a football field, on average, if stretched out).

-Some cells comprising the membranes have cilia (small finger-like projections) that help keep microorganisms out of the lungs.

-Goblet cells in the respiratory and intestinal epithelium secrete mucus to maintain the moistness and integrity of the mucosal membrane and often impart a slightly acidic pH, which is why alpha-streptococci, thriving in acidic conditions, are the dominant member of the normal flora in the respiratory tract.

Normal Flora of Mucous Membranes

-Dependent on site of mucous membrane

-Normal flora in this area must be able to survive low pH (e.g., respiratory tract: streptococci; genital tract: lactobacilli)

SKIN INFECTIONS

Modes of Infection

-Breach of intact skin

-Skin manifestation of systemic disease

-Toxin-mediated skin damage

-Many skin infections are multibacterial, caused by several organisms working together (e.g., diabetic foot sores and tropical ulcers)

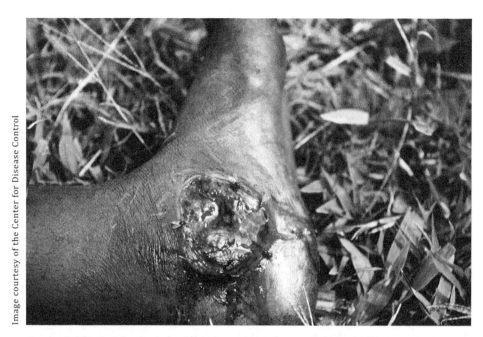

Image courtesy of the Center for Disease Control

FIGURE 13.2   *Tropical ulcer with a multibacterial etiology*

COMMON CAUSES OF BACTERIAL SKIN INFECTIONS

1. ***Staphylococcus aureus***

-Gram-positive cocci in clusters, nonmotile, nonspore forming, facultatively anaerobic

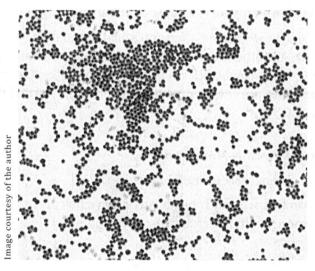

Image courtesy of the author

FIGURE 13.3   Staphylococcus aureus, *Gram's stain*

-Three important species of staphylococcus to know

    Staphylococcus aureus (primary pathogen)

    Staphylococcus epidermidis (normal flora on skin)

    Staphylococcus saprophyticus (primary pathogen in UTI of young women)

-Major cause of skin infection

-May have capsules made of polysaccharides; form biofilms

-*S. aureus* produces coagulase (differentiates *S. aureus* from other staphylococci) converts soluble fibrin in plasma to insoluble fibrin protein. This protein can surround the bacterial focus of infection and prevent phagocytes from reaching the organisms

-Some strains produce yellow colonies on BAP ("yellow or golden staph"); many are beta-hemolytic on blood agar

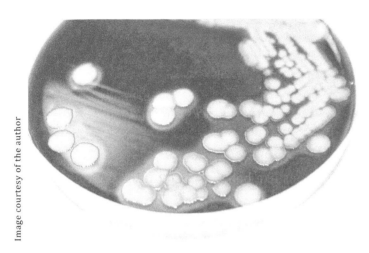

Image courtesy of the author

FIGURE 13.4 Staphylococcus aureus *culture on a blood agar plate showing beta-hemolysis*

-Produce many toxins and enzymes as virulence factors. Examples include:

- Exfoliative toxin: in scalded skin syndrome; destroys cell junction attachments

- Membrane-damaging toxins like leucocidin: destroys WBC

- Catalase—breaks down hydrogen peroxide produced by neutrophils

- DNase: breaks down DNA

- TSST-1: toxic shock syndrome toxin—superantigen effects

- Protein A: Fc receptor on surface of *S. aureus*

Impetigo

-Can be caused by *S. aureus* alone or in combination with Group A streptococcus.

-Impetigo is a superficial skin infection of the epidermal layer of the skin— it is usually seen in small children and is infectious from person to person. It is often seen around the mouth on the face but can present anywhere on the skin surface.

-Treatment of uncomplicated impetigo can usually be done topically and by keeping the area clean with soap and water.

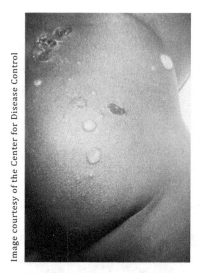

FIGURE 13.5   *Impetigo on the buttocks of a child*

-*Staphylococcus aureus* is well known as a causative agent for skin and soft tissue infections like boils but also causes systemic, life-threatening infection.

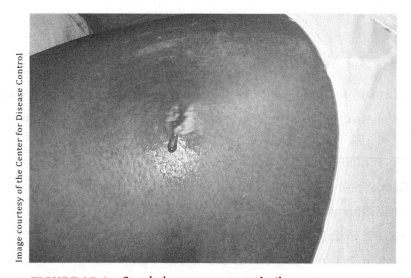

FIGURE 13.6   *Staphylococcus aureus boil*

Toxic Shock Syndrome (TSS) caused by the superantigen of *S. aureus*

-Life-threatening, multisystem effects caused by elaboration of a Type 1 exotoxin, TSST-1

-Generally starts with a localized infection with a toxin-producing strain of *S. aureus,* and the disease is due to the systemic spread of the exotoxins, not the bacterium

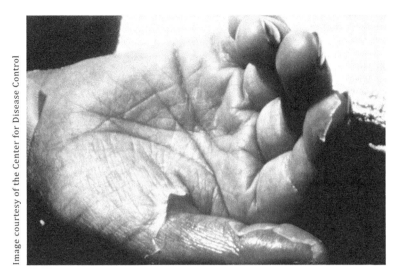

Image courtesy of the Center for Disease Control

FIGURE 13.7 *Skin desquamation due to exfoliative toxin in toxic shock syndrome*

-Mechanism of pathogenicity: TSST-1 is a superantigen, capable of activating huge numbers of T cells, which produce and release massive amounts of cytokines, causing all the pathology associated with the disease

-Symptoms: fever, vomiting, sunburn-like rash, eventual shock

-First identified in conjunction with tampon use—now known to be common in all surgeries where gauze packs the wound

-Often in combination with scalded skin syndrome, where the skin peels off (desquamates) due to an exfoliative toxin

-Prompt IV antibiotic treatment necessary

Staphylococcal boils and abscesses

-Staphylococcal boil or furuncle is a typical, uncomplicated skin infection causing painful lesions—this can be a result of an external or internal infection

-If external infection, the bacterium is capable of spreading to the bloodstream and causing septicemia, leading to septic shock; if internal, then the abscesses usually originate from foci of bacteria that have been spread systemically

Abscess: localized lesion with accumulation of pus anywhere in the body; may be caused by one type of bacterium, like *S. aureus,* or may be polymicrobial in nature with many different bacterial species contributing.

2. *Streptococcus pyogenes*

-Gram-positive cocci in chains, nonmotile, facultatively anaerobic

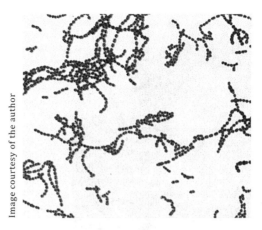

FIGURE 13.8   Streptococcus *species, Gram's stain*

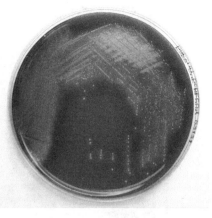

FIGURE 13.9   Streptococcus pyogenes *on blood agar plate, beta-hemolytic*

-Can produce capsules made of hyaluronic acid

-Also called Group A streptococci or GAS, or beta-hemolytic streptococci (Group A)

-Hemolysis is due to production of streptolysin, a hemolysin that breaks down sheep red blood cells in culture media

-*S. pyogenes* is typed or grouped on the basis of cell wall antigens

Lancefield's grouping: based on cell wall group carbohydrate antigens

-Produces many toxins and enzymes as virulence factors

- M protein inhibits phagocytosis and aids the adherence of bacteria to host cells

- Spe, erythrogenic toxin: rash seen in "scarlet fever" both are super-antigens

- Streptokinase: dissolves blood clots, allowing bacteria to spread

- Hyaluronidase: breaks down connective tissue

- Deoxyribonuclease: degrades DNA

- Proteases (e.g., IgA protease): degrades IgA, which is on mucosal membranes traps bacteria in mucus, and prevents bacteria from attaching to the host cells and infecting

-Causes impetigo, erysipelas, cellulitis, flesh-eating disease (necrotizing fasciitis), and other syndromes not related to skin infection like pharyngitis

-Erysipelas is a *Streptococcus pyogenes* infection in the skin and must be treated promptly and effectively so as not to spread to deeper layers or systemically

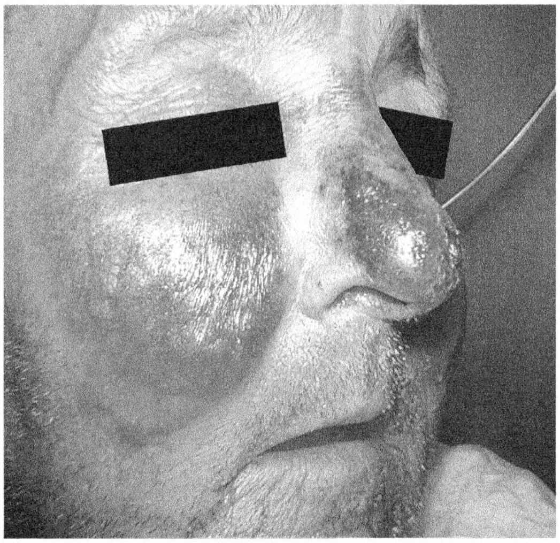

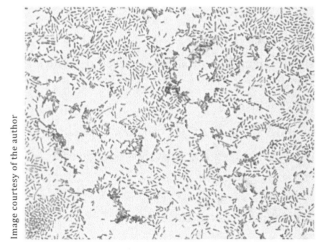

FIGURE 13.10 *Erysipelas (a type of cellulitis)*

Image courtesy of the Center for Disease Control

3. *Pseudomonas aeruginosa*

-Gram-negative, aerobic, nonspore-forming bacillus, motile and found in water and soil

-Produces exotoxins and contains endotoxin in the cell wall

-Many virulence factors: proteases, toxins, hemolysins, phospholipase C

-Often an opportunistic pathogen (e.g., in burned skin)

-Difficult to treat (naturally resistant to many antibiotics)

Image courtesy of the author

FIGURE 13.11 Pseudomonas aeruginosa, *Gram's stain*

-Produces a blue–green iridescent pigment called pyocyanin (results in blue–green pus)

    Pyocyanin may be a virulence factor, damaging neutrophils

-Colonizer of lungs in cystic fibrosis patients

-Can produce capsule (loosely organized = slime layer)

-Cause of "swimmer's ear:" external otitis, dermatitis (self-limiting rash) in swimmers and hot tubbers

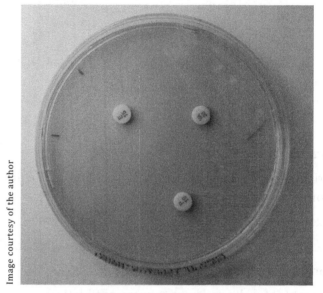

Image courtesy of the author

FIGURE 13.12   *Pyocyanin produced by* P. aeruginosa *in culture*

4. *Propionibacterium acnes*

-A Gram-positive, anaerobic, diphtheroid bacillus, which is often a causative organism for acne

-Most common skin disease

-Multifactorial blockage in channels transporting sebum to surface

-Secondary infection drives the pustular skin disease (could be with *S. aureus*)

5. Mycobacterial diseases of the skin

-*M. tuberculosis*

-*M. leprae*

-*M. marinum* (ulcers following trauma in water)

-*M. ulcerans* (Buruli ulcers)

-Must stain with acid-fast stain, also called Ziehl-Neelsen stain because the Gram's stain does not penetrate the waxy cell walls.

-Acid-fast bacilli, aerobic, nonmotile

-Production of granulomas or tubercles

-Extended treatment periods with a cocktail (combination) of antimicrobial agents

COMMON CAUSES OF VIRAL SKIN INFECTIONS

1. Warts

-Caused by papillomavirus or human papillomavirus (HPV) (DNA, nonenveloped)

-Tumor growth; most growths are benign

-Transmitted by direct contact

-STD = genital warts; certain genotypes are associated with cervical, penile, and anal cancer (types 16, 18)

-Plantar warts: flat, usually on sole of foot

-Cutaneous warts on hands

-Flat warts on surface of skin

-Most warts disappear spontaneously after 3–5 years

2. Molluscum contagiosum

-Poxvirus, DNA, enveloped, also called "water warts"

-Infects epidermal cells to form fleshy wart-like lesions

-Swimming pools are great for transmission because virus is resistant to chlorine

-Resolves spontaneously

3. Orf

-Poxvirus, DNA, enveloped

-Zoonotic virus associated with goats and sheep

-"Contagious pustular dermatitis"

4. Hand, foot, and mouth disease

-Caused by coxsackie virus, an enterovirus, RNA, enveloped

-Vesicular lesions on skin, buccal mucosa, and tongue

-Usually disease of childhood

5. Herpes viruses

-Eight herpes viruses infect humans

-DNA virus, enveloped

-Most significant characteristic of the members of the group is the ability to become **latent** in nerve ganglion and reactivate at a later time

HSV-1: cold sores—usually

HSV-2: genital herpes (STD)—usually

HHV-3: chickenpox/shingles (also called varicella zoster virus)

HHV-4: Epstein–Barr virus (EBV)

HHV-5: cytomegalovirus (CMV)

HHV-6: roseola (mild disease of childhood)

HHV-7: sometimes causes roseola, otherwise unknown

HHV-8: Kaposi's sarcoma associated in AIDS

HSV-1

-Very common, >90% of the population has been infected, most in childhood

-Transmitted by direct contact

-Cold sores

-Lesions contain virus

-After the primary infection, there is latency in nerve ganglia (usually trigeminal ganglia in the head); stress triggers reactivation to the same dermatome

-Herpes gladiatorum: wrestlers, lesions on body (many must take antivirals for life)

-Herpes whitlow: occupational disease in healthcare workers (usually a finger lesion)

-Complications: herpetic encephalitis and keratitis

Image courtesy of the Center for Disease Control

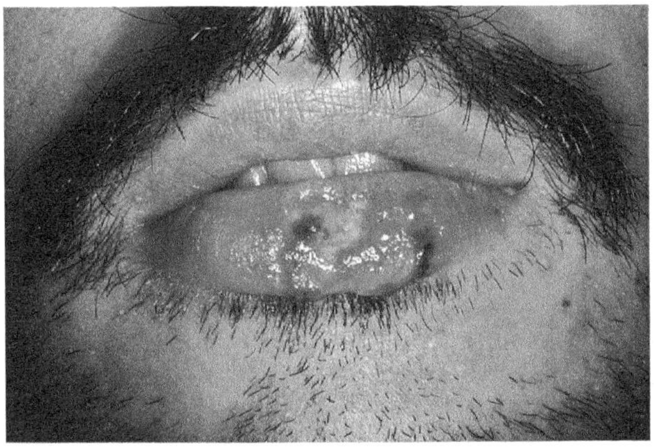

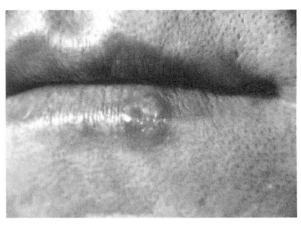

FIGURE 13.13 *Herpes cold sore in a HIV patient*

Image courtesy of the Center for Disease Control

FIGURE 13.14 *Herpes cold sore in a healthy person*

Chickenpox and shingles

-Caused by HSV-3 or varicella zoster virus, enveloped DNA virus, one serotype

-Severe infections in immunocompromised

-Transmitted by airborne transmission, very infectious, lesions contain virus

-Acquired as a respiratory infection; develops to typical vesicular rash with lesions in different stages

-Establishes latency in nerve ganglia near spine dorsal root ganglion: shingles or herpes zoster is the name given to the reactivation of the virus; typically appears in a "belt" of lesions on one dermatome

Image courtesy of the Center for Disease Control

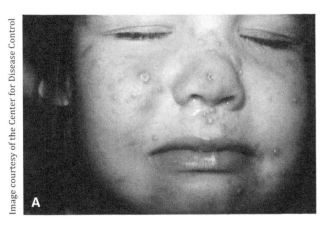

FIGURE 13.15a *Chickenpox and*

Image courtesy of the Center for Disease Control

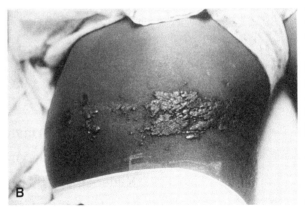

FIGURE 13.15b *Shingles*

Measles (roseola)

-RNA, Paramyxoviridae, enveloped, one serotype

-One of the most infectious viral diseases—infection by airborne route

-Infection starts with respiratory infection, progresses to rash

-Rash not infectious, probably a result of immune complex formation

-Vaccination effective (MMR)

-Macular rash with "Koplik's" spots in oral cavity (Koplik's spots are red, white, and blue lesions seen in early stages of measles)

-Complications: middle ear infections, pneumonia, encephalitis, blindness

-Severity of disease increases with vitamin A deficiency, so the disease can be life-threatening, especially in populations with malnutrition

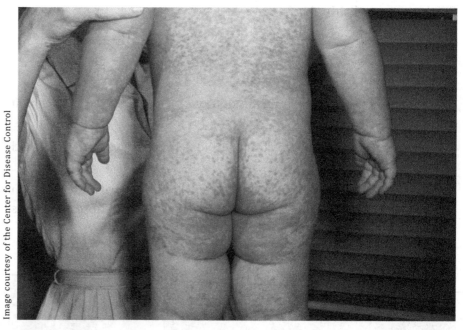

Image courtesy of the Center for Disease Control

FIGURE 13.16   *Measles rash*

7. Rubella (German measles)

-RNA, Togaviridae, enveloped, one serotype

-Milder disease than measles

-Macular rash

-Complications: rare in children

   Adults: encephalitis

   Pregnant women: fetal development of congenital rubella

8. Fifth disease/parvovirus B19/erythema infectiosum/slapped cheek syndrome

-Parvovirus, DNA, nonenveloped

-Mild rash disease of childhood; usually no complications in children

-Pink lacy rash; cheeks become very red, which is usually the first noticeable sign in children

-Major complication: TAC (transient aplastic crisis) in pregnant women. Parvovirus has a tropism for nucleated red blood cells, and it invades and destroys these cells in the bone marrow. This means that the mother's hemoglobin can drop 30%–40% very quickly, and the fetus will not be getting oxygen This leads to stillbirth/spontaneous abortion.

COMMON CAUSES OF FUNGAL SKIN INFECTIONS

-Types of fungal infections (also called mycoses or tineas)

    Superficial

    Cutaneous

    Subcutaneous

    Systemic

    Opportunistic

1. Superficial mycoses: confined to outer layers of skin, do not invade

    example: *Malassezia furfur*—causes tinea versicolor or pityriasis versicolor

        "black piedra"—nodular infection of hair shaft

2. Cutaneous or dermatophytic: infect only skin, hair, or nails; infect the superficial keratinized tissue

-Three different types of keratin-loving fungi

    Epidermophyton

    Trichophyton

    Microsporum

-These three cannot grow at 37 °C or in the presence of serum, so this may be why they stay in the outer layers of the skin

-Often zoonotic (e.g., *Microsporum canis*)

-Arthrospores adhere to keratin, germinate, and invade, producing keratinase to break down this waterproofing protein in the skin

-Tinea (ringworm) is characterized by annual scaling, itching patch, raised margin

    Tinea capitis: ringworm of the scalp

    Tinea corporis: ringworm of the body

Tinea cruris: ringworm of the groin ("jock itch")

Tinea pedis: ringworm of the feet ("athlete's foot")

Tinea unguium: infection of the nails

3. Subcutaneous

-Fungi that cause subcutaneous mycoses are usually found in soil and on plants

-Usually introduced by trauma (e.g., rose thorn)

-Lesions usually become granulomatous and spread via the lymphatics

-Usually remain in subcutaneous area, but some of the fungi can spread further to cause systemic infection

a. *Sporothrix schenckii* infection

- Widespread in nature

- Occupational hazard of gardeners

- Disseminated infection in immunocompromised individuals

  - **"Dimorphic,"** meaning a fungus at ambient temperatures and a yeast at body temperatures

b. Chromoblastomycosis

- Caused by any of five different fungi—often cause chronic granulomatous lesions

4. Systemic

-Dimorphic fungi included here; each are geographically restricted

-Four primary systemic mycoses

Coccidioidomycosis: *Coccidioides immitis*: soil mold SW United States, Canada, South America

- Infection is usually self-limited

Blastomycosis: *Blastomyces dermatitidis*: origin not really understood

- Chronic lung infections, and develop granulomatous and suppurative infections in the lungs, then can disseminate to the rest of the system

Histoplasmosis: *Histoplasma capsulatum*: soil, avian habitats with guano

- Occurs worldwide, but incidence varies and most cases are in the United States

- Disease can mimic tuberculosis

Paracoccidioidomycosis: South American blastomycosis, endemic in Canada and South America

- Initial lesions in lung (granulomas) can spread and lead to chronic progressive lung disease when systemic

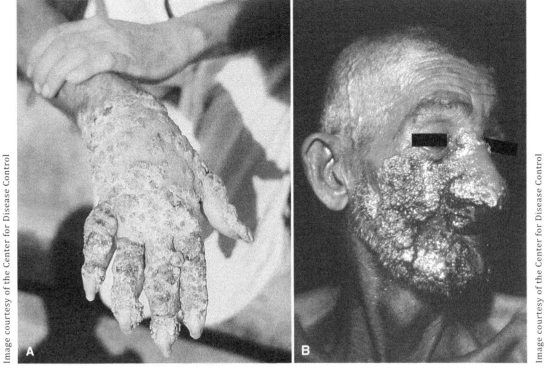

Image courtesy of the Center for Disease Control

Image courtesy of the Center for Disease Control

FIGURE 13.17a and 13.17b *Chromoblastomycosis caused by* Paracoccidioides braziliensis

5. **Opportunistic**

   a. ***Candida* species**: most common yeast causing systemic mycosis

   - Found as normal flora on skin and in the intestine

   - Changes in mucosal pH or after antibiotics in adults

   - Newborns susceptible as low amounts of normal flora

   - Immunocompromised can develop systemic infection

   b. ***Cryptococcus neoformans***: characterized by a thick polysaccharide capsule

   - Large numbers in pigeon feces

   - Usually infects immunosuppressed

   - *Cryptococcus neoformans var gattii* can infect immunocompetent

   c. **Aspergillosis**: caused by Aspergillus species (fumigatus, flavus, niger, terreus)

   - Occurs worldwide

   - Inhaled conidia may germinate in lungs and invade tissues

   - Can also cause allergic reactions

   - Formation of fungal balls in cavities (e.g., in damaged lung tissue)

d. **Mucormycosis**:

- Often infect diabetics and severely burned patients

e. ***Pneumocystis jiroveci***: causes pneumoniae in immunocompromised patients (e.g., people with AIDS)

COMMON CAUSES OF PARASITIC SKIN INFECTIONS

-Many parasites can cause skin lesions

-Hookworms burrow through skin (dermatitis)

-*Leishmania*: several different species of parasite

Diseases due to Leishmania: visceral, cutaneous, and mucocutaneous

-Duck *Schistosoma*: "swimmers' itch" (even in Alberta!)

-*Onchocerca*: filarial (nematodes) live in subcutaneous nodules

-Myiasis: eggs laid by dipteran flies on skin hatch, and larva burrow, which cause lesions (can become secondarily infected with skin flora)

-Arthropods: ticks, lice, and mites also can cause small lesions that become infected with skin flora

Device-Related Infections

Devices like catheters, pacemakers, artificial joints, and intravenous lines all increase the risk for a patient to become infected. One of the most common sources of infection is the skin—the normal flora on the skin, especially *Staphylococcus epidermidis.* Often the infection is introduced during the implanting of the device.

Biofilms form easily on artificial surfaces of devices and are impossible to remove with antibiotic treatment; often the device must be removed to clear the infection with antibiotics. Although antibiotics will penetrate through a biofilm, for some unknown reason, they do not affect the bacteria within a biofilm. Leukocytes on the other hand, do not have the ability to get into the biofilm and phagocytose organisms. This makes the biofilm impervious to chemotherapy and to the immune system, allowing an infection to continue to exist in the body.

Remember that biofilms are not static—bacteria are continually leaving the biofilm, which can spread an infection.

Vascular Grafts

Vascular grafts are often taken from another part of the same patient and can be infected—often at the time of surgery. An example is coronary artery bypass graft (CABG). Infection can result from:

1. Intraoperative contamination

2. As an extension from an adjacent infected tissue

3. Hematogenous seeding (bloodstream infection seeds the new tissue graft)

    - The most common organism infecting a vascular graft is *S. aureus.* This is usually a very aggressive infection.

Intravenous Catheter

Peripheral and central venous catheters are common areas for infection to occur. Here, the needle and the tubing will remain in place for an extended period of time. There are four common sites where infection can occur:

1. Microbial contamination of the infusate (not common due to rigid quality control, but it does happen)

2. Hub: tubing connector to the needle apparatus

3. Microbial contamination at the insertion site

4. Hematogenous infection from the bloodstream infecting the insertion site

Blatant signs of infection are seen in only about half of the cases proved infected.

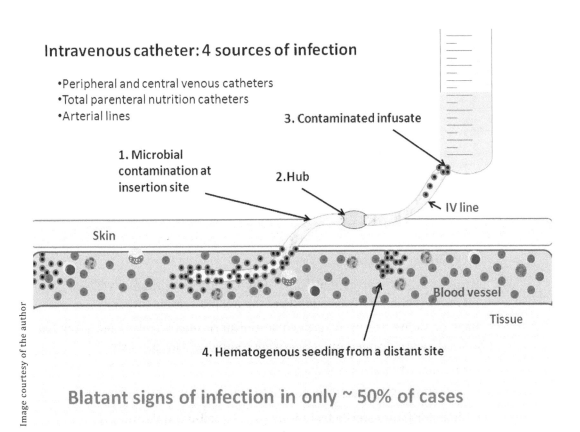

Image courtesy of the author

FIGURE 13.18   *Sources of infection associated with a vascular catheter*

Dialysis

Dialysis is a filtration method by which toxic wastes are removed from the blood in patients with renal (kidney) failure.

-Two major methods

    Hemodialysis

    Peritoneal dialysis

a. Hemodialysis

-Major infectious risks are due to contamination of the equipment; the bloodborne infections like HIV, HCV, HBV

-In-hospital procedure; blood is directed through a dialysis machine and "cleaned" several times a week

-Very time consuming; patient is in the hospital for hours each time

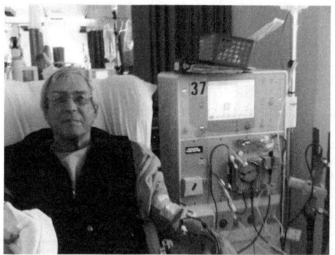

© Anna Frodesiak, Creative commons

FIGURE 13.19   Hemodialysis

b. Peritoneal dialysis

-Patients have a permanent "port" (giving access to the body cavity) and can manage their dialysis outside of the hospital (ambulatory)

-Bags of saline are used to perfuse the peritoneal cavity, then after five hours they are drained out, effectively removing a lot of wastes

-Problems with peritoneal dialysis

    Infection of the "port" with skin bacteria, leading to peritonitis

    Risk for faulty sterile technique (due to self-administration)

    Reduction in opsonins due to the peritoneal washing

-Infection is usually due to skin bacteria entering the abdominal cavity:

 Staphylococcus epidermidis

 Staphylococcus aureus

 Streptococcus species

 Bacillus species

 Gram negatives

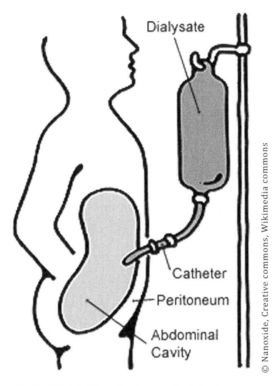

FIGURE 13.20   Peritoneal dialysis

-Patients on circulating ambulatory peritoneal dialysis (CAPD) often get infections, sometimes as many as one every two months

-Approximately 70% get infections during the first year, and most are within the first six months

-Peritonitis is the major complication of peritoneal dialysis, but prognosis for peritonitis in dialysis patients is good: <1%

Peritonitis

-Inflammation/infection of the peritoneal cavity

-Dominant symptom: moderately severe abdominal pain

-Pain is aggravated by motion, even breathing!

-Other symptoms: anorexia, nausea, vomiting, fever, abdominal distention

-Major complication: development of an intraperitoneal abscess—these are usually polymicrobial and involve both aerobes and anaerobes like *Bacteroides* species

Trivia: Harry Houdini died of peritonitis

-Complications occur more often in children

Abscesses

a) **Skin**: usually *S. aureus*

b) **Peritoneal**: usually as a result of dialysis; usually polymicrobial

c) **CNS** (central nervous system)
    - Embolization of organisms from a distant site (e.g., from endocarditis)
    - Spread from a nearby focus of infection (i.e., middle ear infections)
    - Complication of surgery
    - Complication of trauma or congenital abnormalities
    - Complication of AIDS (e.g., *Toxoplasma gondii*)

d) **Lung**
    - Often caused by oral microflora, e.g., Nocardia, Mycobacteria or anaerobes
    - Localization depends on organism (aerobic or anaerobic)
    - Result: cavitation and destruction of lung tissue (necrotizing pneumonia)

e) **Liver**
    - Often caused by amoebae (only *Entamoeba histolytica*)
    - Characteristically no pus; somewhat immunologically privileged site
    - *Echinococcus granulosum* hydatid cysts
    - Bacterial liver abscesses are often polymicrobial

f) **Tonsillar abscesses**
    - Often *S. pyogenes* (GAS), also oral flora
    1) Peritonsillar abscesses: also called quinsy
    2) Retrotonsillar abscesses: dangerous if not treated quickly due to propensity to spread infection to the brain
    - Draining and antibiotics are used to control spread of infection further

g) **Osteomyelitis**
    - Infection/abscess of the bone
    - Three sources of infection
    - Nearby site of infection

- After trauma (e.g., skull fractures)

- Circulating microbes

- Most common cause of osteomyelitis coming from the blood is *S. aureus*

- Most common cause of osteomyelitis coming from a nearby site is polymicrobial (mix of Gram negatives and Gram positives)

- Difficult to treat; bone is hard to get antibiotics into

- Long treatment periods, sometimes up to a year

Acute osteomyelitis

- Often end of long bones, typically children

- Bone lesions very painful

Chronic osteomyelitis

- Usually with necrotic bone fragments

- Surgery necessary and prolonged antibiotics

- Amputation of limbs can be an end result to stop spread!

Wounds

Five Types of Wounds

1. Incised: produced by a sharp object (e.g., surgery)

2. Puncture: penetration of sharp object (e.g., nail, bite)

3. Lacerated: tissue is torn

4. Contused: caused by a blow that crushes tissue

5. Burns

1. **Incised**: surgical infections with contamination of the surgical site during operation or infection of the stitches after surgery

   - Associated with hygienic conditions in the operating room, immune status of the patient, and the competence of the surgeon and OR staff

   - Not uncommon to have patients' own normal flora infecting a surgical site

     Upper body: mainly *Staphylococcus aureus*

     Lower body: primarily fecal flora (Gram negatives and enterococci)

   - Common to use preoperative and peroperative antibiotic therapy for "dirty surgery" (i.e., abdominal surgery)

   - Wound abscesses: often the abscess is bounded by a thick, fibrin-containing wall shielding the organisms; often have to be surgically drained because antibiotics do not penetrate well and diffuse poorly in infected or damaged tissue

2 & 3. Punctures and Lacerations

- Can often be anaerobic in nature due to the deep penetration of the wounding object (nail or teeth)
- Bites can be punctures (e.g. cat bites, snake bites) or lacerations (human bites, dog bites)

Bite infections

- Usually polymicrobial
- Most common symptom is localized cellulitis at the site
- Purulent discharge is common, often gray and foul-smelling (indicating the presence of anaerobes)
- More severe in ~10% of individuals: with fever, regional lymph node swelling, and lymphangitis
- Puncture bite wounds (e.g., cats and snakes) are more often infected

Spider bites

- Can become infected; toxin is injected, which damages the tissues, which become easily infected

Snake bites

- 8000 Americans are bitten by snakes/year
- Venom can cause tissue necrosis, and infection can easily develop
- *Pseudomonas aeruginosa* is a very common cause of snake bite infection, but other Gram negatives, like *Salmonella* species, coagulase negative; staphylococci are also common

Human bites

- Often infected, more often than animal bites
- Both aerobic and anaerobic bacteria are implicated (oral flora is very diverse)
- *Eikenella corrodens* is an important pathogen in human bite infections

---

Tetanus or "Lockjaw"

-More than 50% of cases are in puncture wounds, caused by *Clostridium tetani,* an anaerobic, Gram-positive, spore-forming bacillus normally found in soil.

-Most important virulence factor is tetanospasmin—an exotoxin.

-Bacteria do not invade but rather stay at the site of injury and produce exotoxins, which diffuse into the central nervous system and peripheral nerves.

-Tetanospasmin blocks release of inhibitory neurotransmitters (glycine and GABA) across the synapse, causing spasms of muscles, which cannot get the signal to relax.

-Death can result from spasms of respiratory muscles, pneumonia, or regurgitating stomach contents into the lungs.

-Neonatal tetanus is still common where traditional practices during childbirth dictate that the umbilical cord either be packed with earth or clipped off with unsterilized instruments.

-Toxoid exists; antitoxin TIG can also be given.

4. **Contused or "closed fist"**—crush wounds or blunt trauma

 - For example, pyomyositis, an acute infection (often caused by *S. aureus*) that affects the skeletal muscles

 - Long duration of vascular insufficiency—damage to tissue leads to increased susceptibility to infection

5. **Burns**

 - Infections result from a disruption in the normal homeostasis, resulting from lack of integrity in the outer integument

 - Mortality rate of burns >40% of the body surface is extremely high

 - Very important to maintain blood flow to affected area

 - Decreased immune responses in large burns (lack of circulation)

 Management of burns: necrotic tissue is a good medium for growth of bacteria and often must be removed surgically

 - Burn areas should be closed as soon as possible, and topical antibiotics should be used prophylactically

 - Hemorrhage, eschar formation, and greenish discoloration indicates infection

 - Often both Gram negatives and Gram positives in mixed infections

 - *Pseudomonas aeruginosa* is a common bacterium infecting burns

Deeper Wound Infections

Cellulitis

 - Acute spreading infection of the deeper layers of the skin

 - Can progress to a bloodstream infection (septicemia)

 - Involves subcutaneous tissues

 - Usually originates from superficial skin lesions (e.g., shaving cuts, puncture wounds like vaccination sites, boils, or ulcers, etc.)

 - Majority of cases is caused by *Staphylococcus aureus* and *Streptococcus pyogenes*

- IVDU (intravenous drug users) often fall victim to this due to lack of attention to sterile injection, plus the fact that many are immunosuppressed

Anaerobic cellulitis: areas of traumatized tissue or poor blood circulation

- Diabetics are prone to cellulitis in the feet
- Causative organisms vary dependent on the type of trauma
- Infections in the lower part of the body are normally caused by fecal flora and by oral flora in the upper part of the body

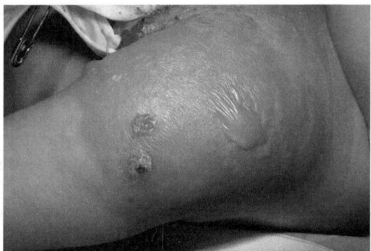

Image courtesy of the Center for Disease Control

FIGURE 13.21   *Cellulitis resulting from a vaccination*

- Foul-smelling exudates
- Marked swelling and gas lead to gangrene (tissue death)
- Signs: red, warm, inflamed tissue, usually painful, development of systemic symptoms like fever, chills
- Prompt IV antibiotics necessary in addition to surgical removal of damaged tissue

Classical Gas Gangrene (anaerobic cellulitis with necrosis)

-It is usually caused by *Clostridium perfringens* (anaerobic, Gram positive, spore-forming bacilli)

-*C. perfringens* spores are normally found in soil but also can be normal in human and animal intestine.

-Gas gangrene is usually a result of traumatized tissue with poor blood supply (anaerobic environment) that has been contaminated with spores of *C. perfringens.*

-Buttocks and perineum are common sites for infection.

-Organisms spread rapidly in subcutaneous tissues and invade deeper tissues, and produce gas as a by-product of metabolism (mostly carbon dioxide). This causes a crackling sound on palpitation

-Alpha toxin destroys tissue cells and leukocytes; collagenase, hyaluronidase, and other enzymes further break down tissue.

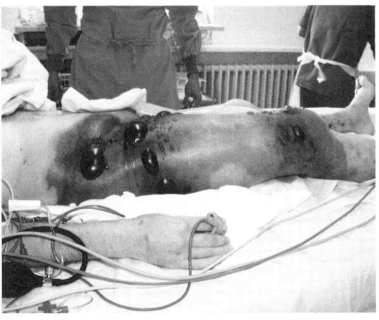

© Engelbert Schropfer, Stephan Rauthe and Thomas Meyer, Creative commons public domain

FIGURE 13.22   Classical gas gangrene

Interested? Want to learn more?

For more reading, several texts online at the U of A library are recommended:

1. Brooks, GF, Carroll KC, Butel JS, Morse SA, editors. Jawetz, Melnick, and Adelberg's Medical Microbiology, 24th ed. Blacklick OH-McGraw Hill; 2007.

2. Ryan KJ, Ray CG, editors. Sherris Medical Microbiology, 5th ed. New York – McGraw-Hill, 2010.

3. Mandell GL, Bennett JE,Dolin R, editors. Mandell, Douglas and Bennett's Principles and Practices of Infectious Diseases, 7th ed. Churchill Livingstone Elsevier, Philadelphia, 2010.

Chapter 14

Eye Infections

Learning Objectives:

1. Describe how infections can disrupt the normal functioning of the eye.

2. Define the different types of infections according to the site of infection (conjunctivitis, keratitis, etc.).

3. List the immune defence mechanisms in the eye.

4. Describe risk factors for eye infections.

5. Identify commonly encountered eye infections, their causative agents, and their clinical appearances.

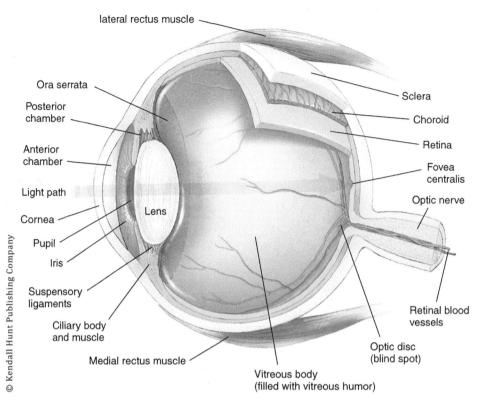

lateral rectus muscle

Ora serrata
Posterior chamber
Anterior chamber
Light path
Cornea
Pupil
Iris
Suspensory ligaments
Ciliary body and muscle
Medial rectus muscle
Lens

Sclera
Choroid
Retina
Fovea centralis
Optic nerve
Retinal blood vessels
Optic disc (blind spot)

Vitreous body (filled with vitreous humor)

© Kendall Hunt Publishing Company

FIGURE 14.1   Eye anatomy

-Infections of the eye can result from an external infection, or internal (i.e., organisms circulating in the blood).

-Outer membrane of eye (conjunctiva) is exposed to external environment and infectious organisms—think of this as the "skin" of the eye.

Definitions

-**Blepharitis**: inflammation of the eyelid margin

-**Dacryocystitis**: inflammation of the lacrimal sac (tear sac)

-**Conjunctiva**: thin layer of mucous membrane covering the eye

- Especially susceptible to infection; few white blood cells
- Vulnerable epithelial surface covered by eyelid (creates warm, moist conditions that bacteria like to grow on)
- **Conjunctivitis**: inflammation of the conjunctiva

-**Cornea**: outermost lens in the eye; clear

- **Keratitis**: inflammation of the cornea
- Contact lens wearers are at higher risk factor for infections because the cornea can get scratched easily and provide a portal of entry for an organism
- **Keratoconjunctivitis**: inflammation or infection of the cornea and the conjunctiva

-**Lens**: focuses light beams from the cornea to the optic nerve

-**Iris**: pigmented area of eyeball

   Iritis (iridocyclitis): inflammation of the iris

-**Sclera**: white part of the eye

-**Uvea**

   - **Uveitis**: inflammation of the middle vascular covering in the eye; often involves the sclera and cornea

-**Retina**: multilayered sensory tissue containing photoreceptors, which change the visual signal into electrical signal for the optic nerve

   - **Chorioretinitis**: inflammatory infiltrates, which can lead to optic nerve impairment

-**Aqueous humor**: vitreous humor in the eye

   - **Endophthalmitis**: infection of the aqueous humor

Barriers to Infection in the Eye

-Eyelid serves as a mechanical barrier to organisms

-Tears flush away organisms

-Tears contain lysozyme, secretory IgA: chemical barriers to infection

Normal Flora of Eye Surface

-The surface of the eye is sparsely populated with usually only a few species of bacteria:

   Micrococcus species (e.g., *S. epidermidis*)—not *S. aureus*

   Alpha-hemolytic streptococci

   Diphtheroids (*Corynebacterium* but not *C. diphtheriae*)

-Interior chamber of the eye should be sterile in a healthy eye

INFECTION OF THE EYELID

-Infection of eyelid is usually with *S. aureus.*

Blepharitis: inflammation (with or without infection) of lid margins

   - Combination of infectious and allergic causes

   - Infection of eyelids, usually involves bacterial invasion of hair follicles

   - Formation of abscesses in severe infection

   - Loss of eyelashes, itching

   - Can be chronic and may be due to the presence of a mite

Stye: infection of eyelid glands and hair follicles (also called hordeola)

   - Infection of the hair follicle with *S. aureus*, development of a staphylococcal pustule

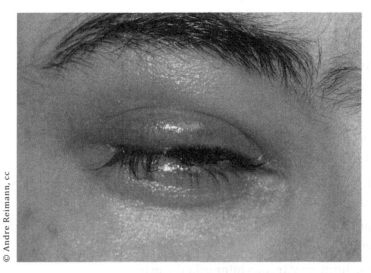

FIGURE 14.2   *Stye or hordeola*

Infection of the Conjunctiva

-Often involves bacteria like *Haemophilus influenzae, Staphylococcus aureus, Streptococcus pyogenes, Streptococcus pneumoniae*

-Intensely red eye associated with a scratching sensation, some photophobia, and blurring of vision from exudates (pus)

-Many bacterial and viral agents causing respiratory tract infection can cause conjunctivitis; also called "pinkeye"

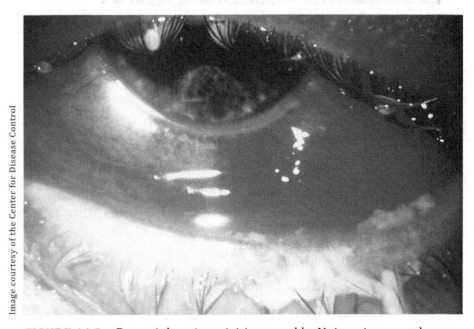

FIGURE 14.3   *Bacterial conjunctivitis caused by* Neisseria gonorrhoeae

-"Inclusion conjunctivitis"—caused by *C. trachomatis* genital serotypes D-K

-Neonatal conjunctivitis (two to four weeks after birth); conjunctivitis caused by *Neisseria gonorrhoeae* characterized by copious production of pus ophthalmia neonatorum *C. trachomatis* can also cause eye infections in combination with respiratory infections, although it usually takes longer for the symptoms to start showing

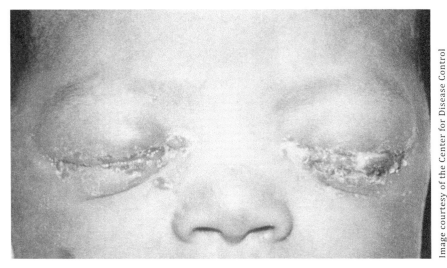

FIGURE 14.4   Gonococcal ophthalmia neonatorum

-Coxsackie virus and some adenovirus subtypes cause acute hemorrhagic conjunctivitis (usually self-limiting)

-*S. aureus* causes a mild conjunctivitis with moderate to heavy exudate, gluing the eyelid shut

-Some microfilaria (e.g., *Loa loa*) migrate in the conjunctiva

-Viral conjunctivitis (e.g., caused by varicella zoster, HSV, measles, adenovirus)

- Usually nonpurulent (a major difference between bacterial and viral conjunctivitis)

-**Acanthamoeba**: protozoan ubiquitous in dust, soil; can cause severe conjunctivitis and deeper infection in contact lens wearers (loss of eye)

-**Trachoma**

- Caused by *C. trachomatis* serotypes A, B, C
- Most common in tropics and subtropics,-transmitted by flies
- Leading cause of blindness in developing countries
- Repeated infections give rise to scarring of the cornea and eyelid
- Eyelashes grow inwards, exacerbating the inflammation

INFECTION OF THE CORNEA (KERATITIS)

-Usual suspects: adenovirus, measles virus, HSV, CMV, VZV, Coxsackie, *C. trachomatis, T. pallidum, S. aureus, S. pyogenes, S. pneumoniae, P. aeruginosa*

-Ulcer formation is often the result of an infectious process in the cornea, leading to scarring and blindness

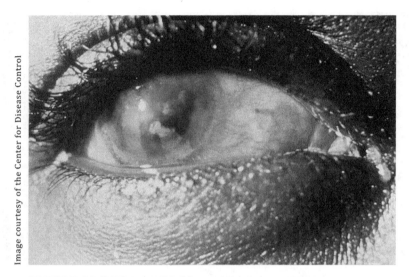

FIGURE 14.5   Interstitial keratitis

-AIDS patients have problems with cytomegalovirus (CMV or HHV-5) keratitis and retinitis

-*Pseudomonas aeruginosa* produce a protease that destroys the collagen holding the corneal epithelium together—very rapid progression and devastation of eye

DEEPER INFECTIONS OF THE EYE

Rubella, HSV, CMV, *Pseudomonas aeruginosa, Toxoplasma gondii, Echinococcus granulosus, Toxocara canis, Onchocerca volvulus*

-Inner areas of eyeball usually site for infections with protozoans and worms

-Organisms that cause corneal ulcers can penetrate deeper and cause intraocular infections

-Prompt diagnosis and treatment important to save eyesight

Ectoparasitic Infections

-Some body lice (e.g., pubic lice) live well in eyebrows and eyelashes

Interested? Want to learn more?

For more reading, several texts online at the U of A library are recommended:

1. Brooks, GF, Carroll KC, Butel JS, Morse SA, editors. Jawetz, Melnick, and Adelberg's Medical Microbiology, 24th ed. Blacklick OH-McGraw Hill; 2007.

2. Ryan KJ, Ray CG, editors. Sherris Medical Microbiology, 5th ed. New York – McGraw-Hill, 2010.

3. Mandell GL, Bennett JE, Dolin R, editors. Mandell, Douglas and Bennett's Principles and Practices of Infectious Diseases, 7th ed. Churchill Livingstone Elsevier, Philadelphia, 2010.

Chapter 15

Upper Respiratory Tract Infections (URTI)

1. Describe the defense mechanisms against infection in the upper respiratory tract.
2. List some common causes of pharyngitis, including the common cold.
3. Describe the cause and pathogenicity of EBV causing infectious mononucleosis.
4. Discuss the pathogenicity of *S. pyogenes.*
5. Discuss the pathogenicity of *C. diphtheriae.*
6. List causes of otitis media and epiglottis.
7. Discuss the cause and pathogenicity of whooping cough.

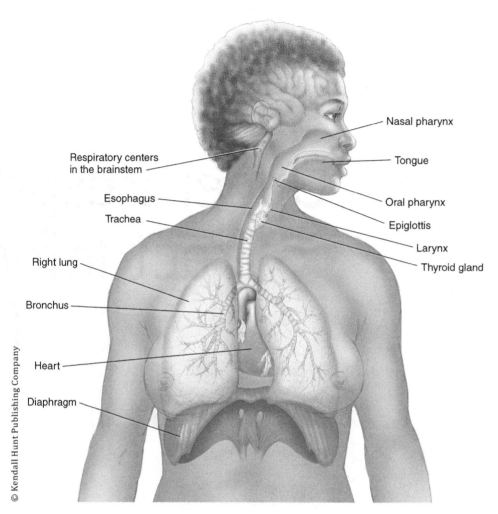

© Kendall Hunt Publishing Company

FIGURE 15.1   Respiratory tract anatomy

Defenses Against Infections in the Upper Respiratory Tract

1. Hairs in nose

2. Upper part of nose contains mucous membrane with cilia

3. Upper part of throat contains mucous membrane with cilia

4. Junction of nose and throat contains lymphoid tissue (tonsils and adenoids in children) that contain macrophages

But, at the same time

- Tonsils can easily become infected and spread through upper tract and to ears

- Adenoids can be infected and enable spread of organisms to ears

Diseases That Are Considered as Upper Respiratory Tract Infections

-Strep throat and complications

-Common cold

-Infectious mononucleosis

-Diphtheria

-Otitis media

-Epiglottitis

-Whooping cough

Normal Flora of the Upper Respiratory Tract

-Alpha-streptococci dominate*

- - *S. epidermidis*, some *S. aureus*, other *Micrococci* sp.

- - *Neisseria* sp.

- - *Haemophilus* sp.

- - Diphtheroids

- - *S. pneumoniae*

- - Low numbers of beta-hemolytic streptococci

- - *Moraxella catarrhalis*

-Numbers of apathogenic bacteria are usually so great that the other potential pathogens cannot establish themselves

-Findings of pathogens such as *N. meningitidis, S. pyogenes, S. aureus, S. pneumoniae* in the throat can be meaningless (transient flora)

-Finding of microorganisms in the sinus is significant (sterile site!)

Bacterial Disease of the Upper Respiratory Tract

Pharyngitis

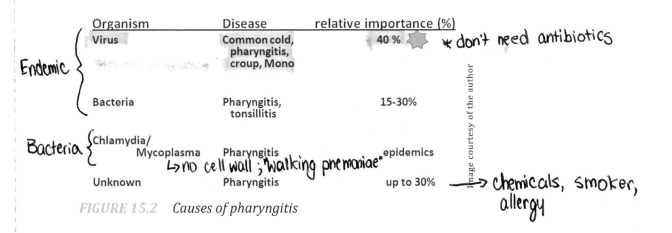

FIGURE 15.2   Causes of pharyngitis

Streptococcal Pharyngitis (Strep Throat)

-Caused by *Streptococcus pyogenes* (GAS or Group A streptococci)—also called beta-hemolytic streptococci

-Strep throat cannot be differentiated from other types of pharyngitis by visual inspection

✱ Need lab tests to prove that *S. pyogenes* is present

Diagnosis: "rapid tests" in doctors' offices and MediCenters OK and reliable if positive, but if negative, then culture must be done in a laboratory (point-of-care test has low sensitivity but high specificity)

-rapid test = filter paper with antibodies (change colour = positive)

Symptoms: sore throat, local inflammation, fever, ± tonsillitis, may have "strawberry tongue," especially in scarlet fever

Complications: scarlet fever, rheumatic fever, Sydenham's chorea, post-streptococcal glomerulonephritis

Treatment: need to treat all cases of *Streptococcus pyogenes* to prevent complications—diagnosis is important! Penicillin is still effective and safe to use

Image courtesy of the Center for Disease Control

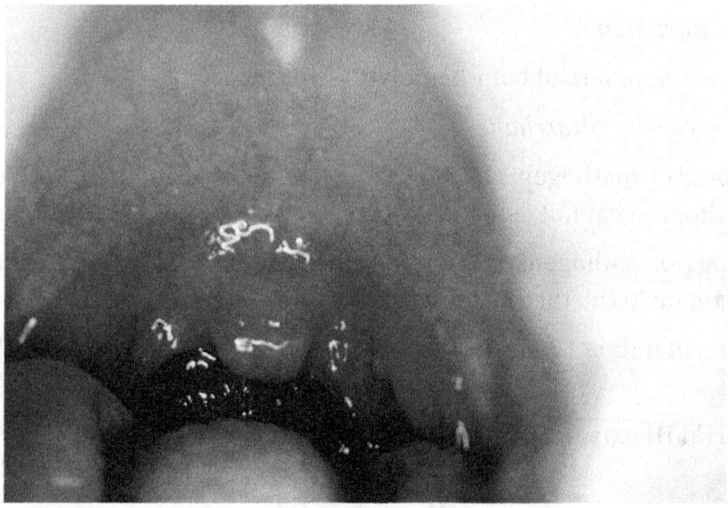

FIGURE 15.3   *Streptococcal pharyngitis*

-can progress to glomerulonephritis or Sydenham's Chorea (flailing movements)

Scarlet Fever

-Caused by *S. pyogenes*

-Pinkish-red rash (sandpaper-like texture) due to erythrogenic toxin

✱ erytho = red
genic = causing

-More than 80 types of Group A strep can cause pharyngitis, but the first infection usually results in Scarlet fever because the patient has no immunity to the erythrogenic toxin

-only get it ONCE, antibodies formed

-Complication of note: rheumatic fever

-Strawberry tongue is due to sloughing off of upper layer of skin from tongue

-can progress to Rheumatic Fever

-Varies in severity

Rheumatic Fever: noninfectious complication of a *Streptococcus pyogenes* infection   **✱ Type III hypersensitivity**

-*S. pyogenes* have M protein in their cell walls, which affords protection against phagocytosis and also aids with adherence to host cells

-M protein is antigenic; antibodies are formed against this after a strep infection

-Anti-M protein antibodies circulate in the blood and mistake the myosin in the heart muscle for *S. pyogenes*, bind the heart muscle cells, and this initiates complement activation leading to inflammation

-Heart valves (especially the mitral valve) and myocardium can be damaged

- Strep A = "PING-PONG" Infections

- easily treatable with penicillin

↳ **can predispose patient to endocarditis (bacteria growing on a biofilm of a heart valve)**

Diphtheria

-Caused by *Corynebacterium diphtheriae*, an aerobic, Gram-positive, pleomorphic bacillus, nonmotile and nonspore-forming

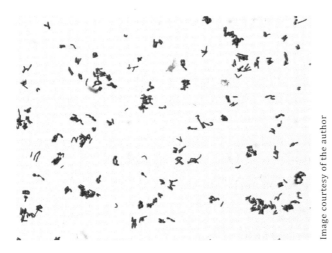

Image courtesy of the author

✱ toxins diffuse out into tissues and has tropism for nerves

FIGURE 15.4   *Gram's stain of* Corynebacterium diphtheriae

-Bacteria do not invade tissues; they produce an exotoxin, which inhibits protein synthesis and is neurotropic

-Once leading cause of mortality in children

-Majority of Canadian cases found in the far north

-Recent epidemic in Russia due to cessation of vaccination program

-Vaccine-effective (toxoid)

Symptoms

- Sore throat   **- white-gray membrane across back of throat (fibrin, dead tissue, bacterial cells, WBC)**
- Fever
- Malaise
- Neck swelling   **("bull neck")**
- Nerve paralysis   **(because of tropism for nerves)**

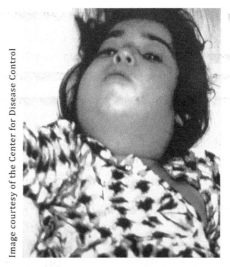

Image courtesy of the Center for Disease Control

FIGURE 15.5 *Bull neck of* C. diphtheriae

Pathogenicity

- Apathogenic unless the bacterial strain has been "lysogenized" or "transduced," meaning the organism is infected with a specific bacteriophage with a gene encoding for the toxin

- White–gray membrane across back of throat (composed of fibrin, dead tissue cells, leucocytes and bacterial cells)

- Three types of bacterial subspecies

    C. diphtheriae gravis

    C. diphtheriae mitis

    C. diphtheriae intermedius

- All types can be apathogenic or pathogenic

- All isolates of *C. diphtheriae* must be tested for toxin production

- Effects of toxin

    - Myocarditis

    - Cardiac failure

    - Polyneuritis

- Toxin interferes with protein synthesis in cells, especially nerve cells

Treatment

- Antibiotics and antitoxin always in combination

Vaccine

- Effective; must have boosters

- Tetanus toxoid usually in combination with diphtheria toxoid (DTaP)

*apathogenic unless lysogenized or transduced by a bacteriophage which transfers a gene that encodes for a toxin

Other Infections

- Cutaneous diphtheria (common in tropics) causes skin ulcers — *causes sores on body*

Whooping Cough (*Bordetella pertussis*)

-Also called "100 day cough"

-Caused by an aerobic, Gram-negative coccobacillus; usually has a capsule

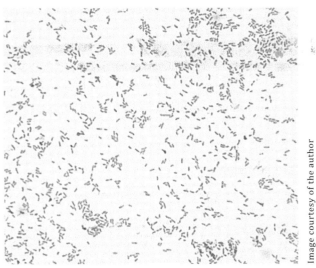

-produces exotoxins
-does not invade, remains in throat

FIGURE 15.6   *Gram's stain of* Bordetella pertussis

-**Symptoms** and stages of disease

- **Catarrhal stage:** starts as a pretty normal looking cold with some coughing and sneezing. This is the most infectious stage for transmission
  - cold like

- **Paroxysmal stage:** gasping cough develops; characteristic "whoop" when gasping for air. Sometimes vomiting, cyanosis, and convulsions if very bad
  - gasping cough
  -100 days

- **Convalescence stage:** healing begins, but cough continues for about three months until the cilia have regenerated again
  -not as severe, but still coughing

-**Pathogenicity**: bacterium produces many virulence factors, which allow it to be a successful pathogen

- Filamentous hemagglutinin: enables adherence to ciliated epithelium
- ✱ Tracheal cytotoxin: inhibits DNA synthesis in ciliated cells *-damages ciliated cells*
- ✱ Pertussis toxin: causes increase in lymphocytes; activation of lymphocytes to cause systemic symptoms like fever *- enters bloodstream and causes systemic effects*
- Adenyl cyclase toxin (reduces leukocyte activity), dermonecrotic toxin (kills tissues around the bacterium), and hemolysin
- Endotoxin (lipopolysaccharide) in cell wall
- Capsule: antiphagocytic

-Bacterium does not invade; after infection (droplet), it resides in the upper respiratory tract and produces the toxins that provide the virulence

Complications: infants are most at risk for serious disease

- Broken ribs

- Pertussis pneumonia

- Oxygen deprivation to the brain (includes convulsions)

-For sound of the cough, go to http://whoopingcough.net/cough-child-muchwhooping.wav

Treatment: antibiotics do not work well and are usually used only to prevent the transmission of whooping cough to others. Usually use macrolide antibiotics

Vaccine: acellular vaccine preparation, which is good, but probably needs boosters

-no antibiotic for paroxysmal stage (have to wait for cilia to regrow)

-children given antibiotics to prevent spread to siblings, etc.

Streptococcus Pneumoniae

-Facultative, anaerobic, Gram-positive cocci in pairs (diplococci)

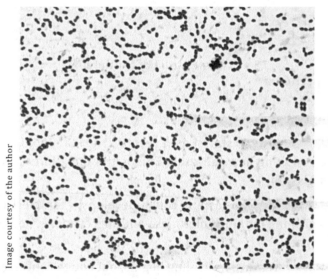

Image courtesy of the author

FIGURE 15.7   *Streptococcus pneumoniae, Gram's stain*

-May be normal flora in the throat

-Alpha-hemolytic colonies on BAP (blood agar plate)

-Colonies often show an indented form due to an autolysin produced—more prominent as the culture ages

-Many virulence factors produced that cause inflammation

-Often encapsulated (polysaccharide capsule) and only pathogenic if encapsulated

-Growth enhanced in 5% CO_2

-Diseases associated with *Streptococcus pneumoniae*:

    Pneumonia

    Otitis media

    Septicemia, bacteremia

    Sinusitis

    Meningitis

    Conjunctivitis

-Increasing problem with resistance to penicillin (not due to production of beta-lactamase)—genetic mutation with the penicillin-binding proteins (PBPs)

-**Vaccine** available—covers many serotypes conjugated vaccine for infants ,2 years and immunosuppressed individuals and polysaccharide vaccine for normal individuals

Haemophilus Influenzae

-Aerobic, Gram-negative bacillus, small, pleomorphic

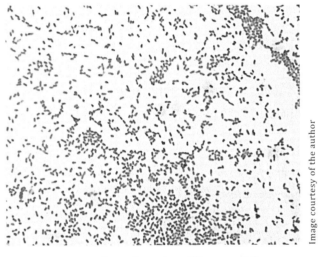

Image courtesy of the author

FIGURE 15.8   *Gram's stain of* Haemophilus influenzae

-Fastidious, needs hemin, NAD, 5% CO_2 for growth

-Often has capsules, typing system based on capsular types (b most important)

-Capsules important virulence factor

-Growing numbers of strains producing beta-lactamase

-Associated diseases:

    Otitis Media

    Meningitis (type b)

    Epiglottis

Pneumonia

Sinusitis

Conjunctivitis

-Vaccine available for the most virulent strain, *H. influenzae* b, very effective in preventing meningitis in children, although there are starting to be some cases of meningitis showing up caused by other serotypes

Moraxella catarrhalis

-Aerobic, Gram-negative diplococci

-Associated with respiratory infections in children

-Part of the normal flora in day care children (>50% of children in day care have *S. pneumoniae*, *H. influenzae,* and *M. catarrhalis* in their nasopharynx)

-Most strains produce beta-lactamase

-Associated diseases:

Pneumonia

Otitis media

Sinusitis

OTITIS MEDIA—MIDDLE EAR INFECTION

-Common complication of URTI

-Infection of the middle ear; most common in children

-Pathogens involved:

Streptococcus pneumoniae
Haemophilus influenzae   } Most common—cause "colds," eye infections, and otitis media; can also spread to lower respiratory tract
Moraxella catarrhalis

Staphylococcus aureus
Streptococcus pyogenes   } Less common
Chlamydia pneumoniae

-Symptoms

- Earache due to buildup of pus inside eardrum

- Complications: deafness

- Further progress of the infection

ACUTE SINUSITIS

-Etiology and pathogenesis similar to otitis media

-Clinical symptoms: facial pain and localized tenderness

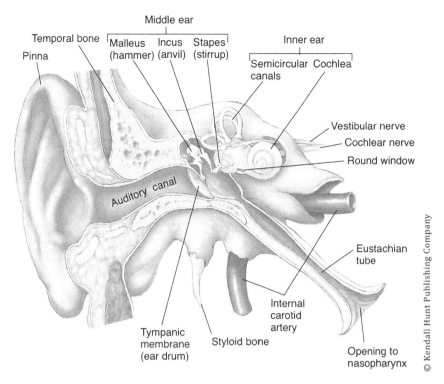

Middle ear

Temporal bone Malleus Incus Stapes Inner ear
Pinna (hammer) (anvil) (stirrup) Semicircular Cochlea
canals

Vestibular nerve
Cochlear nerve
Round window

Auditory canal

Eustachian
tube

Internal
carotid
artery

Tympanic
membrane
(ear drum) Styloid bone Opening to
nasopharynx

© Kendall Hunt Publishing Company

FIGURE 15.9 *Ear anatomy*

-Complication: abscess formation (often caused by anaerobic bacteria)

-Causative organism can be isolated from an aspirate of pus from the sinus

ACUTE EPIGLOTTITIS

-Most often seen in young children, usually due to *H. influenzae* (Gram negative bacilli)

-Typical sign is children lean forward to breathe and drool

-Bacteria spread from nasopharynx to epiglottis, cause severe inflammation, and swell, closing airways

-Life-threatening; call for help to intubate!

Viral Diseases of the Upper Respiratory Tract

COMMON COLD

-More than 200 different viruses can cause a cold, so immunity not usually developed

-50% of colds caused by rhinoviruses (>113 serotypes) ✳grows @ 33°C

-Fifteen percent to 20% of colds caused by corona viruses

-Other viruses, like adenovirus, coxsackie, etc. can also cause "colds"

-spread by direct contact

-Can easily spread to middle ear, lower respiratory tract, and sinuses

- Symptoms: sneezing, wheezing, nasal secretions (coryza), congestion, usually no fever

-No vaccines available; no effective antiviral treatment available yet

-Transmission by hands (direct contact) is most important!

Rhinovirus

-Picornaviridae, RNA, nonenveloped virus

-Survival outside of body for extended periods

-not in lower respiratory tract
-can trigger asthma

-Grow best at 33 °C

-Transmission: direct contact

-Low infective dose (1 virion)

-No antivirals, no vaccine, only symptomatic relief with nose spray, over-the-counter drugs

Corona Virus

-Coronaviridae, RNA, nonenveloped

-SARS CoV causing a frightening epidemic was an animal corona virus (from a civet cat) that had jumped the species barrier. This disease started in China and was imported to Canada; many people died of a severe lower respiratory infection

-No vaccine; no antiviral

-significant pathogen in cattle; can go into middle ear & lower resp.

LATENT

Epstein–Barr virus: (HHV-4)

-Major cause of infectious mononucleosis (IM) (kissing disease)

-DNA virus, enveloped

-Site of latency: B lymphocytes

-Most people have an infection in childhood that is not severe; the older the patient, the more severe the disease is likely to be due to the immune system being more prepared and more mature to take on intruders

-Virus causes systemic effects on cardiovascular and lymphatic systems

-Virus sheds intermittently in saliva throughout life

Symptoms: fever, sore throat, swollen lymph glands, general weakness, extreme fatigue, enlarged spleen

Diagnosis: screening test

-cold symptoms carry on for months and months

-heterophile = weird antibodies that agglutinate other mammals RBC

- "Heterophile" antibodies (antibodies that are not specific for EBV but rather agglutinate RBC from other species of animals) are produced in IM. Test for the presence of these antibodies—MONOSPOT

Virus-specific tests: usually test for antibodies to the specific viral proteins that regulate the replication of the viral particle.

Complications: ampicillin rash can develop if you are monospot positive and are given ampicillin or another beta-lactam. This is not only a rash but a syndrome with high fever, etc.

-B cell lymphomas like "Burkitt's lymphoma," nasopharyngeal carcinoma (Burkitt's is the most common childhood cancer in Africa and has an association with malaria endemic areas)

Treatment: no antiviral, no vaccine; risk of splenic rupture with activity; bed rest and fluids

★should NEVER treat with Ampicillin or Penecillin

Laryngitis and Tracheitis

-Spread of infection from upper respiratory tract down to larynx (voice box) and trachea

Adults: laryngitis: hoarseness

tracheitis: hoarseness and burning, retrosternal pain

Children: croup: swelling of the mucous membrane

- Larynx and trachea constructed of nonexpandable rings of cartilage,

- Narrow passages—obstruction

- Parainfluenza virus (RNA) common cause of croup in children characterized by a seal-like barking cough

Interested? Want to learn more?

For more reading, several texts online at the U of A library are recommended:

1.   Brooks, GF, Carroll KC, Butel JS, Morse SA, editors. Jawetz, Melnick, and Adelberg's Medical Microbiology, 24th ed. Blacklick OH-McGraw Hill; 2007.

2.   Ryan KJ, Ray CG, editors. Sherris Medical Microbiology, 5th ed. New York – McGraw-Hill, 2010.

3.   Mandell GL, Bennett JE,Dolin R, editors. Mandell, Douglas and Bennett's Principles and Practices of Infectious Diseases, 7th ed. Churchill Livingstone Elsevier, Philadelphia, 2010.

Chapter 16

Lower Respiratory Tract Infection (LRTI)

Learning Objectives:

1. Discuss *Mycobacterium tuberculosis* pathogenicity, latent infection, and active disease.
2. Describe pneumonia caused by *S. pneumoniae* and its pathogenicity.
3. Identify and discuss characteristics of some viral causes of LRTI: RSV, Parainfluenza, and Influenza A.
4. Define antigenic shift and antigenic drift in Influenza A.

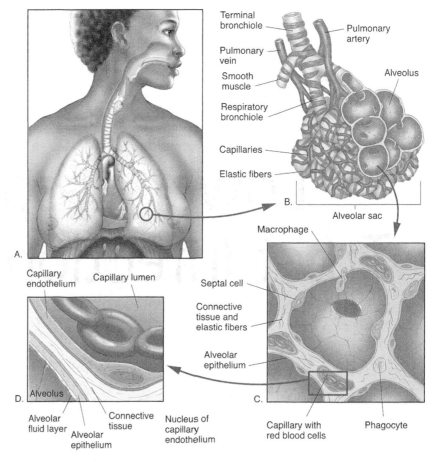

FIGURE 16.1   *Anatomy of the respiratory tract*

Defenses Against Infection in the Lower Respiratory Tract

*lower infections tend to be more severe

1. Particles trapped in larynx, trachea, and larger bronchial tubes are moved upward by action of cilia (so-called "ciliary elevator").

2. Microorganisms reaching lung are usually ingested by macrophages.

3. IgA antibodies in secretions attach to bacteria and trap them in mucus

Infections are usually more serious in the lower respiratory tract than upper respiratory tract infection and disseminate to the bloodstream relatively easily.

-Choice of antimicrobial therapy is important based on the causative organism and may be life-saving.

-Infections are divided into:

    acute: acute bronchitis ; acute exacerbations of chronic bronchitis

        bronchiolitis

        pneumonia

chronic: tuberculosis, aspergillosis, lung abscesses, empyema, infections associated with cystic fibrosis, parasites

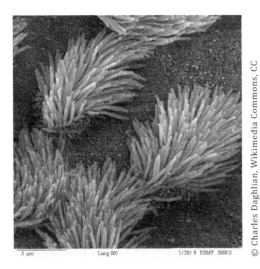

FIGURE 16.2   Ciliated tracheal epithelium

- CROUP:
- common in children
- swelling of mucous membrane
- parainfluenza virus common cause

Acute Bronchitis

-Inflammatory condition of the tracheobronchial tree

-Usually associated with infection (bacteria and virus)

-Usually prominent cough

Bronchiolitis

-Disease restricted to children <2 years

-Bronchioles of children are very small in diameter; if cells lining them are inflamed and swollen, the passage of air to alveoli is restricted

-Infection results in necrosis of epithelial cells, leading to peribronchial infiltration, which may spread to lung and give interstitial pneumonia

-Seventy-five percent caused by respiratory syncytial virus (RSV)

Cystic Fibrosis

-Genetic disease with pancreatic insufficiency, abnormal sweat chloride, and production of viscous bronchial secretions

-Secretions cause stasis in lungs, predisposes to infection

-Common causes of infection in CF:

    S. aureus

    P. aeruginosa

    H. influenzae

Lung Abscess

-Endogenous process caused by a mixture of aerobes and anaerobes leads to necrotizing pneumonia (*Bacteroides* and *Fusobacterium* prominent)

-Most common cause is aspiration of gastric juices as a result of altered consciousness

Pleural Effusion and Empyema

-Pleural effusion (fluid) found in 50% of pneumonia cases

-If organisms spread to pleural space, a purulent exudate or "empyema" results

-Most often caused by *S. aureus*, Gram-negative bacilli, and anaerobes

Mycobacterium tuberculosis (tuberculosis)

-Slender, acid-fast bacilli (stained with Ziehl-Neelsen) grow slowly and in clumps (Note that *M. tuberculosis* is genetically a Gram positive, but the Gram's stain will not penetrate the thick, waxy cell wall)

-Very resistant to drying and chemicals due to thick lipid layer in cell wall

-Contain sterols in cell wall in addition to peptidoglycan

-Capable of intracellular growth in macrophages for evading host defense

-Produce enzymes and other substances that induce inflammation and help *M. tuberculosis* survive in the lysosome

-Transmission: airborne

-Ten percent of world's population is infected (not all develop illness)

-TB is responsible for 5%–6% of all deaths worldwide

Three things possible after *M. tuberculosis* exposure (infection):

1. Latent infection where few TB organisms enter macrophages and remain latent there. No activation of macrophages
2. Primary tubercle forms, but the immune system can stop replication
3. Miliary infection: spread of active infection—this happens especially in immunocompromised individuals

[handwritten margin note: -Primary Tubercle: ⌐>often in lungs, and host walls off the infection in a "tubercle"*]*

Clinical TB Disease

-CMI usually controls infection but is also responsible for the pathology

-Primary Infection is often in the lungs. The host walls off the infection in a "tubercle," which consists of mostly macrophages in a granuloma

- If infection is arrested at this point by the host defenses, the tubercle becomes calcified ("Ghon complex") and is visible on X ray

- If the host defenses cannot contain the bacilli, disseminated infection results

- Miliary infection: may be directly disseminated from a primary infection or may be a reactivation of a latent infection

- Characterized by spread of tubercles in tissues
- Earlier called "consumption"
- Symptoms: weight loss, fever, night sweats, chronic cough, hemoptysis, lethargy *(active TB infection)*

TABLE 16.1 *Comparison of a TB Infection and a TB Disease*

TB Infection (Latent)	TB Disease (Active)(in Lungs)
MTB present	MTB present
Tuberculin skin test positive	Tuberculin skin test positive
Chest X ray normal	Chest X ray usually reveals lesion
Sputum smears and cultures negative	Sputum smears and cultures positive
No symptoms	Symptoms: cough, fever, weight loss
Not infectious	Infectious before treatment
Not defined as a case of TB	**Defined as a case of TB**

Risk factors for clinical tuberculosis

- Presence of another infection (e.g., HIV)
- Physiological and environmental stress (e.g., malnutrition)
- Depressions of the immune system (e.g., elderly patients)

Laboratory Diagnosis

-Finding of acid-fast rods in sputum, urine, tissue

-Culture: six weeks for a negative culture, usually two to three weeks for a positive culture

-PCR used for diagnosis; must do susceptibility testing to determine drug regimen

Immunity

-Assessed by use of tuberculin test (PPD or Mantoux) (skin test). A positive PPD only indicates exposure to a *Mycobacterial* species

-BCG vaccine: Bacillus Calmette-Guérin, strain of *M. bovis*—this is a very poor vaccine in adults, but it can be used with some success in children who live in high-risk situations

Interferon Gold Test: new test said to be able to differentiate between a latent and an active TB infection. Blood is taken from the individual, and the T lymphocytes are isolated from the other blood cells. They are then stimulated with PPD, and the interferon gamma cytokine secreted from sensitized lymphocytes measured

Treatment

-Growing problem with multidrug resistance

-Mixture of drugs used to treat in attempt to reduce development of resistance

*Type IV hypersensitivity

- quantiferon Gold test to check for activated T-1 lymphocytes

-not very effective

-Multiple drug regimens used to prevent the development of drug resistance

-Isoniazid, rifampicin, pyrazinamide, ethambutol, streptomycin

-**MDR-TB** and **XDR-TB** are part of a growing problem

MDR-TB defined as resistant to isoniazid and rifampicin (first-line drugs)

XDR-TB resistant to first- and second-line drugs

-Prolonged treatment (as long as a year)

-Patient not infectious while on drugs, provided the organism is susceptible to them *(about ~2-3 weeks)*

Pneumonia ("The Old Man's Friend")

Typical pneumonia: classically caused by *S. pneumoniae*; responds to penicillin treatment

Atypical pneumonia: caused by other organisms; penicillin-resistant

-Microorganisms gain entrance to lungs by inhalation; only particles 5 microns in diameter and smaller will be able to reach the alveoli

-Lungs can be seeded by a systemic infection in the blood

-Pneumonia is the most common cause of infection-related death

-Causes of pneumonia in adults and children differ:

Adults: mainly bacterial

Children: mainly viral

Streptococcus pneumoniae* Pneumonia or *"Pneumococcal Pneumonia"

-Caused by *Streptococcus pneumoniae*, facultative, anaerobic, Gram-positive diplococci with polysaccharide capsules

-Most common cause of community-acquired pneumonia, involves alveoli and bronchi

-Can affect even previously healthy individuals, sometimes associated with URTI

-About 50% with pneumonia get dissemination to the bloodstream

Symptoms

-Fever, blood-tinged sputum, breathing difficulties, chest pain

-Often disseminates to the bloodstream and causes bacteremia, septicemia

-BACTEREMIA = SPREAD TO BLOOD

Treatment

-Penicillin, macrolides, resistance-emerging

Vaccines

-Vaccines: polysaccharide and conjugate vaccines available

Pneumonia Caused by *Haemophilus Influenzae*

-Aerobic, Gram-negative coccobacillus

-Typically strikes patients with immune defects, diabetes, alcoholism, poor nutrition, cancer, splenectomy

-Symptoms same as pneumococcal pneumonia

Treatment

-Second-generation cephalosporins because some strains of *H. influenzae* produce beta-lactamase

Pneumonia Caused by *Moraxella catarrhalis*

-Aerobic, Gram-negative diplococci

-Patients with immune defects like cancer at higher risk

-Not common

ATYPICAL PNEUMONIA

-Includes pneumonia caused by *Mycoplasma pneumoniae*, Chlamydia *psittaci, Chlamydia pneumoniae, Legionella pneumophila, Coxiella burnetii*

-Typically slower onset and tendency to chronicity

-Often occur in outbreaks, epidemics, or as zoonoses

Pneumonia Caused by *Mycoplasma pneumoniae*

-Very small organisms, cannot stain with Gram's stain (because no cell wall) (genetically belong to Gram positives)

-Causes "walking pneumonia," pneumonia that looks terrible on an X ray, but the person is still walking and behaving relatively normal

-Can be responsible for 15%–40% of pneumonia, depending on the year and situation

-Often affects school-aged children and teenagers

-P1 protein on organism responsible for adhesion

-Can cause neurological complications

Symptoms

-Low-grade fever, cough, headache

-May have erythema skin manifestations

Diagnosis

-Serology, PCR (culture very poor)

Treatment

-Tetracyclines, macrolides, no vaccine available

- RSV:
  - RNA, enveloped
  - causes tissue damage by syncytia formation
  - risk factor: prematurity
  - passive immune response

Pneumonia Caused by *Chlamydia psittaci*

-Very small infectious particle (elementary body) 0.3 μ (probably Gram negative but cannot be seen in a normal Gram's stain)

-Obligate intracellular parasite

-Zoonosis: birds most common reservoir, especially parrots

-Varying severity, from life-threatening pneumonia to a mild pneumonia, depending on the strain

Symptoms

-Fever, headache, chills, mucus production

-Subclinical infections common

Diagnosis

-Serology, PCR (culture difficult, also need a Class 3 lab (high risk))

Treatment

-Tetracycline, macrolide

-No vaccine available

Pneumonia Caused by *Chlamydia (Chlamydophila) pneumoniae*

-Infectious particle = elementary body (see *C. psittaci*)

-Obligate intracellular organism, can grow in macrophages, smooth muscle cells, endothelial cells, lymphocytes

-Transmitted by droplets, often epidemics transmitted person-to-person

-Majority of people have at least one infection with this organism in a lifetime; however, pneumonia does not develop in most

-When it causes pneumonia, this is usually a mild disease

-Symptoms resemble *Mycoplasma pneumoniae,* with the addition of fatigue

-Subclinical pneumonia and chronic pharyngitis common

-Complications can be serious

Laboratory diagnosis

-Serology, PCR (culture poor and not done by many labs)

Treatment

-Tetracyclines, macrolides

Pneumonia Caused by *Legionella pneumophila*

-Gram-negative bacillus, cause of "Legionnaires' disease," "Pontiac fever"

-Can grow in macrophages

-Suspected airborne transmission; occurs in outbreaks

-Commonly found in water (reservoirs, plumbing of buildings, air-conditioning units)

-Relatively resistant to chlorine and temperatures <55 °C

Symptoms

-High fever, cough, signs of pneumonia

Laboratory diagnosis

-Culture, PCR, serology, urine antigen detection

Treatment

-Macrolides

-No vaccine

Pneumonia Caused by *Coxiella burnetii*

-Gram-negative, small coccobacillus, obligate intracellular

-Zoonosis

-Often transmitted by ticks in animals, and human infection is contracted by ingesting contaminated dairy products or inhalation (goats, sheep)

Symptoms

-Fever (1–2 weeks), chills, chest pain, headache

Laboratory diagnosis

-Serology, PCR

Treatment

-Tetracyclines

-No vaccine

Other Bacterial Causes of Pneumonia

Usually as secondary infections or in immunocompromised (e.g., elderly in nursing homes and auxiliary hospitals)

Gram-positive:	*S. aureus*
	S. pyogenes
Gram-negative:	*Pseudomonas* sp.
	Klebsiella pneumoniae

Viral Causes of Lower Respiratory Tract Infections

RSV (Respiratory Syncytial Virus)

-RNA virus, Paramyxoviridae, enveloped

-Causes damage to lungs because of syncytia formation and the resulting inflammation

-Transmitted primarily by direct contact

-Significant pathogen in infants and children <5 years; infants <1 year are most at risk for life-threatening pneumonia, but it can occur in elderly patients

-Occurs in outbreaks and epidemics, late winter and early spring every year

-Major risk factor for acquiring RSV is prematurity

Symptoms

-Coughing, wheezing, difficulty breathing

Laboratory diagnosis

-Direct FA test, culture, PCR

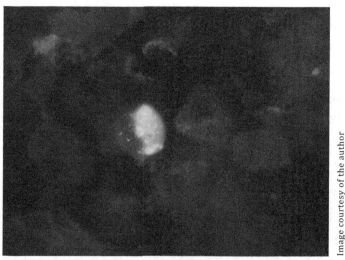

Image courtesy of the author

FIGURE 16.3   DFA (direct fluorescent antibody) test for RSV

Treatment

-None effective; ribavirin sometime given as a last resort, but no evidence exists for use. No vaccine but monoclonal Synagis can be given monthly to prevent high-risk babies from getting RSV

Influenza A Virus

-RNA, Orthomyxoviridae, enveloped, segmented genome

-Typing done by characterizing the H (hemagglutinin) and N (neuraminidase) glycoproteins that project from the surface of the envelope

-Three subtypes of Influenza virus, A, B, and C:

  Influenza A: eight segments of RNA; antigenic drift and shift; has subtypes 16 H, 9 N

  Influenza B: eight segments of RNA, no antigenic shift; no subtypes

  Influenza C: seven segments of RNA, no antigenic shift; no subtypes

-Influenza A can occur in epidemics and pandemics

-Strains of Influenza A are named for type, location of isolation, serial number, year, and subtype of H and N (e.g., A/Johannesburg/33/94/[H3N2])

·A has subtypes, B &c do NOT

Influenza A

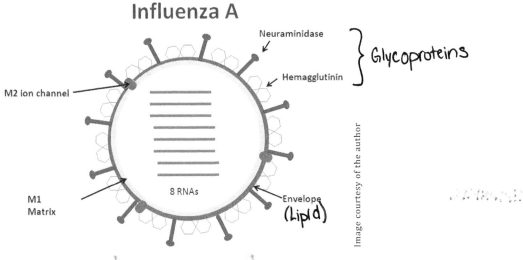

Image courtesy of the author

FIGURE 16.4   *Influenza virus diagram*

-Small infectious dose, incubation one to three days

-Virus is viable on hard surfaces for 24 to 48 hours

-Transmission is mainly droplet, but there is now a question about possible airborne transmission

Symptoms

-Chills, fever, malaise, headache, cough, sore throat, and muscle aches

-Symptoms more severe in smokers due to lack of well-functioning ciliated respiratory cells

Diagnosis

-First few cases in a community diagnosed with help of laboratory tests (serology, culture, PCR, direct FA)

-Clinical diagnosis after it is established that the epidemic has started

Treatment

-**Amantadine**: sometimes used for prophylaxis, but there is growing resistance to this drug, and the side effects are disturbing. It blocks the M2 ion channel in the viral particle and prevents the virus from uncoating and releasing its RNA in the host cell

-**Neuraminidase inhibitors** (oseltamivir and zanamivir): much better and more effective with less side effects. Inhibit the release of viral particles from the host cell

Vaccine

-New vaccine strains needed for yearly vaccine; vaccine good if it matches the H and N type of the circulating strain.

-Virus is produced in eggs for mass production—egg allergies are a contraindication for vaccination unless there is a cell culture produced vaccine available at the clinic

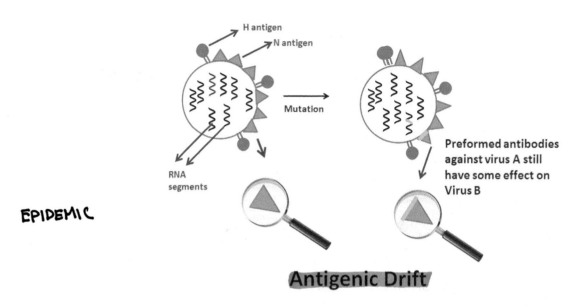

EPIDEMIC

FIGURE 16.5   *Antigenic drift*

Small changes (mutations) in the glycoproteins, making the virus a bit different but still recognizable by the immune system (cross-immunity)

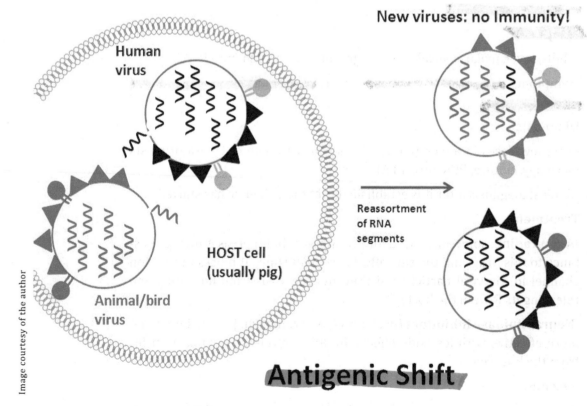

PANDEMIC

Image courtesy of the author

FIGURE 16.6   *Antigenic shift*

Major change in antigenicity, change of one whole segment of RNA, new strain created, risk for pandemics because no one has immunity to this new strain

-Rare occurrence because two different viruses must infect the same cell

Pandemic: disease occurs in more than one continent at the same time

-Three to four pandemics every 100 years

caused by "antigenic shift"

-Significant mortality rates (often due to secondary infections and comorbid conditions, not primarily to the Influenza disease itself)

-Global spread of disease in six to nine months

-Pandemic does not mean severe disease —it describes the spread of the disease

Epidemic: spread of disease in a specified area

-Due to antigenic drift

caused by "antigenic drift"

-Annual occurrence in temperate zones during the winter

-30,000 deaths/yr in the United States attributed to every epidemic

-Nosocomial infection is common, especially in institutions (e.g., nursing homes)

Pneumonia Due to CMV (Cytomegalovirus or Human Herpesvirus 5)

-DNA virus, Herpesviridae, enveloped

-Can cause serious pneumonia

-Results in nuclear inclusions and large swollen cells (cytomegaly)

-Chronic infection, lifelong latency after an infection in macrophages and T lymphocytes

-Virus is shed at intervals in blood, urine, saliva, semen, cervical secretions, and breast milk

-About 50% of population has antibodies and so have been infected at some time in their lives

-Transmitted by direct contact (kissing, etc.), sexual contact, blood, transplanted tissue

-Cause of ~10% of infectious mononucleosis in healthy individuals (but no heterophile antibodies produced, so the monospot will be negative)

-Complications: pregnancy, cytomegalic inclusion disease in neonates if mother has the primary infection while pregnant, transplant patients, immunosuppressed individuals (e.g., HIV)

Fungal Diseases of the Lower Respiratory Tract

Histoplasmosis

-Caused by *Histoplasma capsulatum*, dimorphic fungus (yeast-like morphology in tissues, filamentous mycelium on agar plates)

-Infection by inhalation of spores from the mycelial form often in bat and bird droppings

Symptoms: similar to tuberculosis (primary lesion in lung) and can also disseminate through the blood and lymph, resulting in lesions in many parts of the body

-Initial symptoms mild and subclinical, few cases are severe (i.e., in immunocompromised)

Treatment

-Amphotericin B or itraconazole

Coccidioidomycosis

-Caused by *Coccidioides immitis*, dimorphic fungus

-Spores in soil in South America and southern United States—frequent occurrence in San Joaquin Valley in California—also called "San Joaquin fever" or "valley fever"

-Forms thick-walled spherules in body, filled with spores

-Most infections subclinical, transmission aerosols (dust storm)

Symptoms

-Chest pain, fever, coughing, weight loss, tuberculosis-type disease can develop in about 1%

Laboratory diagnosis

-Isolation of organism from tissue or fluids

Treatment

-Amphotericin B, ketoconazole, itraconazole

***Pneumocystis jiroveci* Pneumonia**

-Caused by *Pneumocystis jiroveci (earlier called carinii)*, opportunist, normal flora in many people

-Disease of immunosuppressed (e.g., HIV patients), high mortality due to this pneumonia

-Very common in immunosuppressed individuals—incidence increasing as the number of this type of patient increases

-Organism found in alveoli in lungs; very difficult to treat in immunocompromised

Symptoms

-Difficulty breathing, coughing

-Often no sputum

Laboratory diagnosis

-Demonstration of the organism in tissue and fluids (e.g., bronchoalveolar lavage (BAL))

Treatment

-Trimethoprim-sulfamethoxazole (best), pentamidine isethionate

Aspergillosis

-Genus contains many species of *Aspergillus* that are ubiquitous in nature

-Some species (e.g., *Aspergillus fumigatus*) can cause a wide variety of conditions including bronchopulmonary aspergillosis, which results from an allergic reaction to the antigen in the lungs

-In patients with preexisting lung cavities or chronic lung disorders, Aspergillus can cause infection—fungal ball forms in lung (Aspergilloma)

-In immunosuppressed patients, disseminated infection is common

-Very difficult to treat, sometimes impossible in immunocompromised

PARASITIC INFECTIONS OF THE LOWER RESPIRATORY TRACT

-Many helminths involve the lung at some stage of their development and may cause a transient pneumonia

   ***examples**: Hookworm

   Ascaris

   Microfilaria: Wuchereria or Brugia

Echinococcus granulosus

-Dog tapeworm; cannot grow to a mature tapeworm in the human

-Localizes in the lung in a large percent of cases and forms a hydatid cyst

-Hydatid cyst contains scolexes (heads) and hooks for new tapeworms; these cysts can grow in size and cause respiratory distress

-Common in northern and rural communities even in Alberta

-Worldwide distribution

-Worms differ in localization of cysts dependent on geographical area—in Alberta they form predominantly lung cysts, but in other countries liver cysts are more common

Paragonimus westermani

-"Oriental lung fluke"

-Even adult parasites live in lung

-Infection by ingesting crustacea with infective metacercariae, which migrate from intestine to lungs

-Adults develop in fibrous cysts that connect with bronchi (where eggs are released)

-Infections cause chest pain, breathing difficulty, and bronchopneumonia if there are large numbers of parasites

Amoebic Causes of Lower Respiratory Infection

-*Entamoeba histolytica*

-Abscess formation, usually associated with liver cysts and disseminated infection

-Can disseminate further to brain

Interested? Want to learn more?

For more reading, several texts online at the U of A library are recommended:

1.   Brooks, GF, Carroll KC, Butel JS, Morse SA, editors. Jawetz, Melnick, and Adelberg's Medical Microbiology, 24th ed. Blacklick OH-McGraw Hill; 2007.

2.   Ryan KJ, Ray CG, editors. Sherris Medical Microbiology, 5th ed. New York – McGraw-Hill, 2010.

3.   Mandell GL, Bennett JE,Dolin R, editors. Mandell, Douglas and Bennett's Principles and Practices of Infectious Diseases, 7th ed. Churchill Livingstone Elsevier, Philadelphia, 2010.

Chapter 17

Upper Alimentary Tract Infections

Learning Objectives:

1. Identify the major defenses to infection in the mouth.
2. Describe the major bacterial species in the mouth contributing to dental caries and periodontal disease and the pathogenesis (e.g., biofilm formation).
3. Describe the pathogenesis of *Actinomyces* species causing "lumpy jaw."
4. Describe the clinical syndrome caused by the mumps virus.
5. Discuss the pathogenicity of *Helicobacter pylori* as a cause of peptic and duodenal ulcers.

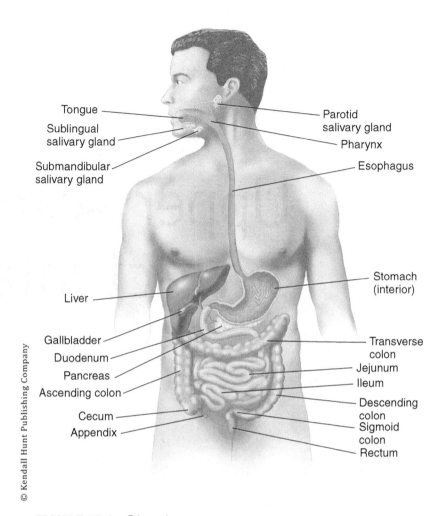

© Kendall Hunt Publishing Company

FIGURE 17.1   *Digestive organs*

Upper alimentary tract: includes mouth, esophagus, stomach

Normal flora of the mouth

-when sick= less saliva

-Age- and dentition-dependent

(if have teeth)

-Rich and varied normal flora in mouth, aerobes and anaerobes

-More organisms per ml than in the large intestine!

***Streptococcus* species are dominant** (mostly alpha-streptococci)

Other species commonly found:

-accumulation of microorganisms
on teeth =dental plaque
(biofilm)

Micrococcus species

Neisseria species

Candida species (yeast)

Anaerobic bacteria including *Fusobacterium, Peptostreptococcus,*

   Actinomyces, Bacteroides

Entamoeba gingivalis

Trichomonas tenax

INFECTIONS OF THE ORAL CAVITY

-Mouth is continuous with the pharynx, but different set of microorganisms due to presence of teeth

-Most of the organisms make specific attachments to the teeth or the mucosal surfaces

-More than 1 L saliva produced per day (flushes mouth, contains secretory IgA, lysozyme, lactoperoxidase, WBC)

-If salivary flow decreased (e.g., dehydration or between meals), there is a fourfold increase in the microbial population in a short time

-Dehydrated patients: mouth is overgrown with organisms; results in BAD BREATH

Bad breath: caused by the waste products of the metabolism of anaerobic oral bacteria

-Anterior (front) of the tongue often gets the flora rubbed off, unlike the posterior section. If you scrape the back of your tongue and smell this, you'll know what your breath smells like to others

Candida Albicans YEAST

-Opportunistic dimorphic fungus

→and in babies

-Common cause of mouth and throat infection in immunosuppressed (e.g., those taking inhalation steroids, chemotherapy, broad spectrum antibiotics, and immune defects or disease—this includes the very young and the very old)

-produces pseudohyphae

-Thrush in mouth (pseudohyphae grow down into the tongue) may spread to the esophagus, which causes swallowing to be painful

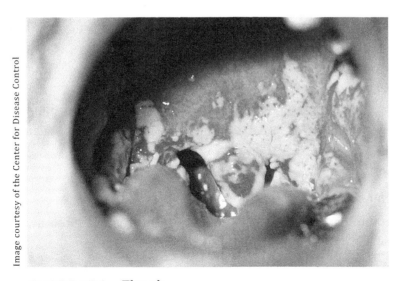

Image courtesy of the Center for Disease Control

FIGURE 17.2   *Thrush*

Dental Caries

-Can lead to tooth decay

-Teeth are unlike any other exterior surface of the body and do not shed surface cells

-Accumulations of microorganisms and their by-products form "plaque" (biofilm)

-Carbohydrates converted to lactic acid within the biofilm, which decreases pH and corrodes the tooth enamel

-More than 300 species of bacteria in mouth—most important cariogenic bacterium is *Streptococcus mutans*

-Bacteria do not attach to clean tooth surfaces

-Within minutes after brushing, a thin layer of protein from the saliva coats the outside of the tooth (pellicle)—bacteria can attach to the pellicle and produce dextran

　　bacteria + dextran (polysaccharide) = PLAQUE (BIOFILM)

-Plaque can be several hundred cells thick and is not permeable to saliva

-Even plaque as thin as 0.1 to 0.2 mm can become depleted of oxygen, which encourages anaerobes and streptococci to grow

-As more plaque accumulates, the worse the breath will be

Mechanism of tooth decay: local acid production dissolves enamel

-Low fluoride levels in enamel make it more susceptible to attack

-If caries develop, bacteria may reach the dentin

-Bacteria that cause "tooth decay" differ from those causing caries

-Bacteria causing tooth decay are usually Gram-positive rods and filamentous bacteria such as *Actinobacillus actinomycetemcomitans*

-When bacteria penetrate pulp, contact is made with nerves and blood vessels (abscess formation)

-If abscess is not treated, soft tissues in jaw and face area can become infected primarily due to anaerobic bacteria

Local "immune" defenses against caries: saliva and crevicular fluid in gingival crevice. Leukocytes and complement are important components

Prevention of dental caries

-Hygienic strategies

　　*examples: tooth brushing, flossing, plaque removal, mouthwash with chlorhexidine, fluoride treatment

Periodontal Disease

- Inflammation and degeneration of supporting structures

- May occur in the absence of caries, but plaque is a major factor

-Cementum covering the roots of teeth attacked by caries as gums recede with age

Gingivitis

-Infection restricted to gums

-Bleeding of gums on brushing

-Bacteria involved are:

  Streptococci sp.

  Actinomycetes sp.

  Anaerobic Gram negatives

Periodontitis

-Progression of gingivitis

-Chronic disease; responsible for 10% of tooth loss in adults

-Symptoms: inflamed gums, bleed easily, may have some pus pockets

-Increased probing depth, deep pockets

-Eventually results in deterioration of bone and supportive tissue, tooth loss

-Many species implicated (e.g., *Porphyromonas* sp., *Actinobacillus* sp.)

Abscess Formation

-Usually polymicrobial, often predominantly anaerobic (e.g., *Bacteroides, Fusobacterium, Peptostreptococcus,* etc.)

-Usually arise with pulpal necrosis

-Abscess contains pus and necrotic tissue—this breaks down bone

-Localized, well-defined swelling and pain

-Can in worst case scenario progress to cellulitis

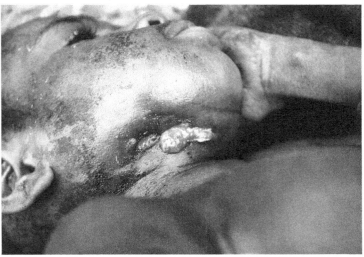

Image courtesy of the Center for Disease Control

FIGURE 17.3   Untreated dental abscess from lower molars

Actinomycosis ("Lumpy Jaw")

-*Actinomyces israelii* is a Gram-positive, filamentous anaerobic rod

-Can be normal flora in the oral cavity

-Causes painful abscesses

-Also causes abscesses in the brain and lung and pelvis

-Abscess formation, healing, and scarring leads to deformation of bone and tissue—hence, "lumpy jaw"

-Tendency to become a chronic infection

-Dental procedures (= wounds) can trigger the infection

Vincent's Disease or Vincent's Angina ("Trench Mouth")

-Also called acute necrotizing ulcerative gingivitis (ANUG)

-Caused by anaerobic bacteria

WORKING TOGETHER {
Anaerobic Gram-negative bacilli: *Prevotella intermedius*
Anaerobic Gram-negative spirochetes: *Borrelia vincentii*

-Severe ulcerative disease with pain; extremely foul breath

*Treated with antibiotics active against anaerobes, plus surgical debridement of necrotic and infected tissue

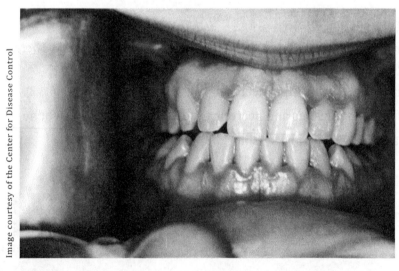

Image courtesy of the Center for Disease Control

FIGURE 17.4   Vincent's angina (with unhealthy gums)

VIRAL CAUSES OF UPPER ALIMENTARY TRACT INFECTIONS

Mumps Infection of the Parotid Gland

-Parotid glands are one of three salivary glands

-Mumps virus is a RNA virus, enveloped, transmitted in saliva

-Most infectious 48 hours before symptoms appear

-Viruses multiply in lymph glands in throat, then invade the parotid glands via the bloodstream as a result of the ensuing viremia

Symptoms

-Inflammation and swelling of the parotid glands, fever, pain on swallowing (either one- or two-sided)

Complications

-Orchitis (inflammation of the testis); oophoritis (inflammation of the ovaries) leading possibly to sterility; pancreatitis

-Encephalitis

- Secretes saliva

- has vaccination, may need booster

- droplet transmission

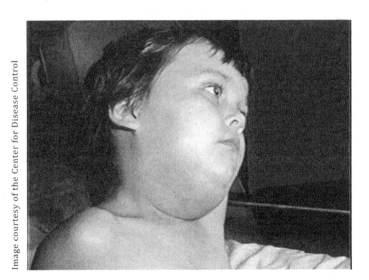

Image courtesy of the Center for Disease Control

FIGURE 17.5   *Mumps*

Diagnosis

-Laboratory confirmation not necessary; clinical diagnosis is adequate

Treatment

-Supportive, no antivirals

Vaccine

-Attenuated, included in the MMR

INFECTIONS OF THE STOMACH

-Stomach is normally protected from infection by high acidity pH <2

Helicobacter pylori

-Cause of peptic ulcer disease (gastric and duodenal ulcers)

-Known for >100 years by pathologists but first cultured in 1982

-Spiral-shaped, microaerophilic, Gram-negative bacterium, motile by polar flagella

-From 30%–50% of world population has antibodies

-Associated with contaminated drinking water and wells but transmission not proven

-Specialized bacterium can survive in acid conditions of stomach

-Main virulence factor: urease enzyme

Pathogenesis

-Stomach mucosa contains cells that secrete gastric juice containing proteolytic enzymes and hydrochloric acid—stomach lined with a thick layer of mucus protecting the stomach lining from acidity

-Bacteria live and move in the thick mucus layer—polar flagella are effective

-*H. pylori* has tissue tropism for the gastric epithelial cells, but more than 90% are in the mucus

-Attachment of the bacterium induces increased gastrin production, which causes increased stomach acidity

-*H. pylori* produces urease and breaks urea from food down to ammonia and carbon dioxide. This increases the pH locally around the bacterium, protecting it from acid

-Ammonia does cause some damage to the lining of the stomach; this attracts neutrophils, and an inflammatory response is induced

-Strains containing the gene "CagA" (or cytotoxin-associated gene) are more virulent and are thought to be able to induce stomach cancer—*H. pylori* is classified by the WHO as a class 1 carcinogen

Treatment

-Combination of antibiotics (to prevent resistance) and anti-HCl agents

Handwritten margin notes:
- has flagella which are very strong that allow it to move in thick mucus

- H. pylori produces large amounts of urease, urea is broken down to ammonia → ammonia causes stomach wall irritation = stomach ulcers formed

Diagnosis

-Serology: if you have antibodies, then you have the bacterium

-Biopsy: often taken during gastroscopy; PCR, culture, urea test

Noninvasive diagnosis: breath test (C^{14} labeled urea ingestion)

- Subject drinks ^{14}C labeled urea; exhaled breath is measured for content of ^{14}C, which would have been split from the urea molecule if urease is present

No vaccine

Interested? Want to learn more?

For more reading, several texts online at the U of A library are recommended:

1. Brooks, GF, Carroll KC, Butel JS, Morse SA, editors. Jawetz, Melnick, and Adelberg's Medical Microbiology, 24th ed. Blacklick OH-McGraw Hill; 2007.

2. Ryan KJ, Ray CG, editors. Sherris Medical Microbiology, 5th ed. New York – McGraw-Hill, 2010.

3. Mandell GL, Bennett JE,Dolin R, editors. Mandell, Douglas and Bennett's Principles and Practices of Infectious Diseases, 7th ed. Churchill Livingstone Elsevier, Philadelphia, 2010.

Chapter 18

Lower Alimentary Tract Infections

1. Differentiate between intoxications and infections with emphasis on individual organisms.

2. Define dysentery and gastroenteritis.

3. Describe the major causes of intoxications and gastroenteritis.

4. Identify some clinical features of viral intestinal infections with norovirus, rotavirus, hepatitis A, and hepatitis E.

Predominant flora of Intestine:

- Gram negatives

- Infection - pathogen multiplies in mucosa or passes through to other systemic organs

- Intoxication - ingestion of preformed toxin

   ⤷ result of both = diarrhea

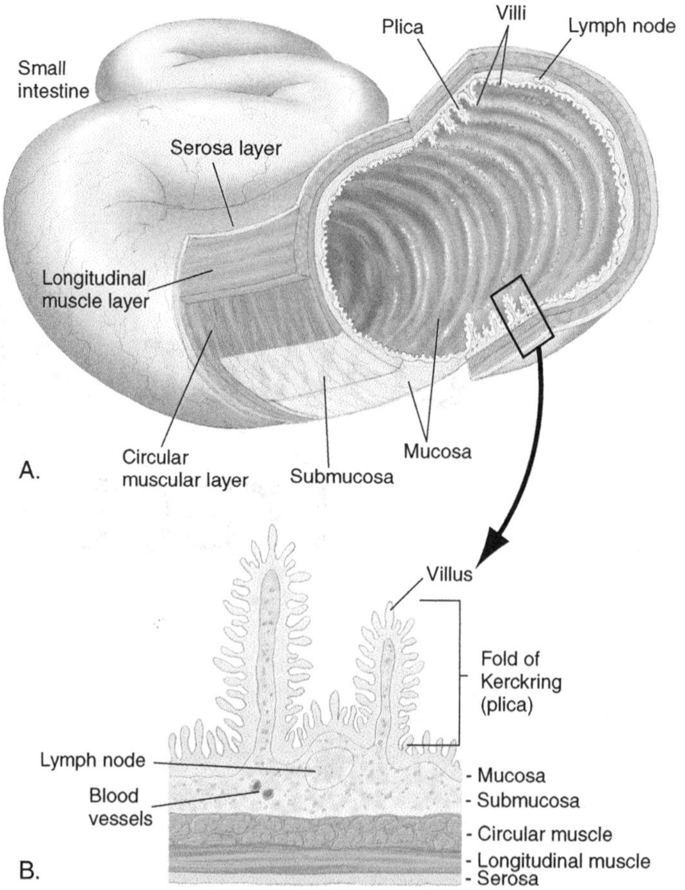

FIGURE 18.1   Small intestine

© Kendall Hunt Publishing Company

TABLE 18.1   Two Types of Gastrointestinal Tract Diseases

Infection	Intoxication
Pathogen multiplies in the body and causes inflammation or produces an exotoxin	Ingestion of a preformed toxin
Fever, usually release of endotoxin	No fever, sudden onset
End result: diarrhea	End result: diarrhea ± vomiting

Note that diarrhea is the major cause of infant mortality worldwide (dehydration)

MAIN PATHOGENIC MECHANISMS OF LOWER ALIMENTARY TRACT (LAT) PATHOGENS

1. Attachment to host cell
2. Cell invasion (some invade lymphatic tissue in intestine)
3. Loss of microvilli (aid in absorption)

4. Release of endotoxin, induction of inflammation

5. Exotoxin production: two basic types

    a. Those that increase the secretion of water and electrolytes from intestine (e.g., *Vibrio cholerae*)

    b. Those that inhibit protein synthesis and cause cell death (e.g., *Clostridium difficile* cytotoxin)

-Remember that many GI pathogens are Gram negative, so they both have endotoxins in their cell walls and produce exotoxins

TABLE 18.2 *Comparison of Dysentery and Gastroenteritis*

Dysentery	Gastroenteritis
Severe diarrhea with blood, pus, and mucus	Diarrhea with no pus, mucus, or blood
± vomiting	± vomiting
Abdominal cramps	Abdominal cramps
Nausea	Nausea
Risk for dehydration	Risk for dehydration
Examples: *Entamoeba histolytica, Shigella dysenteriae*	Examples: *Vibrio cholerae, Cryptosporidium* sp.

✳ ✳ -Dysentry = neutrophils (pus)

- Gastroenteritis = inflammation of the stomach

TABLE 18.3 Intoxications

Cause	Common?	Time to Blast Off	Main Clinical Symptoms	Characteristic Foods
Staphylococcus aureus	Very common	2–4 hr	Vomiting	Meats, salads, custards
*Bacillus cereus**	Uncommon	3–6 hr	Vomiting and diarrhea	Rice, meat, vegetables
*Clostridium perfringens**	Very common	8–22 hr	Vomiting and diarrhea	Meat stews, vegetables
Clostridium botulinum	Uncommon	5–16 hr	Neuromuscular paralysis	Improperly canned goods

✳ most common

- produces spore

*Note that *Bacillus cereus* can cause intoxication or an infection, as can *Clostridium perfringens,* although infections are rare.

Staphylococcus aureus

-Produce exotoxins called enterotoxins; these are heat stable (tolerate boiling for 30 min) and resistant to enzymatic destruction in the gut

Staphylococci grow quickly and easily in food:

    - Salt tolerant, osmotically stable due to the thick cell wall

    - Fairly high resistance to heat (60 °C) for 30 min

    - Temperatures in food "kept warm" are conducive to growth

(typically exotoxins are destroyed by heat)

- Custards, gravies, cream pie, and ham are often sources
- Adequate refrigeration will prevent growth

Staphylococcal enterotoxin

- Triggers vomiting response
- Causes abdominal cramps
- Usually occurs in two to four hours after ingestion
- Usually complete recovery within 24 hours
- No lasting side effects

Bacillus cereus

-Aerobic, Gram-positive bacillus, spore forming

-Heating food may not kill the spores, which then can germinate and produce actively metabolic vegetative cells that produce toxin

-Common in rice dishes

-Self-limiting disease

-Food-associated disease can have two forms:

1. Diarrhea: from production of enterotoxin in the gut (takes 8 to 16 hours for infection)

2. Vomiting: due to ingestion of enterotoxin in food (one to six hr)

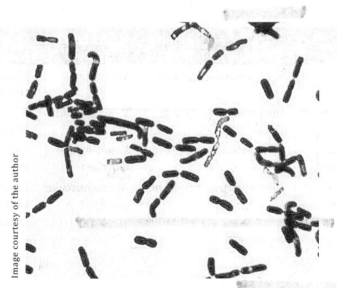

FIGURE 18.2   Bacillus cereus *Gram's stain*

Clostridium perfringens

-Anaerobic, Gram-positive bacillus, spore forming

-Widespread in nature

-Characterized by intense abdominal cramps and diarrhea 8 to 22 hours after ingestion

-grows in intestinal tract and produces exotoxin

-Production of enterotoxin

-Meat stews often associated; boiling of meat stew removes oxygen from the stew, and if spores of *Clostridium* are there, they can germinate and grow into vegetative bacteria

-most cases mild

-Two types of disease:

1. Diarrhea from ingestion of toxin

    - Self-limiting disease

2. Infection: necrotizing enteritis in certain patients who lack trypsin (some south sea islanders) = PigBel

    - Often fatal disease

Clostridium botulinum

-Ingestion of preformed toxin

-Toxin diffuses into the central nervous system, causing paralysis

-Will be discussed further in Chapter 22

LOWER ALIMENTARY TRACT INFECTIONS

TABLE 18.4   *Infections of the GI tract*

Organism	Clinical Symptoms	Pathogenic Mechanism
Salmonella, enteric types	Dysentery	Invasion
Salmonella typhi	Enteric fever* (typhoid)	LPS; bloodstream spread
Shigella	Dysentery	Invasion, cytotoxin
Campylobacter	Dysentery	Inflammation
E. coli EHEC	Watery diarrhea	Cytotoxin
C. difficile	Dysentery	Cytotoxin and enterotoxin
C. perfringens	Watery diarrhea	Enterotoxin
B. cereus	Watery diarrhea	Enterotoxin
Vibrio cholerae	Watery diarrhea	Enterotoxin
Rotavirus	Watery diarrhea	Mucosal destruction
Norovirus	Watery diarrhea	Mucosal destruction
Giardia	Watery diarrhea	Inflammation
Entamoeba histolytica	Dysentery	Invasion
Cryptosporidium	Watery diarrhea	? (probably inflammation)

} Gram negative rods

-gas gangrene

} viral gastroenteritis

Salmonella: two major groups causing very different types of diseases

a) *Salmonella enterica* species (more than 2000 types): causes gastroenteritis (diarrhea)

-usually animal-human

b) *Salmonella typhi*: causes enteric fever or typhoid fever, a type of septicemia (blood stream infection)

-only human disease

Salmonella enterica species

-Facultative, Gram-negative bacilli, motile, nonspore forming

-Common commensals in the GI tract of animals and on the skin of reptiles *(e.g., turtles, snakes)

-normal flora on skin on reptiles

-*Salmonella enterica* is the group name, and then each serotype has its own name (e.g., *Salmonella typhimurium* and *Salmonella enteritidis*)

-Incubation period 12 to 36 hours, fecal–oral transmission, zoonotic

-Need large amounts of bacteria to cause an infection because the bacterium is easily inactivated by the low pH of the gastric acid

-Invade by being taken up in the microfold cells of the Peyer's patches and transported to the lymphatic system

-disease runs it course, immune system heals the body

-Meat products, eggs, poultry are the usual sources; however, it can be a water contaminant, and there have been outbreaks from green salad onions, alfalfa sprouts, watermelon, etc.

-*S. enteritidis* can infect chickens (that do not get sick)—but the eggs the chickens lay can have bacteria in the yolk

-Usually not treated with antibiotics unless it spreads to the bloodstream

-antibiotics may prolong shedding

-Antibiotic treatment of *Salmonella* gastroenteritis tends to cause a prolonged shedding of bacteria—patient remains infectious for a longer time

Salmonella typhi: typhoid fever or enteric fever

-Transmitted only from human to human (fecal–oral), no animal reservoir

-Characterized by high fever, usually >40 °C, headache, bloodstream infection

-Diarrhea may start in second or third week but is not the main characteristic

-Causes septicemia (enteric fever)

-Bacteria invade through intestinal mucosa and enter phagocytes

-Bacteria multiply rapidly in phagocytic cells and disseminate through lymph and blood

-antibiotics: ex. ceftriaxone

-After recovery it is relatively common with a carrier state:

   *example: Typhoid Mary: a cook in the early 1900s who had not been ill with *S. typhi* but nursed a brother who died of typhoid fever. She harbored *S. typhi* in her gall bladder for more than 50 years and infected more than 50 people during her life.

-Treatment is ALWAYS done with IV antibiotics

Shigella species

*infection, not intoxication

-Facultative, anaerobic, Gram-negative bacilli, nonspore forming, nonmotile

-Only a human pathogen; transmission person-to-person (fecal–oral)

-Four species:

Shigella dysenteriae (type A)*

Shigella boydii (B)

Shigella flexneri (C)

Shigella sonnei (D)

-Severity of infection depends on the infecting strain; more virulent strains contain a plasmid essential for attachment and entry of bacteria into cells

-Production of cytotoxin (called Shiga toxin)

-One to two days of incubation; symptoms: intense abdominal pain, diarrhea, and fever

-Treated with antibiotics

Campylobacter jejuni

-Facultative, anaerobe, Gram-negative bacillus, gull wing-shaped bacilli, motile

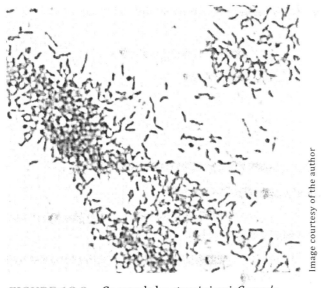

Image courtesy of the author

FIGURE 18.3 Campylobacter jejuni *Gram's stain*

-Fecal–oral transmission

-Most common cause of bacterial gastroenteritis in North America (food borne illness)

-Found in poultry and also other animals' intestinal tracts; has been found in unpasteurized milk among other foods

-Between 80% to 90% of chicken in grocery stores have *C. jejuni* on skin

-No exotoxins but endotoxins (LPS) and cause inflammation of the intestine   -disturbs reabsorption = diarrhea

-Symptoms: abdominal cramps, diarrhea that may be bloody, headache, malaise, fever

-IBD= inflammatory bowel disease

-Self-limiting disease, not usually treated with antibiotics unless severe

-Complications IBD and Guillain–Barré syndrome

Escherichia coli Gastroenteritis

-Facultative, Gram-negative bacilli, motile

-Most strains of *E. coli* are harmless commensals in the intestine

-Pathogenic strains of *E. coli* have acquired genes for virulence factors like special fimbriae for attachment to intestinal cells or exotoxins

-Major types:

Enterotoxigenic *E. coli* (ETEC)

Enteroinvasive *E. coli* (EIEC)

Enteroaggregative *E. coli* (EAEC)

Enteropathogenic *E. coli* (EPEC)

Enterohemorrhagic *E. coli* (EHEC)

Enterohemorrhagic *E. coli* (EHEC or *E. coli* O157:H7)

-Increasing importance in North America and the rest of the developed world—also known as "hamburger disease"

-O157:H7 = inhabits animal intestine, eg. cow

-Best known serotype is O157:H7 (remember the O antigen is part of the LPS, and the H antigen is from the flagella), but there are other serotypes causing the same disease (e.g., the recent large outbreak in Germany with O104)

-Inhabits animal intestine (e.g., cows)

-Fecal contamination of meat in packing plants

-Low infective dose (10 organisms)

-hemorrhagic colitis = inflammation of intestine with blood

-Produce a verotoxin or Shiga-like toxin that causes hemorrhagic colitis and hemolytic uremic syndrome

-Fecal–oral transmission; undercooked hamburger and other meats; can also contaminate water (recent outbreak in the United States associated with spinach)

-Disease is usually self-limiting in adults, but children and elderly can get complications (like HUS)

-treatment: antimicrobials in severe cases

-Treatment: usually rehydration, supportive care, seldomly antibiotics

HUS (Hemolytic Uremic Syndrome)

-Blood is seen in the urine due to kidney failure

-young & old at HIGH risk

-From 5% to 10% of children infected with EHEC get HUS

-Mortality rate ~5%

-found in poorly handled meat, poultry, raw alfalfa sprouts

-Treatment: supportive care, sometimes dialysis, no antimicrobials because you don't want any more toxins to be released from the bacteria because this may make the situation worse

Vibrio cholerae

-Facultative, Gram-negative, comma-shaped bacillus, motile

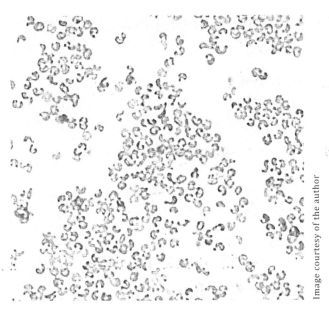

FIGURE 18.4   Vibrio cholerae *Gram's stain*

Image courtesy of the author

-Two main serotypes causing epidemics: classic El Tor and O139

    O139 is causing the ongoing pandemic

-Bacterium survives high pH and high salt concentrations

-Killed by gastric acid; need large numbers of bacteria to get disease

-Produce an exotoxin (enterotoxin) that causes a secretory diarrhea (watery with mucus flecks = rice water diarrhea), up to 20 L/day

-Fecally contaminated water main source (fecal–oral)

-Treatment: rehydration, glucose, and electrolytes are imperative! Antibiotics are secondary and mostly of use for prophylaxis.

- can have >20 L fluid loss/day
- heat labile
- global pandemic = rides on hulls of ships

VIRAL GASTROENTERITIS

-Infections occur worldwide, in both developing and developed nations

-In developing nations, nonbacterial gastroenteritis is a major cause of infant death

-Not clinically distinguishable from other gastroenteritis

-Viruses are specific to humans

-Fecal–oral transmission

-Two main types are rotavirus and norovirus, but there are other small RNA viruses like sapovirus that also are emerging as problems

- 90% cases cause by rotavirus or Norovirus

Rotavirus Gastroenteritis

-RNA virus, nonenveloped

-Most common cause of viral gastroenteritis in children, most are <2 years

-incubation 2-3 days (handwritten)

-Incidence in developed countries = incidence in developing countries, but severity is higher in developing countries due to the other basic problems with nutrition, health

-Often a nosocomial infection

-Mechanism of pathogenesis: inflammation of the intestinal mucosa with damage to the villi

-Symptoms: low-grade fever, diarrhea, vomiting (usually one week's duration)

-Complications: dehydration

-No antivirals

-New vaccines: RotaTeq™; Rotarix™

→will reduce mortality from diarrhea (handwritten)

Norovirus Gastroenteritis

-RNA virus, nonenveloped

-Causes major outbreaks of viral gastroenteritis in all ages

-Responsible for up to 2/3 of all cases of "food poisoning"

-Pathogenesis similar to rotavirus except that it probably uses some blood group antigens for attachment, and it has been found that about 10% to 20% of people infected do not get ill (secretor status seems to be predictive)

-sudden onset=
NO PRODROME;
all of a sudden
have symptoms, no
build up (ex. vomitting,
no nausea) (handwritten)

-Symptoms: no prodrome, nausea, abdominal cramps, diarrhea, vomiting for one to two days

-Self-limiting

-Complication: dehydration

-"Cruise ship virus"

-No vaccine

PARASITIC DISEASES OF THE GASTROINTESTINAL SYSTEM

Protozoan diseases (e.g., *Giardia lamblia, Cryptosporidium, Entamoeba histolytica*)

   - Diarrhea is a major feature of all protozoan intestinal infections

Metazoan (helminthic) diseases: (e.g., tapeworm, roundworms)

   - Usually no diarrhea

DISEASES OF AUXILIARY ORGANS

Hepatitis

-Inflammation of the liver (does not have to be infectious)

-Hepatitis A, B, C, D, E (main types of viral hepatitis—these are from different viral families, and only the name is similar)

-CMV and EBV can also cause infectious hepatitis

✱ Hepatitis A

-RNA virus, nonenveloped

✱ Fecal–oral transmission, often contaminated water, mollusks

-Virus has a high degree of resistance to chlorine **(because of nonenveloped)**

-Incubation period two to four weeks

-Symptoms: nausea, fever, anorexia, vomiting, jaundice

-Usually sudden onset, but 50% of infections are subclinical

-Pathogenesis: multiplication of the virus in the intestinal epithelium, blood stream spread, localization in the liver where the virus damages cells

-Virus exits via the biliary system to feces for excretion

-Diagnosis: test for IgM antibodies to HAV

-No antivirals

✱ Supportive care, self-limiting, NO CHRONIC DISEASE unless there is immunosuppression

-Vaccine: good vaccine exists—lifelong immunity

Hepatitis B, C, D—will be discussed in the cardiovascular and lymphatic infection chapter 23 (bloodborne infections)

✱ Hepatitis E

-RNA virus, nonenveloped

✱ Fecal–oral transmission, probably contaminated water

-Endemic in poor areas with poor sanitation (e.g., India and southeast Asia)

✱ NO CHRONIC DISEASE

-Complication: pregnant women have a 20% mortality if they contract HEV

Interested? Want to learn more?

For more reading, several texts online at the U of A library are recommended:.

1. Brooks, GF, Carroll KC, Butel JS, Morse SA, editors. Jawetz, Melnick, and Adelberg's Medical Microbiology, 24th ed. Blacklick OH-McGraw Hill; 2007.

- acute infection

-jaundice = sign of damaged liver

-Virema= virus in blood

HEP B:
-enveloped DNA virus
-transmission- bloodborne disease, STI
-can cause both chronic and acute disease
-vaccine available

HEP C:
-can lead to liver cancer
-enveloped RNA virus
-transmission- blood borne
-acute & chronic (acute patients 80% become chronic)
-no vaccine available
✱ EGCG of green tea prevents attachment to host cell ↳

2. Ryan KJ, Ray CG, editors. Sherris Medical Microbiology, 5th ed. New York – McGraw-Hill, 2010.

3. Mandell GL, Bennett JE, Dolin R, editors. Mandell, Douglas and Bennett's Principles and Practices of Infectious Diseases, 7th ed. Churchill Livingstone Elsevier, Philadelphia, 2010.

HEP D:
- enveloped RNA
- coexists with HBV to cause disease

Chapter 19

Urinary Tract Infections

Learning Objectives:

1. Describe the components of the urinary tract.
2. Identify the levels of urinary tract infection according to the organ affected.
3. Explain how asymptomatic urinary tract infections can cause disease.
4. Identify the main causes of urinary tract infections in different populations.
5. List parameters used in the urine sediment test for demonstrating kidney damage.
6. Determine important considerations for collecting representative specimens.

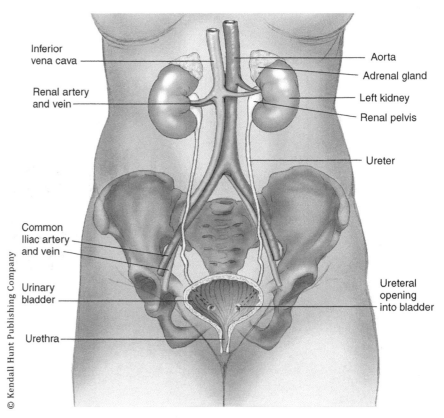

FIGURE 19.1   Urinary tract

Definitions

Urethritis:	infection of the urethra *-most superficial infection*
Cystitis:	infection of the urinary bladder
Ureteritis:	infection of the ureters
Pyelonephritis:	infection of the kidney

URINARY TRACT INFECTIONS

-One of the most common sites of bacterial infection

-More common in females

-Majority of infections are acute and uncomplicated (e.g., cystitis, urethritis)

-Most common type of nosocomial infection (catheter-related); biofilms often implicated

-Severe infections with complications affect kidney function

-Usually acquired by ascending route from outer genitalia through urethra to bladder, then through ureters to the kidney, but systemic infections can also cause UTI

-Kidney infections are the most severe form of urinary tract infection, and bacteria can easily spread to the bloodstream from the kidney, causing sepsis

-asymptomatic UTI:
↳presence of significant numbers of bacteria in absence of symptoms
↳can cause complications (scarring) in kidneys of young children and in pregnant women

URINE

-Wastes removed from blood in kidney (filtration)

-Bladder: urine storage

-Valves control backflow of urine from bladder to ureters

-Urine is normally low pH (~4.5–6.0), has some antimicrobial properties and is normally sterile

-Flushing of urine through system is a mechanism of defense against infection

-Analysis of cell content, osmolality, protein and glucose content, and presence of "casts" important for determination of complicated infection (urinary sedimentation test)

-Casts are protein "molds" of the renal tubules and, depending on the type of cast, will have different significances (some normal or benign disorders and some signaling severe damage)

TABLE 19.1 Bacterial Factors and Host Factors Contributing to UTI

Bacterial Factors	Host Factors
Capsular antigens	Renal calculi
Hemolysins	Ureteric reflux (valve abnormalities)
Urease	Tumors
Adhesion to epithelium	Pregnancy, stress
Intracoital colonization	Neurological problems
	Prostatic hypertrophy
	Short urethra in women
	Catheterization

TABLE 19.2 Common Causes of Urinary Tract Infection

Outpatients	Inpatients
E. coli (80%)	E. coli (40%)
CNS (8%)	Other enteric bacteria (25%)
S. aureus	Gram positives (16%)
Enterococci	Proteus mirabilis (11%)
Strep Group B	Candida sp. (5%)

Symptoms of Lower Urinary Tract Infection

-Painful urination (dysuria)

-Urgency and frequency of micturition

-Catheter-related infections are usually asymptomatic

-Cloudy urine due to WBC (white blood cells) (pyuria) and bacteria (bacteruria)

Symptoms of Upper Urinary Tract Infection

-Fever and same symptoms as for lower UTI

-May have lower back pain

-Asymptomatic infection can occur with both lower and upper urinary tract infections

Urethritis

-Usually transient infection/inflammation

-Usually self-limiting, usually *E. coli*

Cystitis

-Usually uncomplicated unless physical abnormalities exist

-Women are 8X more often affected than men (length of urethra, proximity to anus)

-1/3 of women affected at least once in a lifetime

-Most infections in women due to *E. coli*; second most common cause is *Staphylococcus saprophyticus*, which is characteristic of infections in young women

-Other common causes are other enteric Gram negatives, Gram positives such as *Enterococcus* sp., *Streptococcus* sp., *Staphylococcus aureus*

-Complications of chronic infection: bladder, prostate damage

-Short courses of oral antibiotics for treatment

Pyelonephritis

-Twenty-five percent of untreated cystitis cases can progress to pyelonephritis

-Symptoms are fever and flank or back pain

-Most common cause is *E. coli*

-Complications: kidney damage, bacteremia, and sepsis

-Serious complications—life-threatening

-Always treated with antibiotics

Hematogenous Spread of Organisms to the Kidney

-Systemic infection can spread to kidney (not common), but a few more common examples are *Salmonella typhi*, *Staphylococcus aureus*, *Mycobacterium tuberculosis*, *Leptospira interrogans*

Leptospirosis (Weil's Disease)

-Caused by a spirochete—*Leptospira interrogans*

-Zoonosis, acquired through contact with contaminated water (dogs and rats)

-Entry through small skin breaks or through mucous membrane

-Incubation one to two weeks

-Symptoms: headache, muscle pain, chills, and fever initially, then fever disappears and reappears a few days later when the kidneys and liver are infected

ASYMPTOMATIC INFECTION

-Presence of significant numbers of bacteria (usually >100,000/ml), called bacteriuria, in absence of any symptoms

-Complications in pregnant women and young children: kidney scarring

CATHETERS:
- often have bacteria, but no symptoms

"SIGNIFICANT" BACTERIURIA

-More than 100,000 bacteria/ml or 10^9/liter midstream urine; normally only one type of bacteria

-"Contaminated urine" (usually not taken as a midstream urine) usually has several species

-Exceptions: catheterized specimens, infants, immunosuppressed patients, urine held in bladder for less than 4 hours

- infection with S. saprophyticus

Urinary Tract Infections in Children

-Reflux occurs in 30% to 50% of children with asymptomatic or symptomatic bacteriuria

-Infants and preschool children have a high risk for renal scarring if asymptomatic infections persist for long periods of time

-Urinary tract infections not uncommonly caused by other types of bacteria seldomly seen in adults

> *examples: Streptococcus pneumoniae*
>
> *Haemophilus influenzae*
>
> *Streptococcus pyogenes* Group A

✳supra-pubic aspiration = needle to take urine for small children (incontinent)

ORGANISMS COMMONLY IMPLICATED IN UTI

E. coli

-Gram-negative bacilli, motile, ± capsule

-Has O (somatic), H (flagellar), K (capsular), F (fimbrial) antigens

-Adhesion: p-fimbriae, which mediate attachment to uroepithelial cells

-Usually susceptible to wide variety of antibiotics

- most common in intestine, causes UTI when enters urinary tract

S. saprophyticus

-Gram-positive cocci, coagulase negative, novobiocin resistant

-Infections in healthy young women

↳ differentiation between epidermidis

316   MEDICAL MICROBIOLOGY

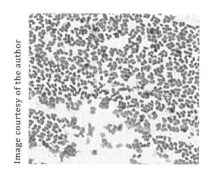

Figure 19.2   Escherichia coli *Gram's stain*

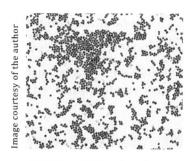

FIGURE 19.3   Staphylococcus saprophyticus *Gram's stain*

Proteus mirabilis

-Gram-negative bacilli, motile

-Normally found in the intestine

-Produce large amounts of urease, ammonium generated from breakdown of urea can cause magnesium and phosphates to crystallize out as "struvite" stones

-Common in UTI of hospitalized patients, catheterized patients

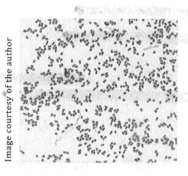

FIGURE 19.4   Proteus mirabilis *Gram's stain*

Enterobacteriaceae sp.

-Gram-negative "enteric" bacilli, ± capsules

-Normal flora in intestine

-Include: *Enterobacter* sp.

Klebsiella sp.

Serratia sp.

-Easily become multiresistant to antibiotics and cause nosocomial infections (e.g., ESBL, or extended spectrum beta-lactamase)

-ICU, neonatal, and extended care facilities are most problematic

Streptococcus agalactiae (Group B Streptococci)

-Gram-positive cocci in chains

-Part of the normal flora in the intestine

-Beta-hemolytic on blood agar but very small zones of hemolysis (You can see the difference between Group A and Group B!)

-Not usual cause of complicated UTI but important if patient is pregnant—neonatal sepsis, meningitis, and respiratory failure could develop in the baby if exposed

* "B" is Bad For Babies

-pregnant women are tested

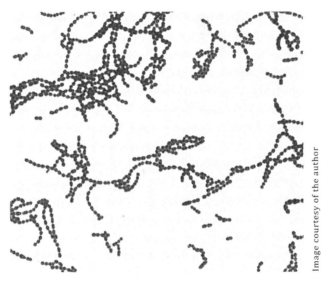

Image courtesy of the author

FIGURE 19.5   Streptococcus agalactiae *(GBS) Gram's stain*

Pseudomonas aeruginosa

-Gram-negative bacillus, motile

-Found in soil, water, intestine

-Opportunist and common cause of nosocomial and catheter-related infections

-Produce endotoxin, exotoxin, extracellular proteases and elastases, and extracellular slime

-Resistant to commonly used antibiotics for UTI

Staphylococcus aureus and *Staphylococcus epidermidis*

-Gram-positive cocci in clusters, differentiated by coagulase test and DNase production

-Often associated with catheterization

-Affinity for growing on catheter surface as a biofilm

Enterococcus faecalis/faecium

-Gram-positive, elongated cocci, often short chains or pairs

-May produce alpha-, beta-, or gamma- (no) hemolysis on BAP

-Common in UTI, normal flora in intestine

-Bile- and salt-resistant

*VRE (vancomycin-resistant enterococci) are a growing problem in health care **HUGE PROBLEM**

-could transfer to staph (MRSA) = double resistance

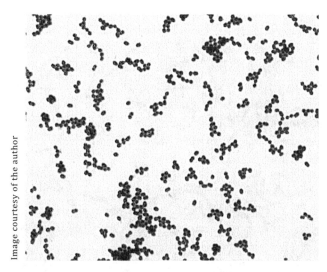

Image courtesy of the author

FIGURE 19.6   Enterococcus faecalis *Gram's stain*

SPECIMEN COLLECTION

-Correct collection and transport important to quantitative culture

-Midstream sample (MSU) in a sterile container

-Incubation in bladder more than 4 hours is best; otherwise note time on requisition

-Babies: bag urine often contaminated with fecal flora

   *Suprapubic bladder aspiration recommended

-Catheterized patients: urine withdrawn from catheter tube with syringe

-*M. tuberculosis*: special instructions, morning urine collected on several consecutive days

-Always refrigerate specimens immediately, and transport refrigerated as soon as possible

-Dip-slide tests OK for uncomplicated cystitis, NEVER for complicated urinary tract infections or infections in children

-Urine esterase can be measured by dipstick (enzyme produced by WBC)

   A positive esterase = presence of WBC and thus infection

-DIPSTICK = enzyme produced by WBC

-Urinary sediments:

Useful for diagnosis of pyelonephritis—presence of protein or RBC casts in urine from glomeruli in kidney, presence of WBC

Interested? Want to learn more?

For more reading, several texts online at the U of A library are recommended:

1. Brooks, GF, Carroll KC, Butel JS, Morse SA, editors. Jawetz, Melnick, and Adelberg's Medical Microbiology, 24th ed. Blacklick OH-McGraw Hill; 2007.

2. Ryan KJ, Ray CG, editors. Sherris Medical Microbiology, 5th ed. New York – McGraw-Hill, 2010.

3. Mandell GL, Bennett JE, Dolin R, editors. Mandell, Douglas and Bennett's Principles and Practices of Infectious Diseases, 7th ed. Churchill Livingstone Elsevier, Philadelphia, 2010.

Chapter 20

Sexually Transmitted Infections

Learning Objectives:

1. List some characteristics bacteria and viruses causing STIs have in common.

2. Describe how STIs are transmitted, and how they can be prevented.

3. Rank the STIs according to their severity regarding location and effect on reproductive health.

4. List major complications from STIs.

5. Identify the major causes of STIs and characteristics of infection.

6. Discern the effects of asymptomatic infection on reproductive health.

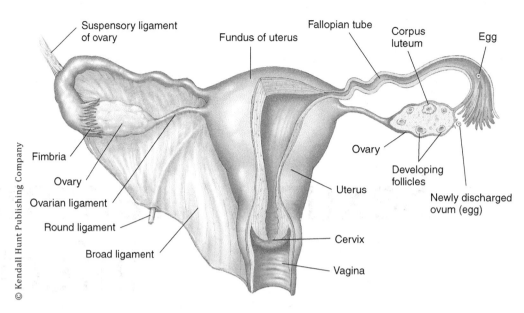

FIGURE 20.1   *Female reproductive tract*

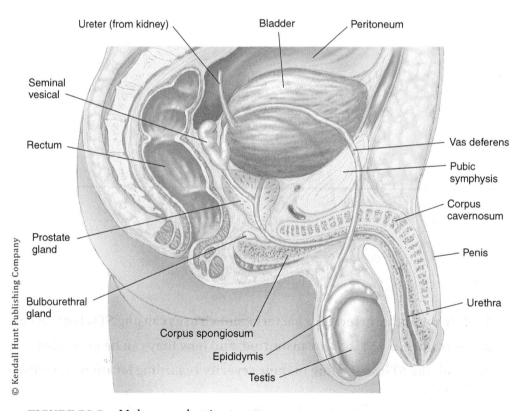

FIGURE 20.2   *Male reproductive tract*

Diseases of the Reproductive Tract Attributable to Sexually Transmitted Infection

PID = pelvic inflammatory disease

   - Infection of the uterus, fallopian tubes, and ovaries

-extreme pain or asymptomatic; causes damage

Cervicitis, vaginitis, urethritis

HIV

Viral lesions due to herpes simplex

Genital warts

Vaginosis

NGU = nongonococcal urethritis (chlamydia-NEW word)

Arthropod infections

SEXUALLY TRANSMITTED INFECTION (STI)

-Most infections of the reproductive tract (but not all) are acquired through sexual contact

-More than 30 infectious agents known to cause STI (e.g., even *Salmonella,* CMV, *E. histolytica* can cause STI)

-Bacterial, viral, and parasitic infections responsible are prevalent world-wide (e.g., *C. trachomatis,* HSV 2, *Trichomonas vaginalis*)

-All can be prevented by careful barrier prevention (e.g., condoms used appropriately)

-No vaccines currently available for STI except for human papillomavirus (Gardasil) (warts)

-STI are of critical importance for fertility and well-being

Characteristics of Agents Typically Causing STI

Fastidious: adapted to spread from humans directly to humans and tolerate inanimate environments poorly, if at all

Conservative: tend to produce negligible symptoms initially

-May produce infection without symptoms but are still infectious

-May persist without infectivity or with intermittent infectivity and symptoms may recur

-May allow reinfection by being poorly antigenic (poor immune response)

Host Factors Important in STI

1. **Principally behavior-oriented factors**

-Number of partners

-Choice of partners

-Frequency of intercourse and intimate contact

-Sites of exposure (type of intimacy)

-Intensity of exposure (including trauma)

-Use of contraception: nonbarrier or barrier

2. **Coexistence of other STI**

-Presence of lesions can allow other organisms to more easily infect because the integrity of the skin and/or mucosal membrane is already disturbed

3. **Site and infectious load of partners infection**

-The higher the infectious dose, the more likely a symptomatic infection will occur

Types of infections involved with STI:

Urethritis (m + f)

Balanitis (m)

Epididymitis (m)

Prostatitis (m)

Vaginitis (f)

Cervicitis (f)

PID or "salpingitis" (f)

Proctitis (m + f)

Eye (infant = ophthalmia neonatorum; adult inclusion conjunctivitis)

BACTERIAL DISEASES OF THE REPRODUCTIVE TRACT

Gonorrhea (*Neisseria gonorrhoeae*)

-characterized by pus
-known as "the drip"

-Aerobic, Gram-negative diplococcus

-Fastidious growth requirements, need 5% CO_2 and complex nutrients in medium

-Do not survive transport media and refrigeration well

-Human pathogen only, reservoir is the human

-Known at least since the ancient Greek times, described by Galen:

gon = semen   rhea = flow (confused pus with semen)

-Prefers mucous membranes; most often infects the genitals but can infect the throat

Transmission

-Transmitted directly from person-to-person; sensitive to drying out

-Not normally contractible from inanimate objects (e.g., toilet seats, etc.)

-Vertical transmission to baby possible

-In males, a single unprotected exposure results in infection 20% to 35 % of the time; in females, 60% to 90% of the time

Incubation period: two to seven days, dependent on infectious dose

Symptoms

-May be symptomatic or asymptomatic (women are more often asymptomatic than men)

-Male: urethral discharge (pus) and dysuria (pain on urination)

Female: vaginal discharge

-Pharyngeal gonorrhea: sore throat

　　Rectal gonorrhea: itching or painful inflammation

Pathogenesis

-Inflammatory and pyogenic (pus-producing) infection, usual site of entry is the vagina or the urethral mucosa but can infect throat, eye, and rectal mucosa

-Adherence of bacteria to nonciliated epithelial host cells mediated by fimbriae (pili) and the Opa surface proteins on the bacterium

-Opa proteins expressed on the cell surface can change their antigens and contribute to the ability of the gonococcus to evade the immune response

-Opa proteins probably also help to "turn off" the T cells

-Bacteria start multiplying after attachment and rapidly spread up the vagina or urethra

-Cell walls of *N. gonorrhoeae* contain LPS (endotoxin)—virulence factor

-Most strains produce IgA protease (breaks down IgA antibodies, which otherwise trap bacteria in mucus, thus allows bacterial adherence to host cells)

-Damage to tissues results from the inflammation that the gonococcus elicits

-Infection is usually localized, but some more virulent strains that are resistant to the bactericidal effect of serum can spread systemically

Complications:

-Rare in men (urethral scarring and sterility if the vas deferens becomes blocked or the testes infected)

-More common in women: PID, infertility, chronic pelvic pain

-Ophthalmia neonatorum in newborns (may result in blindness if not treated)

-Systemic disease in both males and females

-Can result in endocarditis, meningitis, monoarticular arthritis with tendinitis, skin lesions, DIC, and even death, but this is rare

Laboratory diagnosis

-Finding of Gram-negative diplococci in white blood cells on direct smear of urethral discharge from men is diagnostic

(handwritten margin notes)

-damage to tissues results from inflammation that gonococcus elicits (no exotoxin)

-inactivate complement

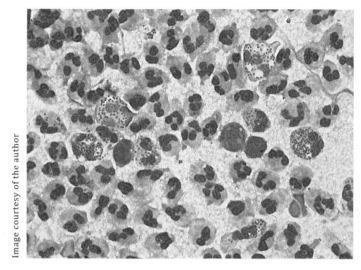

Image courtesy of the author

FIGURE 20.3   *Stained pus from a gonorrheal infection showing intracellular diplococci and many neutrophils*

-culture is most common test

-Culture, PCR, DNA probes

-Serology (looking for serum antibodies) usually not helpful

-Antibiotic susceptibility must be done because there is an increasing problem with beta-lactamase producing strains and resistance to antibiotics

-Antigen typing of strains often done for epidemiological investigations

Treatment: ciprofloxacin, ceftriaxone commonly used

-used to use penicillin (now resistant)

-Increase in prevalence of beta-lactamase producing *N. gonorrhoeae* and other resistant mutants

-partner tracing and treatment important

No vaccine available

-LPS in cell wall
-most common STD

Chlamydia trachomatis

-Gram-negative type of bacterium, not visible by Gram's stain

-Obligately intracellular: cannot produce its own ATP and is dependent on the host cell for energy

-Unique developmental cycle with an infectious form (EB)—elementary body and a metabolically active form (RB) reticulate body

-infectious form is NOT treatable (try to target RB)

-EB is not actively metabolizing and so cannot be targeted with antibiotics

-Three species of Chlamydia infect humans

C. psittaci (zoonosis from birds; resp. infection)

C. pneumoniae (resp. infection, associated with cardiovascular diseases)

-have to live in host cell to replicate

C. trachomatis	A-C	cause trachoma
	D-K	cause genital infections
	LGV 1-3	cause lymphogranuloma venereum

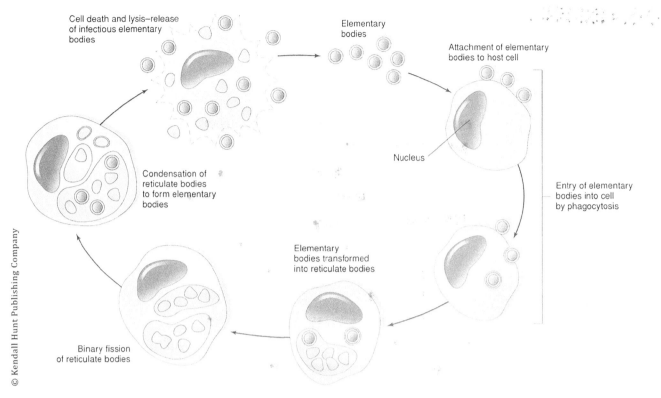

Cell death and lysis–release of infectious elementary bodies

Elementary bodies

Attachment of elementary bodies to host cell

Nucleus

Entry of elementary bodies into cell by phagocytosis

Condensation of reticulate bodies to form elementary bodies

Elementary bodies transformed into reticulate bodies

Binary fission of reticulate bodies

© Kendall Hunt Publishing Company

FIGURE 20.4 *Chlamydia developmental cycle*

Transmission:

- Sexual contact

- Majority of infections are asymptomatic, especially in women

- Vertical transmission to fetus

Pathogenesis

- Elementary bodies (EBs) enter host through break in mucosal membrane

- EBs bind to host cell receptors (e.g., heparan sulfate) and are endocytosed

- EBs internalized in a vacuole (called the chlamydia vacuole)—this does not fuse with the host lysosomes and is thus protected from the enzymes in lysosomes

- Site of infection determines disease

- *C. trachomatis* produces no toxins; mechanism for production of disease is the induction of inflammation, which can spread to the fallopian tubes

-D-K = ENDEMIC

- Serotypes D-K infect only columnar and transitional epithelial cells including eyes
- LGV strains are very invasive and cause systemic disease, including endocarditis

Genital Infection with *C. trachomatis* D-K:

-Endemic worldwide; most common bacterial cause of STI

-Highest frequency in 15- to 25-year-olds

→ More than 50% asymptomatic (women)

-PID >50% asymptomatic (salpingitis)

- Consequence: ectopic pregnancy

Scarring of fallopian tubes

Infertility

Peritonitis and sometimes hepatitis

-Causes NGU (nongonococcal urethritis), epididymitis in men

-Can cause proctitis in either sex

Complications for the Neonate

-Acquired by vertical transmission

-First symptoms are eye infection and failure to thrive (about one month after birth)

-Can cause systemic infections with severe pneumonia

-Suspected that chlamydia acquired early in life can pave the way for chronic lung diseases in adulthood

Laboratory diagnosis

-Culture in cell cultures, DNA probes, PCR (urine and secretions)

-Serology not helpful

Treatment

-Tetracycline or macrolides (e.g., azithromycin)

-No development of resistance to antibiotics

-Partner tracing and treatment is important

Immunity

-No effective immunity; bacterium is poorly antigenic

-Antibodies produced are not protective

-Usually antibodies are not produced in simple infection

No vaccine

- antibiotics that will penetrate host cell membranes

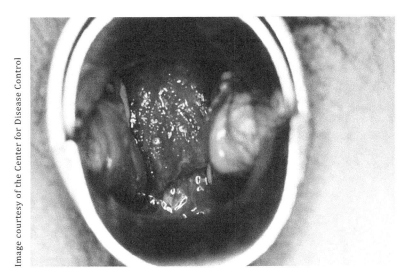

Image courtesy of the Center for Disease Control

FIGURE 20.5   *Inflammation and erosion of the cervix due to* C. trachomatis

LGV (Lymphogranuloma venereum)

-Serious disease (Africa, Asia, South America)

-Occurs sporadically in Europe, North America, Australia

-Caused by *C. trachomatis* L1, L2, L3

-Systemic infection

-Primary lesion is an ulcerating papule at site

-Incubation one to four weeks

Symptoms: lesion, fever, headache, myalgia, inguinal buboes containing replicating chlamydia

Complications: lymphoid spread of disease to rectum—proctitis

- Pain, hepatitis, pneumonitis, meningoencephalitis

- Abscesses form in lymph nodes

- Chronic granulomatous reactions in lymphatics resulting in anal fistula or elephantiasis of genitals

Diagnosis and Treatment

-Same as for *C. trachomatis* D-K

No vaccine

Haemophilus ducreyi (Soft Chancre or Chancroid)

-Aerobic, Gram-negative bacilli

-Seen most frequently in tropics

-Occurrence associated with drug use in developed countries

Clinical features

Painful, nonindurated genital ulcers, and local lymphadenitis

Complications: lesions are important for transmission of HIV

Treatment: macrolides, trimethoprim-sulfa, or ceftriaxone

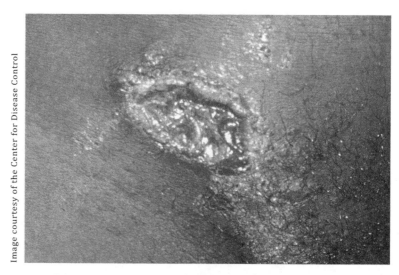

Image courtesy of the Center for Disease Control

FIGURE 20.6   Chancroid due to H. ducreyi

Syphilis *(Treponema pallidum)*

-Spirochete, Gram-negative helix (not visible in Gram's stain)

-Cannot be cultured in vitro (in the lab)

-Known for hundreds of years—reports from 1500s in Europe

-Prevalence low but increasing; often found with other STI

-Closely related to other *Treponema* species causing tropical diseases (primarily skin diseases)

> *examples:*   *T. pertenue* (yaws)
>
>   *T. carateum* (pinta)

-Incubation period usually three weeks

Clinical disease

Three stages of disease

> A. Primary stage: - Initial sign is chancre (painless), which is highly infectious
>
>   - Bacteria enter blood and lymph
>
> B. Secondary stage: -Occurs weeks after the chancre disappears
>
> - Characterized by rash on skin and mucous membranes; rash can have many different appearances—"The Great Imitator"
>
> - Rash itself is very infectious
>
> Latent period: -May last months or years or stay latent forever
>
> C. Tertiary stage: -Fifty percent of patients reach this stage, chronic stage, CNS complications, chronic granulomatous lesions

[handwritten margin notes:]

-risk population = homosexuals, drug users

-highly infectious (hard chancre)

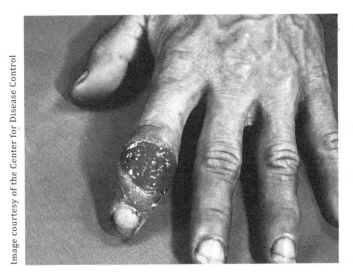

FIGURE 20.7   *Primary chancre of syphilis*

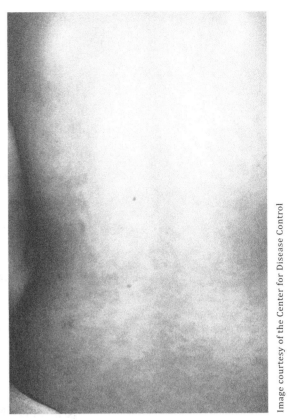

FIGURE 20.8   *Rash of second stage syphilis*

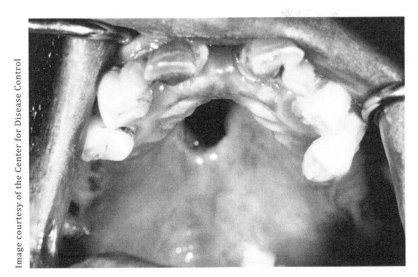

FIGURE 20.9   *Granulomatous lesion ("gumma") shown as a hole in the hard palate*

Pathogenesis

-Portal of entry: minute breaks in skin or on mucous membranes

-Poorly antigenic bacteria due to lipid layer in cell wall; only dead *Treponema* can activate the immune system and induce antibody formation

-Inflammatory responses cause "gumma" formation, lesions that are not painful but cause extensive tissue damage

Complications

- Aortic aneurysm
- CNS damage (paresis), blindness, seizures, dementia
- Congenital syphilis

Laboratory diagnosis

-Serology: several tests used to detect antibodies at different stages of disease

1. RPR: screening test (e.g., blood donors)
   - Detects 70% to 80% of 1° syphilis
   - Nontreponemal test: detects reagin antibodies formed in response to the lipid antigens
2. FTA-ABS: detects late-stage syphilis
   - Treponemal test
3. ELISA/MHA: used for confirmation testing

Treatment: penicillin is drug of choice; no resistance!

Immunity: no known immunity

No vaccine

NONSPECIFIC DISEASE ENTITIES OF THE REPRODUCTIVE TRACT:

Nongonococcal Urethritis

-Any inflammation of the urethra not caused by *N. gonorrhoeae*

-Most commonly caused by *C. trachomatis* but *Ureaplasma urealyticum* also a common cause

Vaginosis

-Most common bacterial infection in fertile women (doesn't have to be a STI)

-No inflammation involved; multiple types of bacteria are involved; many are anaerobic bacteria

-Characterized by a thin frothy vaginal discharge that smells "fishy"

-Often asymptomatic

-Diagnosed by smear and finding of "clue cells," which are epithelial cells covered with adherent bacteria

-Treatment: usually metronidazole

PID (Pelvic Inflammatory Disease)

-Extensive bacterial infection of the female reproductive system

-Usually involvement of the cervix, uterus, fallopian tubes, ovaries

-Can spread to peritoneal cavity and cause liver damage (hepatitis)

-More than 50% of cases are asymptomatic and may have sequelae resulting in infertility, ectopic pregnancies, etc.

-Most cases are caused by *Chlamydia trachomatis*

-also caused by N. gonorrhea

VIRAL DISEASES OF THE REPRODUCTIVE TRACT

Herpes Simplex (HSV)

-DNA virus, enveloped

-Genital herpes simplex usually caused by Type 2 but can be caused by HSV-1

-infection for life

-Incubation one week; primary lesions are vesicles that break down to form shallow ulcers, causing pain and discomfort in the genital area and on urination

-Chronic infection; latent infection in dorsal root ganglia; reactivation

-Most infectious when vesicles are apparent

-Little or no cross-immunity between HSV-1 and HSV-2

-Acyclovir used to treat reoccurrences

-Complications: encephalitis or disseminated herpes in fetus

-still infectious when blisters aren't apparent

-primary infection with HSV 2 often causes aseptic meningitis

-both 1 & 2 cause genital infection, but 2 more common

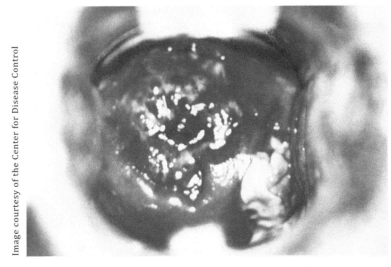

Image courtesy of the Center for Disease Control

FIGURE 20.10   Herpes simplex 2 infection of the cervix

Human Papillomavirus (HPV)

-DNA virus, enveloped

-Cause genital warts

-More than 60 different types of HPV

-Certain serotypes are associated with anal cancer, cervical cancer, and penile cancer (e.g., Types 16, 18)

-Warts of the genital tract may be either flat (must be visualized by painting acetic acid on mucus membranes) or raised ("condylomata acuminata")

-Vaccine—best known is called Gardasil; targets Types 6, 11, 16, 18

-Warts removed by lasers, medication

Human Immunodeficiency Virus (HIV)

-Discussed in Chapter 24

Interested? Want to learn more?

For more reading, several texts online at the U of A library are recommended:

1. Brooks, GF, Carroll KC, Butel JS, Morse SA, editors. Jawetz, Melnick, and Adelberg's Medical Microbiology, 24th ed. Blacklick OH-McGraw Hill; 2007.

2. Ryan KJ, Ray CG, editors. Sherris Medical Microbiology, 5th ed. New York – McGraw-Hill, 2010.

3. Mandell GL, Bennett JE, Dolin R, editors. Mandell, Douglas and Bennett's Principles and Practices of Infectious Diseases, 7th ed. Churchill Livingstone Elsevier, Philadelphia, 2010.

Chapter 21

Neonatal, Perinatal, and Congenital Infections

Learning Objectives:

1. Explain why the newborn and young infant are very susceptible to infection.
2. List common causes of congenital infections.
3. Identify the effects of common infectious diseases in the neonate.
4. Describe preventative measures for congenital infection.

Definitions

Neonate: infant from birth to four weeks of age

Perinatal present either before or after birth ($\pm$ 2 months)

Congenital: present at birth; may be acquired at birth or have been acquired in utero

- Infection during pregnancy, some microorganisms enter bloodstream, establish infection in the placenta and then invade the fetus

- Fetus may die, spontaneously abort, or survive, often with abnormalities

- Striking feature of these infections is the lack of symptoms in the mother

- Infection in the mother is usually a primary (first-time infection) rather than a reactivation of an infection

- Fetus cannot protect itself immunologically from infection, immature cell-mediated immunity and can only produce IgM antibodies in the perinatal period

PERINATAL AND CONGENITAL INFECTIONS

HSV-1 and HSV-2

HIV-1 and HIV-2

Hepatitis B and hepatitis C

Varicella-zoster virus

Papillomavirus

CMV

Rubella

Group B streptococcus (*Streptococcus agalactiae*)

Listeria monocytogenes

Chlamydia trachomatis

Neisseria gonorrhoeae

Signs of Congenital Infection

-Intrauterine growth restriction (IUGR) -small, doesn't thrive

-Blueberry muffin rash -hemorrhagic splotches

-Jaundice -dark yellow - severe (bilirubin toxic to brain cells)

-Hydrops- water in brain

-Presence of blisters

-Thrombocytopenia

-Intracranial calcifications

Handwritten margin notes:

- Host Factors:
  - immature immunity
- breached skin barrier (birth = traumatic)

- fetus infected in utero or at birth

BACTERIAL INFECTIONS AFFECTING THE NEONATE

Congenital Listeriosis

-*Listeria monocytogenes* infection can cause a mild, influenza-like illness in the pregnant woman, a more severe systemic illness or be totally asymptomatic

-Bacteremia in mother infects the placenta and then fetus

-Causes abortion, premature delivery, neonatal septicemia, pneumonia with abscesses or granulomas

Streptococcus agalactiae (Group B Streptococci)

B = BAD FOR BABIES

-Baby is infected during birth by the vaginal canal if mother is colonized with Group B streptococci

-Leading cause of neonatal meningitis and sepsis in the infant, very rapid onset (can be within one day)

-Infection can be early onset (one to seven days after birth) or late onset (7 to 12 days after birth)

-Early onset; more common, and risk factors are prematurity and prolonged rupture of membranes (PROM)

-Mortality of babies with accompanying meningitis is about 50%!

-Pregnant women are screened for Group B strep before delivery (in developed nations) and treated with beta-lactam antibiotics before and during delivery to prevent infection

-No vaccine

-portal of entry = respiratory tract

-more susceptable to damage in prematurity

-late onset infection is usually acquired by mother/nurses/visitors in the hospital

Congenital Syphilis (Treponema pallidum)

-Syphilis transmitted to fetus via placenta, usually latent phase of syphilis disease in the mother

-Severe damage to many tissues

-Mental development deficiencies

-Nerve system damage

-Abnormalities due to tissue damage (e.g., perforation of hard palate)

-Facial deformities

-"Hutchinson's teeth"—characteristic abnormality

↳front teeth are "notched", with space

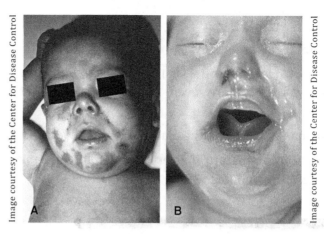

FIGURE 21.1a and b   Congenital syphilis

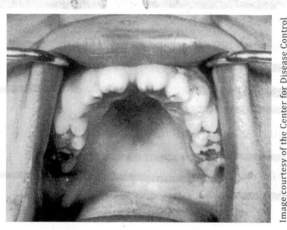

FIGURE 21.2   Hutchinson's teeth in congenital syphilis

Congenital Gonorrhea and Chlamydia

-Chlamydia infections usually begin as an eye infection then progress to pneumonia **(few months after birth)**

-Gonorrhea: ophthalmia neonatorum in newborns

-All babies in developed nations receive erythromycin eye drops at birth to prevent these eye infections, which could damage sight permanently

Gram-Negative Meningitis (e.g., with *E. coli*)

-Uncommon but does occur

Neonatal Tetanus

-Preventable by immunizing mothers and educating about hygienic care of newborns

· can progress to pnemonia, meningitis, or sepsis

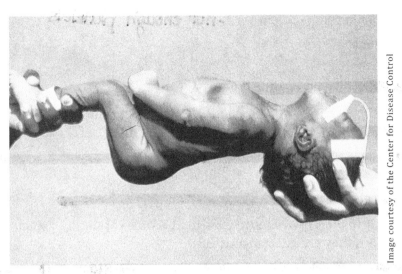

FIGURE 21.3   *Neonatal tetanus (note rigidity)*

Image courtesy of the Center for Disease Control

Staphylococcal Infections

-From mother and other care givers (scalded skin syndrome, etc.)

VIRAL INFECTIONS AFFECTING THE NEONATE

Herpes Simplex

-DNA virus, enveloped

-Pregnant women with a primary herpes infection often lose the baby to spontaneous abortion

-When a mother has vesicles evident, she may have a cesarian to prevent skin exposure of the baby to HSV

-Risk to infant is a disseminated herpes infection, encephalitis

-Can be due either to HSV-1 or HSV-2

-if Herpes is recurrent, she is less likely to pass infection to baby (has antibodies)

-first infection causes most problems in unborn babies (no antibodies)

↳ inflammation of brain tissue (↑mortality)

CMV

-DNA virus, enveloped, HHV-5

-Most common congenital infection

-About half of the babies who are already infected at birth with CMV do not show the effects of the damage until later in life, up to 15 years of age

-Clinical features of severe CMV congenital infection:

- Severe mental retardation
- Spasticity **- nerve system development damaged**
- Eye abnormalities
- Hearing defects
- Hepatosplenomegaly

- some kind of problem with learning

- Thrombocytopenic purpura -not enough platelets
- Anemia

Congenital Hepatitis B and C

-HBV is a DNA virus, enveloped; HCV is a RNA virus, enveloped—both are bloodborne viruses

-The earlier in life an infection occurs, the greater the chance that it will become chronic

-Chronic infection = increased chance to develop liver cancer

-From 70% to 90% of neonates with HBV become chronic as compared to about 10% if they are infected after birth

-To prevent chronicity with HBV, babies are vaccinated at birth and given HB-Ig

-No vaccine or treatment for HCV

-vaccination of newborns in developing/undeveloped countries is goal of WHO

Congenital HIV

-RNA, retrovirus, enveloped

-Infants have poor weight gain, susceptibility to sepsis, developmental delays, lymphocytic pneumonitis, oral thrush, enlarged lymph nodes, hepatosplenomegaly, diarrhea, and pneumonia

-Some infants develop AIDS within the first year

-If mothers do not get their HIV treated while pregnant, there is a 25% chance that the baby will be HIV+, but if she does get treated, then the risk of a HIV+ infant is <1%

-Breast-feeding is not encouraged for HIV+ women unless it is a necessity (e.g., in a developing nation with scanty food supplies). Women are recommended to stop breast-feeding by six months of age (developing world)

- age 1 = evident that there is problem

* only in Western world ($ for antivirals)

-elective cesarians

Congenital Rubella

-Fetus particularly susceptible when mother in first trimester—heart, brain, eyes, and ears are formed in first trimester, and an infecting virus will affect development

-Fetal death common when infection occurs in first month

- 26% abnormalities when infection in second month
- 18% abnormalities when infection in third month
- 7% have abnormalities when infection is in fourth month
  (source: WHO)

-25% of children with congenital infections develop Diabetes type 1, but causality not proven

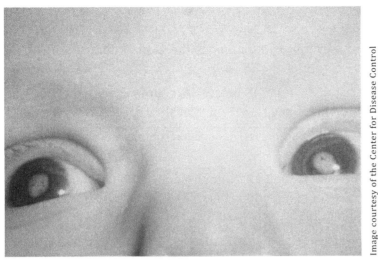

FIGURE 21.4   Cataracts in congenital rubella

PROTOZOAL INFECTIONS AFFECTING THE NEONATE

Congenital Toxoplasmosis

-Results from acute, asymptomatic infection of pregnant women   *- some stillbirths*

-Clinical features of the fetus

- Convulsions

- Microcephaly

- Chorioretinitis *-eyes infected*

- Hepatosplenomegaly

- Jaundice and later hydrocephaly

- Mental retardation and defective vision

-Infection first trimester: 14% of fetal death or abnormality

-Infection third trimester: 59% of fetal death or abnormality

Congenital Malaria

-Often spontaneous abortion

-Severe anemia

MATERNAL INFECTION

Puerperal Fever or "Childbed Fever"

-Usually caused by *Streptococcus pyogenes* Group A but can also be caused by *Clostridium perfringens*

-Major cause of sepsis (childbed fever) and death before the 19th century

-Semmelweis first showed that the doctors and nurses infected the women in labor and directly after the birth by poor hygienic practices

Interested? Want to learn more?

For more reading, several texts online at the U of A library are recommended:

1.   Brooks, GF, Carroll KC, Butel JS, Morse SA, editors. Jawetz, Melnick, and Adelberg's Medical Microbiology, 24th ed. Blacklick OH-McGraw Hill; 2007.

2.   Ryan KJ, Ray CG, editors. Sherris Medical Microbiology, 5th ed. New York – McGraw-Hill, 2010.

3.   Mandell GL, Bennett JE, Dolin R, editors. Mandell, Douglas and Bennett's Principles and Practices of Infectious Diseases, 7th ed. Churchill Livingstone Elsevier, Philadelphia, 2010.

4.   Kliegman R. Nelson Textbook of Pediatrics. 19th ed. Saunders Elsevier, Philadelphia, 2011.

Chapter 22

Central Nervous System (CNS) Infections

Learning Objectives:

1. Identify the major route by which CNS infections occur.
2. List the most common causes of acute and chronic meningitis.
3. Differentiate meningitis from encephalitis.
4. Describe tetanus and botulism and the mechanisms of pathogenicity.
5. Discuss the diseases caused by poliovirus, leprosy, rabies, and West Nile fever.
6. Identify BSE as a TSE, and discuss how the agent can cause irreversible brain damage.

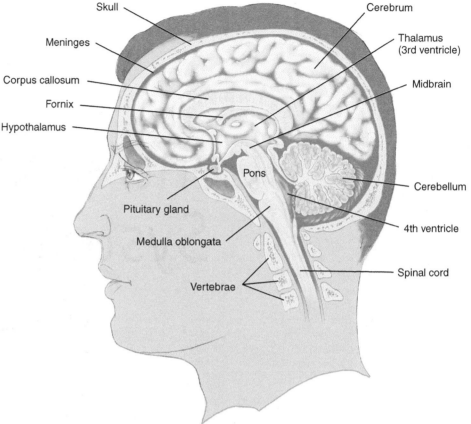

FIGURE 22.1   *Anatomy of the brain*

Central and Peripheral Nervous Systems

-Brain and spinal cord, both enclosed by bone

-All nerves in the body connected to spinal cord

    Motor nerves (CNS):   carry messages from central to peripheral

    Sensory nerves (PNS):   carry messages from peripheral to CNS

-Axons: long extensions of nerve cells; transmit impulses (bundles of axons make up the nerves)

-Ganglia: small bodies containing sensory nerve cells located near spinal column (but outside of it)

-Motor nerve cells: located in the spinal column

-Encephalitis: generalized inflammation or infection of the brain

-Meningitis: inflammation or infection of the meninges

-Meninges: three membranes covering the surface of the brain and spinal cord

Outer membrane:	dura mater
Middle membrane:	arachnoid
Inner membrane:	pia mater

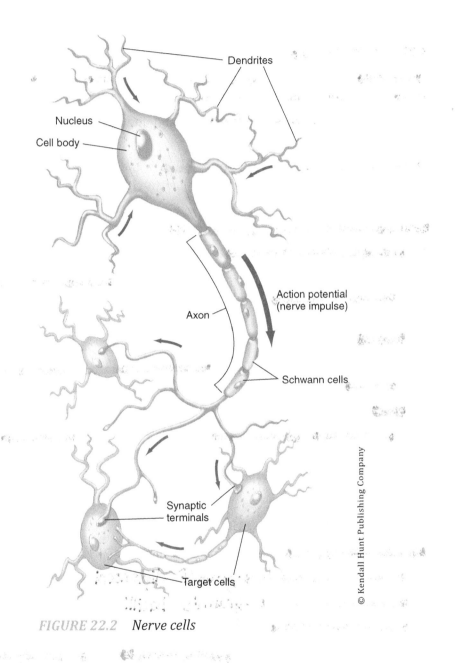

FIGURE 22.2   *Nerve cells*

Cerebrospinal Fluid (CSF)

-Fills the four ventricles in the brain

-Flows between the arachnoid and the pia meninges, cushions the spinal cord

-Sterile in normal conditions

-Usually 100 to 160 ml volume

-should be clear in normal person

-Has low levels of complement and antibodies and very few phagocytic cells

-"Ultra-filtrate" of blood

-Bacteria can multiply very quickly; CSF is a good nutrient source

Blood–Brain Barrier

-Cell layer that allows the passage of some molecules to pass from the blood to the CSF but prevents others

-Only lipid-soluble drugs can cross the blood–brain barrier (e.g., chloramphenicol)

-cannot use penicillin to treat meningitis (can't cross barrier)

-Inflammation can change the permeability of the blood–brain barrier so that some drugs that normally cannot penetrate are able to do so

Routes Microorganisms Take to the CSF

1. Bloodstream and lymphatics

    - Chief source of CNS infections, but organisms must pass through the blood–brain barrier (some viruses can pass through unhindered; e.g., polio)

2. Nerves

    - Some viruses can travel up the axon cytoplasm and travel along nerve bundles (e.g., rabies, HSV)

3. Bone

    - Skull fractures, osteomyelitis (infection of the bone), mastoiditis

Diseases of the CNS

BACTERIAL MENINGITIS

-Three bacterial species cause the majority of cases (70%)

   Streptococcus pneumoniae -gram ⊕ diplococci

   Haemophilus influenzae -gram ⊖ bacilli

   Neisseria meningitidis

-All of the aforementioned can produce capsules and evade phagocytosis (capsule is the most important virulence factor for bacteria causing meningitis)

-General symptoms of meningitis

   ± sore throat

   Fever, headache

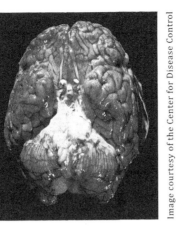

Image courtesy of the Center for Disease Control

FIGURE 22.3 *Bacterial meningitis (autopsy photo)*

Irritability

Neck stiffness

± photophobia

Reduced alertness

Loss of consciousness, confusion

PYOGENIC MENINGITIS (ACUTE RESPONSE)

- neutrophils = POS

-Neutrophils are the dominant leukocyte in the CSF for this acute disease

-CSF has elevated protein levels and decreased glucose levels

-Usually a "positive" Gram's stain (evidence of bacteria) and/or positive culture

-Caused by *S. pneumoniae, N. meningitidis, H. influenzae,* and *S. agalactiae*

↳ only in babies

Streptococcus pneumoniae Meningitis

-Very high mortality rate, more common in children but can affect any age

-Most common bacterial cause of meningitis in the elderly

-Often acute onset

-From 20% to 30% mortality in treated cases

-Type of bacterial meningitis with the highest complication rate, 15% to 20% sequelae in treated cases

- highest complication rate of all meningitis

-Has capsule and produces IgA protease; very good at inducing inflammation

-Vaccines available

 Adults: vaccine to polysaccharide capsular antigens

 Children: vaccine is a conjugated polysaccharide

Neisseria meningitidis Meningitis

-Many serotypes; main types are A, B, C, Y, and W-135

-Mostly B and C in North America

-Virulence factors: capsule, IgA protease, endotoxin, pili, etc capsule, IgA protease, endotoxin, and pili

-Infections characterized by acute onset, skin rash (petechiae, ecchymoses)

-Thirty percent of patients develop disseminated intravascular coagulation (DIC), endotoxinemia, and shock

-Most severe cases: Waterhouse–Friderichsen syndrome with bleeding into the brain and adrenal glands

-No vaccine for type B yet; good vaccines available for C and A

-Mortality 100% if untreated, 10% if treated

-Less than 1% sequelae if treated in time

Haemophilus influenzae Meningitis

-Serotype b most common cause of meningitis

-Before a vaccine was developed, this was the most common cause of meningitis in children <5 years of age

-Infants <4 months protected by maternal antibodies, but these disappear, and there is a window of susceptibility until they produce their own IgG antibodies to the organism

-Onset usually insidious (days)

-Virulence factors: capsule, IgA protease, pili, endotoxin, OMPs

-Five percent mortality in treated cases but 9% with sequelae

Streptococcus agalactiae Meningitis

-Bacteria usually acquired at birth from the mother

-Fifty percent mortality in neonates

-Most common organism causing neonatal meningitis

-Difficult to diagnose meningitis in an infant; signs are poor feeding, lethargy, vomiting, diarrhea, respiratory distress, sometimes bulging fontanelle

-Complications severe in those who survive

Approximately 30% have cerebral or cranial nerve palsy, epilepsy, mental retardation, or hydrocephalus

CHRONIC GRANULOMATOUS AND LYMPHOCYTIC MENINGITIS

-Predominant cell is the mononuclear cell (macrophage/lymphocyte)

-CSF protein may be moderately increased

-CSF glucose may be moderately decreased

-"Negative" Gram's stain (no bacteria seen) and "negative" culture as a common finding, but this is a "false negative" because the numbers of organisms to be reliably detected are too small

>   *example: *M. tuberculosis* and *L. monocytogenes* are present in only small numbers and are difficult to see on a stained smear of CSF

Listeria monocytogenes

-Important cause of meningitis in immunocompromised adult or pregnant

-Intrauterine infection of infants (crosses placenta)

-Not uncommon in farm workers

-Very difficult to diagnose—often very few bacteria

-CNS complications severe

-Increased % of monocytic cells in CSF

Mycobacterium tuberculosis Meningitis

-Focus of infection is elsewhere

-Usually associated with acute miliary tuberculosis

-Gradual onset but presentation variable in terms of symptoms

-Complication: bacteria in the vertebrae destroy the intravertebral disks to form epidural abscesses, which compress the spinal cord and lead to paraplegia

-Difficult to diagnose unless patient is known to have TB

-Characteristic fibrin clot in CSF sometimes seen in vitro

FUNGAL MENINGITIS

-Seen most often in patients with compromised immune systems, chronic meningitis

-*Coccidioides immitis* and *Cryptococcus neoformans* most common causes, followed by *Histoplasma capsulatum*

-Cryptococcus usually transmitted by bird droppings

-Slow onset; may take weeks

-Diagnosis may be difficult (few organisms), usually monocytic infiltration of phagocytes

-Treatment difficult

Cryptococcus neoformans

-Encapsulated yeast

-Associated with pigeon droppings

-Inhalation of *C. neoformans* may cause only lung infection but may disseminate in immunocompromised

-May cause a chronic meningitis

-Treated with amphotericin B and flucytosine

-High mortality rate even in treated cases (30%)

PROTOZOAL MENINGITIS

Naegleria fowleri or *Hartmannella* Species

-Reach meninges through the nose

-Usually contracted by swimming in contaminated lakes (bird poop)

-Almost always fatal

VIRAL MENINGITIS

Viruses are the major cause of "acute aseptic meningitis syndrome"

-Characterized by a lymphocytic pleocytosis **(LOTS = PLEOCYTOSIS)**

-Difficult to diagnose the viral agent

-Usually self-limiting but differs according to virus type

-Most cases caused by enteroviruses and HSV

Causative viral organisms

    Enterovirus 85% to 95% of all

    Arbovirus (e.g., St. Louis encephalitis)

    Mumps virus

    Lymphocytic choriomeningitis virus (LCV)

    Herpesviruses

    HIV

- abrupt onset [handwritten annotation in left margin]

OTHER MICROBIAL DISEASES OF THE NERVOUS SYSTEM

Tetanus or "Lockjaw"

-Caused by *Clostridium tetani*, an anaerobic, spore-forming, Gram-positive bacillus

-Ubiquitous in soil

-Symptoms caused by a neurotoxin, tetanospasmin (bacteria do not invade and remain at the site of injury)

-Toxin enters the CNS via peripheral nerves or blood

-Tetanospasmin (toxin) blocks the relaxing of muscles causing spasms

-Release of neurotransmitters that would block the firing of the nerve causing overactive nerve impulses that are not stopped in the normal manner

-Death usually from spasms of respiratory muscles

-Vaccine good, part of the DPT

-Most of the cases in North America are >50 years due to lack of boosters

-Temporary protection against tetanus in acute situations by administration of tetanus immune globulin (TIG)

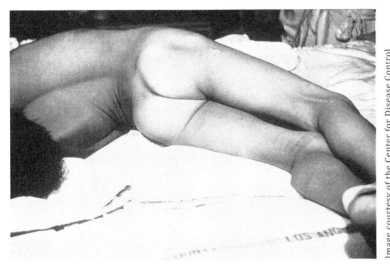

Image courtesy of the Center for Disease Control

FIGURE 22.4   Adolescent with opisthotonos (severe muscle spasms) due to tetanus

Botulism

-Caused by *Clostridium botulinum*, an anaerobic, spore-forming, Gram-positive bacillus

-Normally found in soil and water sediments

-Cause of food poisoning, often in canned vegetables with low acidity

-Different strains of *C. botulinum* produce different toxins:

Type A toxin:	most virulent, western United States
Type B toxin:	most European strains and eastern United States
Type E toxin:	from strains in water sediments

-Most potent bacterial toxin produced; inactivated by boiling

-Clinical symptoms: progressive flaccid paralysis 1 to 10 days, nausea, double vision, difficulty swallowing, general weakness

Pathogenesis

-Production of a neurotoxin, botulinum toxin

-Flaccid paralysis due to the effect of the toxin blocking the release of acetylcholine; this block results in a lack of ability to fire the nerve impulses

Infant botulism

-Many cases associated with ingestion of honey

-Infants do not have a good protective gut flora <1 year

-Symptoms: lethargy and constipation

-Treatable with no ill consequences if diagnosis made in time

-Treat with anti-toxin, botulinum immune globulin (BIG)

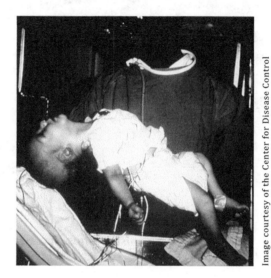

FIGURE 22. 5   Infant botulism

Botox

Cosmetic uses

- Minute amounts of toxin administered under the skin can remove frown lines and wrinkles

- Paralysis of the peripheral nerves

Therapeutic uses

- Many neurological conditions are treated with Botox

- Blepharospasm, strabismus, hemifacial spasm, spasmodic torticollis, hyperhidroses, urinary retention, etc.

✳ Leprosy

-Caused by *Mycobacterium leprae* or Hansen's disease

-*M. leprae* can grow in peripheral nervous system

-Preferential growth at 30 °C

-Person-to-person transmission, death from complications

-Two main forms of disease:

Tuberculoid form (neural form): regions of skin lose sensation (usually immunocompetent individuals)

Lepromatous form: progressive, skin nodules, malformations, necrosis of tissue (e.g., lion-face due to necrosis of nose)

-Diagnosis

  - Acid-fast bacilli in smear from tissues

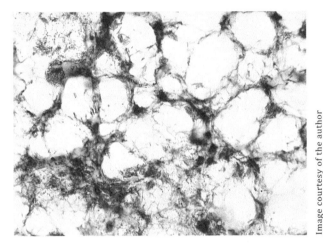

FIGURE 22.6   Skin sample with red stained Mycobacterium leprae, *ZN staining*

Image courtesy of the author

  - Lepromin test (injection of leprae antigens into skin)—helpful only in early stages

-Treatment of leprosy

  Dapsone (sulfa preparation), rifampicin, and clofazimine

-Vaccine: sometimes BCG is used, some effect but not very efficacious

VIRAL DISEASES OF THE NERVOUS SYSTEM

Poliomyelitis

-RNA, enterovirus, nonenveloped

-Fecal–oral: disease initiated by ingestion of poliovirus (nonenveloped, very hardy virus)

-Virus survives in water for extended periods of time

-Most cases are asymptomatic, <1% result in paralysis

-Virus multiplies in the throat and small intestine, then invades through the microfold cells in the Peyer's patches of the lymphatic system; moves to blood, then the CNS

-death of motor neurons
-typically in contaminated water

-When viremia is persistent, the virus infects the CNS and kills the anterior horn motor nerve cells

-Was once a mild disease of childhood, but since the beginning of the 1900s, our standard of living has improved a lot so that the children are no longer getting this disease

-If adults and older children are infected, they usually have a much more serious course of infection due to the more mature immune system

·POST POLIO SYNDROME = cause unknown but usually affects same muscles and nerves as primary infection

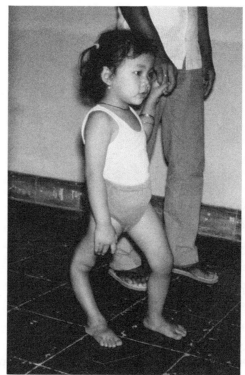

FIGURE 22.7   Polio-affected child

Image courtesy of the Center for Disease Control

Symptomatic Polio Disease

1. Abortive poliomyelitis

-Most common form, minor flu-like illness

2. Nonparalytic poliomyelitis

-Aseptic meningitis, has minor flu-like symptoms plus stiff neck and back

3. Paralytic poliomyelitis

-Major illness, flaccid paralysis

-First symptoms are usually severe myalgia in one limb, motor or sensory disturbances, then weakness in the limb

-Two types of paralytic polio

    a. Bulbar: involves one or more cranial nerve centers, including the respiratory center in the medulla oblongata

    b. Spinal: about 1/3 of cases affect the lower limbs

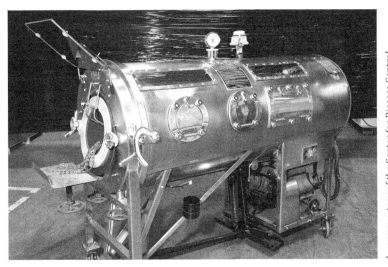

-tropism = GI tract

-mechanically breathing

FIGURE 22.8   *Iron lung (Emerson respirator) for treatment of bulbar polio*

PPMA or PPS

-Post-polio muscle atrophy of post-polio syndrome (many years later, same muscle groups are affected

Treatment of polio: no antiviral

-Supportive treatment—bed rest, no exercise

-Vaccines

    - Salk: IPV (inactivated polio vaccine), recommended by CDC

              1954, inactivated virus, need boosters

    - Sabin: OPV (oral polio vaccine)

              1963, oral vaccine containing three strains of poliovirus, living attenuated, better immunity but chance of virus reverting to wild-type

Rabies (Hydrophobia)

-Zoonotic viral disease (enveloped RNA virus), can infect all species of mammals

-Virus usually contracted by bite of rabid animal

-Rabies can also penetrate an intact mucus membrane

-Death always results from infection if treatment not initiated quickly, and high mortality even if treated with immune globulin

-Virus travels slowly up the peripheral nerves to the CNS, eventually causes encephalitis

-Average incubation is 30 to 50 days

-Two types of rabies: furious and paralytic

-First symptoms

> Sore throat, headache, fever, discomfort at site, muscle spasms and convulsions (swallowing muscles often spasm and sight of water can trigger spasms)

-Raccoons account for most of the rabies cases in the wild, skunks, bats, foxes also common

-Vaccine

> - Indications for vaccination are exposure to virus, either in a laboratory or in the wild (e.g., bite)

> - Five to six injections during 28 days

> - Passive immunization usually provided simultaneously with immune globulin harvested from humans

-If disease develops, mortality is almost 100%

Arboviral Encephalitis

-Mosquito-borne viruses (all RNA)

-Symptoms

> Chills, headache, fever, mental confusion, and coma

-Humans and horses frequently affected

> EEE = eastern equine encephalitis

> WEE = western equine encephalitis

-St. Louis encephalitis, California encephalitis, La Crosse strain, West Nile virus, Japanese B encephalitis, etc

-Monitored by use of "sentinel" animals (rabbits or chickens) except West Nile, where dead crows are collected and tested

West Nile Virus

-RNA, enveloped

-Family Flaviviridae

-First isolated in 1937 in West Nile province of Uganda

-Outbreaks are known in Israel, Romania, South Africa, Asia, and North America in humans and horses

-1999: WNV appeared in New York with 62 cases and 7 deaths

-2000: spread to other states in New England

-2001: spread to Canada

-Since: WNV has been isolated from crows in all provinces of Canada

-Alberta 2003—July was the first positive test

-Disease spread along the migratory birds' routes

-Majority of cases are asymptomatic and mild; only 15% to 20% of people bitten by an infected mosquito get any symptoms at all

-New disease symptomology and progression: never seen before **polio-like** disease (North American strain of virus has been shown to be different than earlier strains in Europe and Africa—maybe more pathogenic?)

-Complicated WNV

- Found mostly in elderly and immunocompromised with preexisting chronic conditions

- Rapid onset of severe headache, high fever, stiff neck, vomiting, drowsiness, confusion, muscle weakness, coma

- Both meningitis and encephalitis

"PROTOZOAL" DISEASES OF THE NERVOUS SYSTEM

Trypanosomiasis

-African trypanosomiasis = sleeping sickness

-Caused by *Trypanosoma brucei gambiense* or *rhodesiense*

- Same disease but different severity (gambiense is milder and slower progressing)

-Trypanosomas are flagellates; transmitted by tsetse fly

-No effective vaccine

- Parasite is capable of antigenic variation

-Treatment difficult—but possible if disease is caught early

-Eradication of vector is the prevailing strategy for control of disease

PRION DISEASE—TRANSMISSIBLE SPONGIFORM ENCEPHALOPATHY

-Caused by a self-replicating protein with no nucleic acids (not "life" form with DNA or RNA)

-Very long incubation times (years)

-CNS damage is slow and progressive; no fever or inflammation

-Spongiform degeneration of the brain

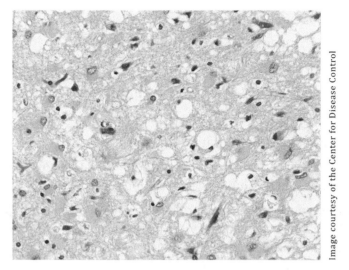

Image courtesy of the Center for Disease Control

FIGURE 22.9   *Spongiform encephalitis in CJD*

-No treatment

-Prions are not living organisms per se and are found to still be active even in formalin after more than 20 years

-Very difficult to inactivate: alkali pH and long autoclaving at 160 °C (2 hours) is the usual method

-Most animal species have a prion disease

Scrapie

- Prion disease of sheep

Kuru

- Prion disease now hopefully extinct, spread by cannibalism, and contact of infected brain tissue to open sores

BSE = bovine spongiform encephalitis (mad cow disease)

-Late 1980s epidemic in England due to feeding cattle with ground sheep containing scrapie prions (>180,000 animals confirmed as diseased)

-Mass slaughter of animals for prevention

-Concern for humans if it can jump the species barrier (see following on vCJD)

-Brain and eye most infectious

-Milk, muscle, and excretions are said to be noninfectious or very low risk

CJD = Creutzfeldt-Jakob disease

-Rare disease, 1 million to 2/million population is the norm

-Has been transmitted by corneal transplants and by athletes ingesting steroid preparations made from human thyroid extracts

[handwritten note:] -affects brain and spinal cord in cattle- abnormal protein causes accumulation of

vCJD = variant Creutzfeldt-Jakob disease

-Has emerged in England after the BSE epidemic (according to WHO statistics, there were 129 cases of vCJD in England between October 1999 and November 2002)

-Alberta has had 46 deaths reported due to CJD since 1999 (increased incidence?)

-Affects younger persons than the classical CJD

-Psychiatric and sensory symptoms are the primary symptoms (different from CJD)

-Diagnosed by MRI

- See plaques of "amyloid protein" (polymer of prion protein)

-No treatment, no cure, no vaccine

Inherited TSE

-Fatal familial insomnia

-Gerstmann-Straussler-Scheinker syndrome

Interested? Want to learn more?

For more reading, several texts online at the U of A library are recommended:

1. Brooks, GF, Carroll KC, Butel JS, Morse SA, editors. Jawetz, Melnick, and Adelberg's Medical Microbiology, 24th ed. Blacklick OH-McGraw Hill; 2007.

2. Ryan KJ, Ray CG, editors. Sherris Medical Microbiology, 5th ed. New York – McGraw-Hill, 2010.

3. Mandell GL, Bennett JE, Dolin R, editors. Mandell, Douglas and Bennett's Principles and Practices of Infectious Diseases, 7th ed. Churchill Livingstone Elsevier, Philadelphia, 2010.

Chapter 23

Cardiovascular and Lymphatic Infections

Learning Objectives:

1. Describe the role of the cardiovascular and lymphatic systems in spreading disease.

2. Identify endotoxin as a major cause of a systemic inflammatory response, and describe the three major activating events.

3. Define lymphangitis, septicemia, and septic shock.

4. Discuss the causative agents and clinical events in anthrax, Lyme disease, plague, and tularemia.

5. Describe the syndromes and causative agents of hepatitis B, hepatitis C, and hepatitis D.

6. Review the cause and clinical symptoms of malaria.

7. Identify yellow fever as the prototype for flaviviruses, and discuss the disease in relation to dengue fever and West Nile fever.

Blood and Lymphatic Systems

-Supply blood (transports oxygen to tissues and CO_2 from tissues) and nutrients to the body's tissue cells, removes wastes

-Heat and cool the body tissues

-Systemic infections: can be carried via these systems to all tissues of the body

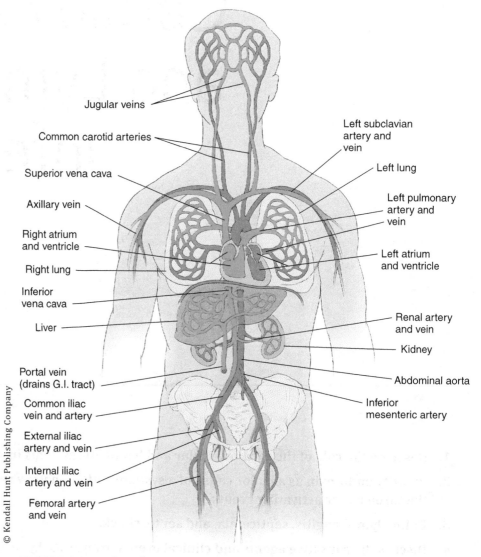

Jugular veins

Common carotid arteries

Superior vena cava

Axillary vein

Right atrium and ventricle

Right lung

Inferior vena cava

Liver

Portal vein (drains G.I. tract)

Common iliac vein and artery

External iliac artery and vein

Internal iliac artery and vein

Femoral artery and vein

Left subclavian artery and vein

Left lung

Left pulmonary artery and vein

Left atrium and ventricle

Renal artery and vein

Kidney

Abdominal aorta

Inferior mesenteric artery

© Kendall Hunt Publishing Company

FIGURE 23.1   Circulation

-Passive circulation of an organism in the bloodstream (no replication specified) is given a name ending in *-emia* that specifies the agent (e.g., bacteremia, viremia, fungemia, toxemia)

-When blood pressure falls due to a septicemia (bacteremia where the organism is actively replicating), the blood flow to vital organs is not sufficient and septic shock results

Heart: - Muscular pump in a fibrous sac called the pericardium

- Left and right sides separated by a septum

- Each side divided into an atrium (receives blood) and a ventricle (discharges blood)

- Heart valves at entrance and exit to each ventricle

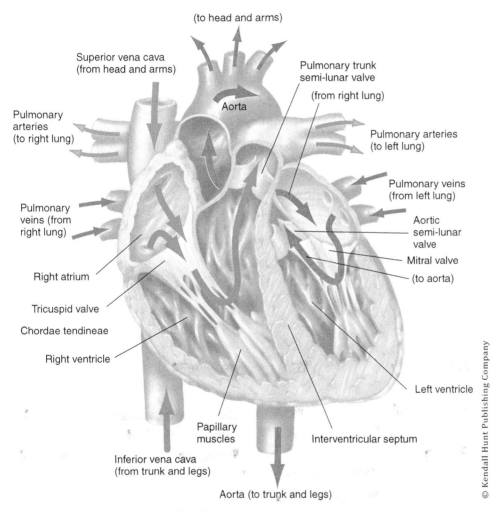

FIGURE 23.2 *Structure of the heart*

Arteries: - Vessels with thick muscular walls, transports oxygenated blood, under pressure

- Subject to atherosclerosis ("hardening of the arteries")

Veins: - Vessels that return to the heart and lungs from the tissues with blood depleted of oxygen; venous system has a series of valves to ensure the blood flows the right way

- Low pressure

Lymphatics: - System of lymphatic vessels begins in tissues as tiny tubes (resemble blood capillaries)

- Lymph or "interstitial fluid": colorless, thin fluid derived from plasma containing some white blood cells that have leaked out of the capillaries to the interstitial tissues
- Lymph vessels take up organisms and waste products for transport
- Valves in lymphatic vessels prevent backflow
- Vessels drain into the lymph nodes, which are tissue clumps with accumulations of phagocytes
- Lymph eventually discharges into a large vein
- Lymphangitis: spread of infectious agent up the lymphatic vessels causing inflammation (e.g., GAS, Sporothrix infections)

Spleen:
- Functions to clean the blood and produce antibodies
- Composed of two types of tissue:
1. Multiple blood-filled passages
2. Lymph tissue
- Patients without a spleen are very susceptible to infection with encapsulated organisms because this is where opsonizing antibodies are made

BACTERIAL INFECTIONS OF THE CARDIOVASCULAR AND LYMPHATIC SYSTEMS

Bacteremia: presence of bacteria in the blood; can be transient and have very few symptoms or progress to septicemia

Septicemia: presence of multiplying bacteria in the blood and elaboration of factors that can induce septic shock (e.g., LPS)

Sepsis: clinical evidence of an infection, plus evidence of a systemic response to infection

Two or more of:

Temperature >38 °C or <36 °C, heart rate >90

Respiratory rate >20/min, WBC >12,000

Sepsis syndrome: sepsis associated with organ dysfunction

Septic shock: sepsis with hypotension despite adequate fluid, plus perfusion abnormalities (e.g., lactic acidosis, oliguria, acute alteration in mental status)

↳ most often due to gram ⊖ infections, often nosocomial

Puerperal sepsis: - Nosocomial infection of the uterus with *S. pyogenes*

    - Progresses to the abdominal cavity (peritonitis) and septicemia

    - Very uncommon with good hygienic procedures

BACTERIAL INFECTION OF THE HEART

-Heart has three layers; inner layer = endocardium (epithelial cells) (this lines the heart and valves)

-Infection of the endocardium = endocarditis

Subacute Bacterial Endocarditis (SBE)

-Chronic-type picture, slowly progressing over months

-Infection of heart valves with bacteria in the bloodstream

-Common, often in persons with abnormal valves

-Characterized by fever, weakness, and heart murmur

-Usually caused by alpha-hemolytic streptococci from the oral cavity or enterococci, CNS (wimpy bacteria)

-Development of "vegetations" on the heart valves (which are really biofilms)

Acute Bacterial Endocarditis

-Rapidly progressive damage to heart valves by pyogenic bacteria

-Usually caused by *S. aureus*

-Often an infection occurring after open heart surgery

Pericarditis

-Inflammation of the heart sac (pericardium); often a complication of viral diseases

-Can be autoimmune

-Purulent pericarditis usually caused by *Streptococcus pyogenes*

Rheumatic Fever

-Sequelae of *Streptococcus pyogenes* (GAS) infection

-Autoimmune complication of streptococcal disease, occurs primarily in ages 4 to 18 years not treated with a beta-lactam

-First symptoms are arthritis and fever following an earlier streptococcal infection

-Damage to heart valves due to immune reaction of host defense to the M protein of *S. pyogenes*

-Ten percent get Sydenham's chorea (earlier called St. Vitus Dance)

BACTERIAL INFECTIONS OF THE BLOOD

How do bacteria get into the blood?

1. Breach of the body's natural first lines of defense (e.g., skin, trauma)

2. Infection and inflammation of tissues

   *examples: perforation/penetration of intestine

   appendicitis

   invasion (e.g., *Salmonella*)

   oral surgery, rift in gums

   kidney infection, lung infection

   catheters

Blood cultures

-Blood specimens are usually taken with a blood culture Vacutainer™-type system, at least one aerobic bottle and one anaerobic bottle taken

-Number of "sets" of blood cultures bottles depends on the clinical question

   *example: SBE (subacute endocarditis) may require as many as six sets of blood cultures over a day because there might not be many organisms free floating in blood

-Take blood cultures from **six different sites and "sticks"**

Most common organisms causing blood stream infections

   Staphylococcus aureus and *epidermidis*

   Streptococcus pneumoniae

   Enterococci *(Streptococcus faecalis)* —mostly found in older people

   Alpha-streptococci

   Gram negatives (e.g., *Escherichia coli* and *Klebsiella pneumoniae*)

Bacteria in the blood leads to **four** different scenarios:

1. Bacteremia that clears spontaneously

2. Bacteremia that seeds other areas of the body and causes focal infections

3. Sepsis

4. Septic shock

Bacterial sepsis

1. "Ordinary sepsis"

   - Caused by many different organisms but commonly *S. aureus* and *E. coli*

   - Often these organisms come from the patient's own body

- Initial events in sepsis
    - Vasodilation
    - Capillary leakage and reduced blood volume
    - Lack of oxygen to tissues
    - Hypotension and hypothermia, acidosis, hypoglycemia

2. "Septic shock"
    - Release of substances that inflame vascular system, such as histamine, serotonin, noradrenaline, plasma kinins
    - Macrophages release IL-1 (causes fever), TNF-α, etc.
    - Complement activation resulting in direct effect in vascular leakiness and chemotaxis of neutrophils
    - Neutrophil activation and degranulation
    - Endotoxin activates the blood clotting system resulting in abnormalities with blood flow leading to organ shutdown
    - From 30% to 35% mortality

* ON FINAL

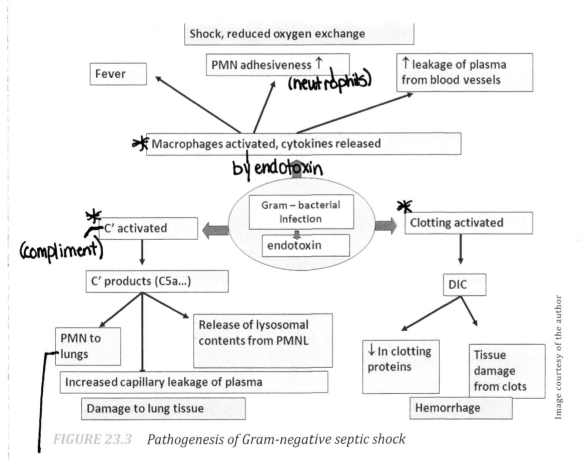

FIGURE 23.3 *Pathogenesis of Gram-negative septic shock*

(neutrophils)

by endotoxin

(compliment)

localizes neutrophils to lungs, releasing granules

Image courtesy of the author

Anthrax

-Caused by *Bacillus anthracis*, an aerobic, Gram-positive, spore-forming bacillus

-Three types of disease

 Cutaneous (most common)

 Pneumonic or inhalation

 Gastrointestinal (very rare in humans)

-Incubation 1 to 10 days, dependent on strain and dose

-Endospores are very hardy and survive for more than 50 years in soil

-Cause disease through toxin production

 Three toxins: protective antigen PA

       edema factor EF

       lethal factor LF

-Must have protective antigen (binding moiety) and at least one of the other factors for toxin to be effective

-Pulmonary anthrax (also called Woolsorters disease) has a high mortality rate

 - Progresses rapidly to damage tissues in lungs; causes hemorrhagic mediastinitis and systemic infection

-Vaccine poorly effective with many side effects

-Treat with antibiotics

-On the list of possible bioterrorism agents

Tularemia (Rabbit Fever)

-Caused by *Francisella tularensis*, a small, pleomorphic, Gram-negative bacillus
-Reservoir is usually rabbits

-Can be acquired by inhalation, ingestion or bites (mosquitoes), or handling of infected carcasses

-Symptoms

 - Local inflammation and ulcer formation at site of infection or pneumonic disease

-Lymph nodes enlarge and may contain pus
Can progress to septicemia, pneumonia, and abscesses through the body

-Low infective dose (10 organisms); untreated, 15% mortality

-Survives for long periods of time intracellularly in phagocytes

-Class 3 pathogen

-No vaccine

-Treat with antibiotics

-On the list of possible bioterrorism agents

Brucellosis

-Caused by *Brucella* sp., small, Gram-negative bacilli

-Three species of *Brucella* cause disease in animals and humans (undulant fever), usually reside in macrophages

-Most common type in North America is *Brucella abortus*

    Reservoirs are elk and bison

-Most common type in the rest of the world *Brucella melitensis*

    Reservoirs are sheep, goats, and camels

-Disease severity is related to infective species; *B. abortus* causes mild disease

-Often transmitted to humans through milk or through minute skin abrasions in people handling animal carcasses

-No vaccine

-Antibiotic treatment

Plague

-Caused by *Yersinia pestis*, a small, Gram-negative bacillus

-"Black death"—decimated world population several times over the ages, often transmitted by rat fleas

-Two types

Pneumonic:	high mortality; bacteria spread systemically and proliferate, causing septic shock and pneumonia; mortality 100% if not treated in the first day
Bubonic:	from flea bite; spreads to lymph and blood; causes "buboes," which are swellings of the lymph glands); mortality 50% to 75% if untreated

-Bacteria live in phagocytic cells and evade host defenses

-Found in wild rodents in North America

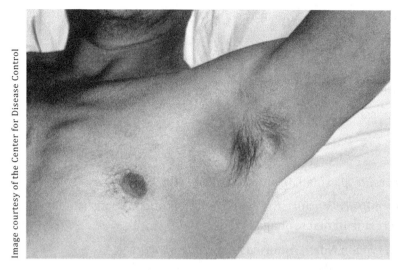

Image courtesy of the Center for Disease Control

FIGURE 23.4   Bubonic plague with a bubo in the armpit

Relapsing Fever

-Most cases caused by *Borrelia recurrentis*, a spirochete, but other species of *Borrelia* can also cause relapsing fever

-Tickborne disease; spread also by lice

-Last great epidemic in WWII—poor hygiene in trenches

-Still endemic in Central America, South America, and East Africa

-Symptoms

- Periods of high fever (when bacteria are circulating in the blood), severe headache, myalgia, arthralgia, lethargy, photophobia and cough, and rose-colored spots

- Hemorrhage is common: conjunctiva, petechiae, hemoptysis (blood in sputum), hematuria (blood in urine)

-Often self-limiting disease (due to production of antibodies in the host)

-No vaccine

-Antibiotic treatment

Lyme Disease

-Caused by *Borrelia burgdorferi*, a spirochete

-First identified in 1975 in Lyme, Connecticut, United States

-Tickborne disease (Ixodes ticks); tick must be attached for 24 hours

-First symptom is often a reddened ring around the site of a tick bite—this is called erythema migrans (bull's-eye rash)

-Not infectious; person-to-person

-If disease is not diagnosed but progresses, serious complications arise: heart damage, facial paralysis, meningitis, encephalitis, dementia, and arthritis are common

-Diagnosis by serology

-Endemic in northeastern United States; also found in Ontario and the maritimes

-No vaccine

-Antibiotic treatment

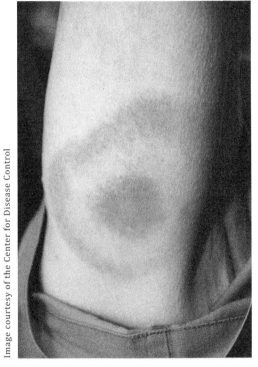

FIGURE 23.5 *Bull's-eye rash of Lyme disease*

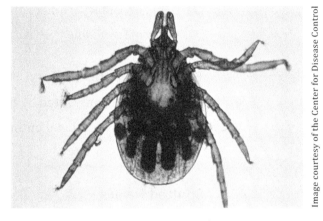

FIGURE 23.6 *Ixodes tick, nymph*

Ehrlichiosis

-Small, coccoid, Gram-negative, obligately intracellular bacteria

-Tickborne, Ixodes ticks

-HE: human granulocytic ehrlichiosis; bacteria live in the neutrophils of the host

-Several species causing disease in animals; horses commonly affected

-No vaccine

-Antibiotic treatment

Typhus

-Caused by *Rickettsia* sp. (intracellular Gram negatives)

-Spread by arthropod vectors; infect endothelial cells of the vascular system

-No vaccine

-Antibiotic treatment

-Epidemic typhus

- Caused by *R. prowazekii*; transmitted by body louse
- High prolonged fever for two weeks, stupor and rash of small red spots
- High mortality if untreated
- Vaccine available

Endemic Murine Typhus

- Sporadic, transmitted by the rat flea
- Texas has occasional outbreaks
- Milder disease type

Spotted Fevers

-Rocky Mountain spotted fever, caused by *R. rickettsii*

-Usually found in the eastern United States, not Rocky Mountains

-Tickborne

-Characteristic rash on palms and sole of feet with fever and headache

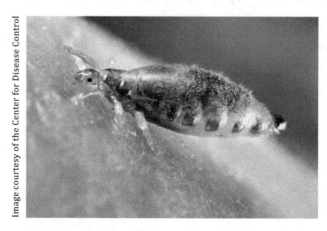

Image courtesy of the Center for Disease Control

FIGURE 23.7   Body louse

-Can be serious and cause kidney and heart failure

-No vaccine

-Antibiotic treatment

Pasteurella Multocida

-Small, Gram-negative bacillus

-Often found in mouths of domestic dogs and cats

-More often acquired from cat bites (bites are deep)

-If untreated, often will result in lymphangitis, developing to sepsis

-No vaccine

-Antibiotic treatment

Cat-Scratch Disease

-Usually caused by *Bartonella henselae,* a tiny, Gram-negative coccobacillus; affects primarily children

-Initial symptoms: papule at infection site, swelling of lymph nodes, malaise, fever

-Usually self-limiting, but can cause serious liver disease

-No vaccine

-Antibiotic treatment

VIRAL DISEASES OF THE CARDIOVASCULAR
AND LYMPHATIC SYSTEMS

Burkitt's Lymphoma

-Caused by EBV (HHV-4); most common childhood cancer in Africa, parts of Asia

-Occurs in same areas as malaria (theory that malaria suppresses the immune system, and this allows latent EBV to activate)

-Treatable with chemotherapy

Viral Hemorrhagic Fevers

-RNA viruses, enveloped

-Most are zoonotic diseases

-First symptoms are fever, chills, headache, nausea, and vomiting

-Followed by jaundice (liver damage)

Yellow Fever

-Classic viral hemorrhagic fever (VHF), RNA virus, enveloped (flavivirus)

-Transmitted by mosquito *(Aedes aegypti)*—a day biter

-Virus causes a hemorrhagic fever syndrome characterized by high viremia, and hepatic, renal, myocardial injury resulting in a high case-fatality rate

-Endemic in tropical South America and sub-Saharan Africa

-Monkeys are the natural host in the wild

- Sylvatic disease (monkey-to-monkey, monkey-to-person by mosquito)
- Urban disease (person-to-person) via mosquito

-Jaundice, fever, chills, nausea

-After three to four days, more severely ill patients with the classical yellow fever disease will develop bradycarditis, jaundice, and hemorrhagic complications

-Fifty percent of patients with severe YF will develop fatal disease

-Diagnosis by serology (finding of antibodies)

-No antiviral treatment

-Vaccine exists: formulated in 1939, attenuated

Dengue Fever

-Dengue fever virus: RNA enveloped, four serotypes, DEN-1 to DEN-4

-Similar symptoms to yellow fever but usually milder

-Transmitted by mosquitoes *(Aedes aegypti)*—day biters

-Endemic in tropics and Caribbean

-Increasing trend: 100 million cases/year worldwide

-Fever, muscle pain, joint pain, and rash

-Also called "breakbone fever"

-Rarely fatal

Dengue Hemorrhagic Fever

-More severe; causes shock within hours

-Thought that it occurs when a person who has had dengue fever with one serotype is infected with another serotype within a year or two of the first infection

-Antibody enhancement of infection

-Found more often in Southeast Asia than anywhere because all four sero-types circulate simultaneously

Other Viral Hemorrhagic Fevers

Ebola: RNA virus, enveloped

- Described 1976 in Africa; reservoir unknown (maybe bats)

- Highly lethal

Lassa: RNA virus, enveloped

- Described 1969; rodent reservoir; arenavirus; high mortality

-The aforementioned are transmitted by contact with body fluids from infected persons and are restricted in geographical location

Hemorrhagic fevers are transmitted by rodents

- Bolivian and Argentinian hemorrhagic fevers

- Hantavirus

Hepatitis

Hepatitis = inflammation **or** infection of the liver

-Caused by both infectious and noninfectious entities

-Infectious causes

Hepatitis A*

Hepatitis B

Hepatitis C

Hepatitis D   These viruses are different viruses, only named
                     similarly
Hepatitis E*

CMV

EBV

*Hepatitis A and E are discussed earlier in the lower alimentary tract infection chapter (Chapter 18)

Hepatitis B

-Enveloped DNA virus

-Tendency to develop a chronic infection, incubation period up to two months

-Typically transmitted by blood and body fluids (transfusions, needle sticks, IDU sharing of needles, coitus)

-Three separate particles found in human blood, but all of them contain the hepatitis B surface antigen (HBsAg)

Dane particle: complete virion

Spherical and filamentous particles: parts of the Dane particle

-Can be transmitted to the baby at birth, who then can have an increased chance to develop liver cancer in their lifetime

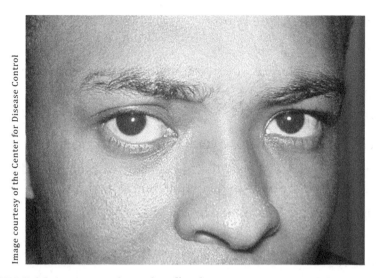

Image courtesy of the Center for Disease Control

FIGURE 23.8   Icteric (jaundiced) sclera in a patient with hepatitis

-Symptoms of hepatitis B (50% of cases asymptomatic): loss of appetite, nausea, low-grade fever, joint pains, jaundice

-Ten percent become chronic carriers, have HBeAg in blood

-Carriers have a high risk of liver disease progressing to cancer (200X higher than the normal uninfected population)

-There are 400 million HBV carriers worldwide

-Vaccination good: WHO has a goal to vaccinate all children

-Antiviral treatment is difficult; lamivudine is best, but there is an increasing problem with resistance

Hepatitis C

-Earlier called "non-A, non-B hepatitis"; seen after blood transfusions; known since 1989

-Enveloped RNA virus, high risk for chronic infection; at least six genotypes

-Long incubation period, 70 to 90 days, so difficult to rule out infection in blood donors with antibody tests: must use PCR

-Symptoms: insidious; symptoms may take years to appear (symptoms same as for hepatitis B)

-Eighty-five percent of infected persons become chronic

Twenty of the chronically infected get liver cancer or cirrhosis as a complication

-There are 100,000 new cases in the United States/year

-Major reason for liver transplantations

-Transmitted mostly by intravenous drug users: dirty needles DU (80%); only slight chance of sexual transmission

-Treatment: not very successful (depends on the genotype)

- Some success with alpha-interferon and ribavirin

-No vaccine

Hepatitis D

-DNA; discovered in 1977

-Hepatitis D needs to borrow the envelope from hepatitis B in order to survive, so it is dependent on the presence of hepatitis B

-Always together with HBV (coinfection)

-Combination of D and B much worse clinically than only B

CMV and EBV Virus (HHV-4 and HHV-5)

-DNA viruses, enveloped, cause hepatitis as a part of a systemic infection

-CMV is most commonly associated with transplant rejection, especially with solid organ transplants

-Transplant recipients are immunosuppressed—best would be if the donor is CMV negative, but the lack of available organs makes this impossible

-Ganciclovir used to prevent CMV infections from donor tissue for the first months after a transplant

-EBV can cause hepatitis but often lymphomas in immunosuppressed

TABLE 23.1   Summary of "Hepatitis Viruses"

	HAV	HBV	HCV	HDV	HEV
Transmission	Fecal–oral	Sexual contact, blood, body fluids, vertical transmission possible	Blood, sexual contact; vertical transmission possible	Blood contact; must have active HBV to get HDV; relatively rare	Fecal–oral, rare in North America
Symptoms of acute Infection	High fever, nausea, fatigue, dark urine, vomiting, jaundice. Symptoms last 1 wk–2 mo	Similar to HAV. 30%–50% develop acute infection (symptomatic) within 4 wk to 6 mo	Similar to HAV though most people with HCV (75%) do not have early symptoms	Similar to HAV though usually more severe	Similar to HAV, but high mortality rate for pregnant women (20%)
Life-long Infection?	No, not chronic; most people clear the virus completely	Yes, but most adults clear the virus; <5% chronically infected. Of these, 15%–20% die of cirrhosis or liver cancer	Yes, but 15%–25% clear the virus, 75%–85% become chronically infected, 5%–20% develop cirrhosis, and 1%–4% develop liver cancer	Yes, when a person is infected with HDV and HBV simultaneously, this is called a coinfection.	No, HEV is not chronic
Vaccine? Treatment?	HAV vaccine Immune globulin shots within 2 wk of exposure to avoid illness. No antiviral	HBV vaccine HBIG to prevent illness or reduce severity. Treatment: alfa-interferon, lamivudine	No vaccine, no postexposure prophylaxis. Pegylated alfa-interferon and ribavirin	Vaccination against HBV prevents HDV infection. No antiviral	No vaccine for HEV; no antiviral except symptomatic relief

Chagas Disease

-Caused by *Trypanosoma cruzi*, a flagellated protozoan

-Also called American Trypanosomiasis

-Transmitted by insect vector "reduviid bug" or "kissing bug"

-Reservoir in rodents, opossums, and armadillos

-Very common in South America, Central America, and parts of the southern United States

-Insect bites human, defecates, and rubs feces into the bite wound

-Most dangerous to children (10% mortality)

-Damage to heart, nerves

-Typical nerve paralysis in eye ("eye of Romana")

-Treatment is difficult

Toxoplasmosis

-Caused by *Toxoplasma gondii*, a protozoan

-Reservoir: domestic cats (have no apparent illness)

-Oocysts are ingested, release sporozoites that invade the host cells, become tachyzoites

-Progress to a chronic form; results in formation of tissue cysts

-Mild symptoms in persons with healthy immune systems

-Most dangerous if pregnant woman is infected: congenital damage to fetus (brain damage and vision problems)

-Loss of immune function (e.g AIDS) allows the reactivation of the tissue cyst

Malaria

-Caused by *Plasmodium* sp., protozoan; vector is the Anopheles mosquito

-Symptoms are chills, fever, vomiting, headache in intervals of two to three days, depending on which of the four species is the infecting organism

-Four species that exclusively infect humans

P. vivax: "benign" malaria

P. ovale

P. malariae

P. falciparum: most dangerous type, "malignant"

- 50% mortality untreated; tendency to cause cerebral malaria

- Highest percentage parasitemia

- Growing problem with development of resistance to drugs

New emergent species: *P. knowlesi* (monkey malaria), especially in southeast Asia; resembles *P. malariae* and can be wrongly diagnosed

-Worldwide prevention measures include mosquito control and use of disinfectant-soaked bed nets

Leishmaniasis

-More than 20 species of *Leishmania* can cause disease, but there are three main species causing disease in humans

> *L. donovani:* "kala azar"; visceral disease in internal organs, often fatal; symptoms resemble malaria
>
> *L. tropica:* "Oriental sore"—skin and mucous membrane lesions
>
> *L. braziliensis:* skin and mucous membrane lesions also called "American leishmaniasis"

-Transmitted by the bite of the sandfly (tropics and the Mediterranean)

-All types cause disfiguring or fatal disease, depending on type

Babesiosis

-Tickborne protozoan, even in United States (northeastern States)

-Symptoms are chills and fever; resembles malaria

-Replication of parasite in the red blood cell

-Most significant effect of infection is anemia

-The same ticks carry Lyme disease (*Ixodes* ticks), so patients may have more than one microorganism causing an infection

HELMINTHIC DISEASES OF THE CV AND THE LYMPH SYSTEMS

Schistosoma

-Caused by a fluke; infection by contact with contaminated water

-Also called "Bilharzia"

-Snail is part of the life cycle: produce cercariae that penetrate the intact skin

-Adult worms live in veins of liver (*S. mansoni*), bladder (*S. hematobium*), or intestine (*S. japonicum*)

> *S. haematobium*: or urinary schistosomiasis, results in inflammation of the bladder and leads to bladder cancer

> *S. japonicum* and *S. mansoni*: intestinal inflammation; liver damage especially with *mansoni*

-Disease manifestations usually result from the host immune response to the eggs

-Adult worms coat themselves with substances from the host that enable them to escape the notice of the immune system

Swimmer's Itch

-Common in Canada and the northern part of United States

-Usually contracted by swimming in infected lakes

-Bird (duck) *Schistosoma* penetrate the outer layer of skin and cause a local allergic reaction but do not penetrate deeper or spread systemically

-Self limiting disease

Interested? Want to learn more?

For more reading, several texts online at the U of A library are recommended:

1. Brooks, GF, Carroll KC, Butel JS, Morse SA, editors. Jawetz, Melnick, and Adelberg's Medical Microbiology, 24th ed. Blacklick OH-McGraw Hill; 2007.

2. Ryan KJ, Ray CG, editors. Sherris Medical Microbiology, 5th ed. New York – McGraw-Hill, 2010.

3. Mandell GL, Bennett JE,Dolin R, editors. Mandell, Douglas and Bennett's Principles and Practices of Infectious Diseases, 7th ed. Churchill Livingstone Elsevier, Philadelphia, 2010.

Chapter 24

HIV and Immunodeficiency

Learning Objectives:

1. Describe HIV as the cause of AIDS.
2. Explain how the HIV virus integrates into the human genome.
3. Identify how the immune system of patients with HIV is compromised.
4. Define opportunistic infections, and describe some of the common indicator infections.
5. Identify elements of HAARTS.
6. List major health risks to healthcare workers.

HIV = Human Immunodeficiency Virus

-RNA retrovirus, enveloped

-Origin unknown; earliest documented case from 1959 in Leopoldville in Africa

-In North America: cluster of cases in Los Angeles county in 1981: first noticed outbreak of HIV disease

-Had been known as "skinny disease" in Africa due to the wasting effects of the disease

-Untreated HIV infection progresses to AIDS (acquired immunodeficiency syndrome)

-No vaccine exists yet; research ongoing

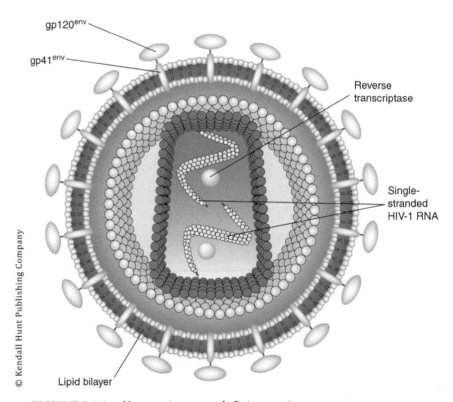

FIGURE 24.1   *Human immunodeficiency virus structure*

Subtypes of HIV

1. HIV-1:   has 11 subtypes (clades); major type of HIV
2. HIV-2:   found in West Africa; much slower infection

-"Global pandemic"

-According to the UN, as of May 2011, 34 million people infected worldwide and 7000 infected every day (half of these do not know they have HIV)

-More than 30 million people have died from AIDS in the past 30 years

-Leading cause of death in sub-Saharan Africa

-Originally thought to be a disease of homosexuals because this was the first group it was found in, but heterosexuals are more numerous, and the rate of disease is increasing at a more rapid rate

- Africa: HIV has always been primarily heterosexual; in some urban areas prevalence is 30% of the population

- Asia, Russia, Middle East: HIV mostly in IDU, prostitutes, and young heterosexual males

Transmission

-Usually bloodborne; also sexual transmission with body fluids; vertical transmission possible

-HIV is enveloped and can be easily inactivated by simple disinfectants (e.g., alcohol) and soaps

Infectivity and Pathogenicity of HIV

-HIV virus contains two strands of RNA, reverse transcriptase enzyme and a glycolipid envelope with protein spikes called gp120

-HIV attaches to the target host cell (human CD4+ T lymphocytes, macrophages, and dendritic cells)

-HIV must attach to both CD4+ and CXCR4 or CCR5 (T cells and macrophages) receptors to gain entry to the cell

-In the host cell, viral RNA is released and transcribed into DNA by reverse transcriptase

-The newly formed viral DNA is incorporated into the human DNA chromosome by the enzyme integrase

-The new DNA formed can either produce more viruses or can remain latent as a provirus, which is not detected by the immune system

-Five percent of individuals never progress to disease

-Can undergo rapid changes in antigenic makeup to help it evade the host defenses, and this contributes to drug resistance (recall that RNA viruses have no proofreading capacity)

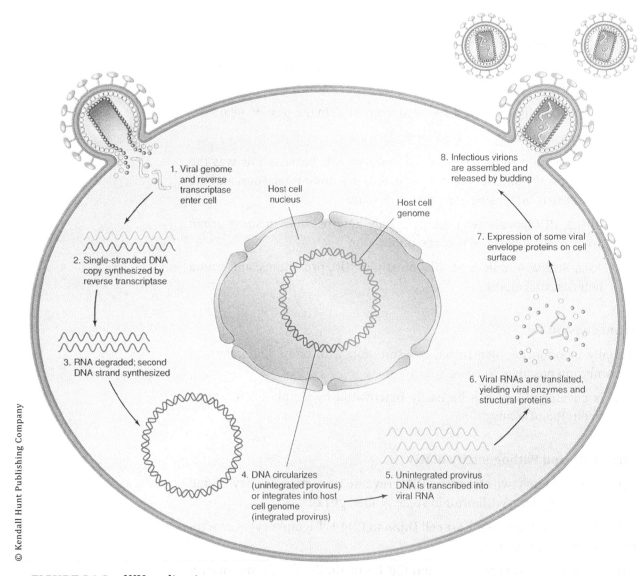

FIGURE 24.2   *HIV replication*

Stages of HIV Infection

Stage A: -Infection can be asymptomatic, subclinical, or may cause chronic swollen lymph nodes

-CD4+ cells: >800/mm3

Stage B: - Called ARC (AIDS-related complex)

-Persistent infections by opportunists like *C. albicans*, VZV, *Cryptosporidium* sp.

-CD4+ cells: 200–800/mm3

Stage C: -Clinical AIDS

-Defined by "indicator conditions" such as *C. albicans* infections of the respiratory mucosa, CMV eye infections, TB, *Pneumocystis jiroveci* pneumonia (PVP), toxoplasmosis of the brain, and Kaposi's sarcoma

-CD4+ cells < 200/mm3

Initial Symptoms of HIV

-Mild, flu-like illness, may go unnoticed

-Most common symptoms are fever, adenopathy, pharyngitis, rash myalgia/arthralgia, thrombocytopenia, leukopenia, diarrhea, nausea

Monitoring of Disease

-Very important as this determines the course of treatment, usually done by two methods:

1. Viral load : number of HIV particles in blood
2. Numbers of CD4+ cells

- Less than 200/mm^3 is indicative of clinical AIDS

(normal CD4+ cells live a few months, but infected CD4+ cells only live two days and are cleared by the immune system)

CLINICAL MANIFESTATIONS OF HIV INFECTION

Oral Disease

-Oral candidiasis: usually caused by *C. albicans* (thrush)

-Results from impaired cellular immunity

-Oral leukoplakia: raised, nonscrapable white lesions usually on tongue caused by EBV (usually asymptomatic)

-Gingivitis and periodontitis: associated with severe pain, bleeding gums, loosening of teeth

-Oral ulcers: HSV-1, HSV-2, CMV

Musculoskeletal Complications

-Polymyositis

   - Myalgia, muscle tenderness, wasting, fatigue

-Pyomyositis

   Skin flora is often found in wound cultures

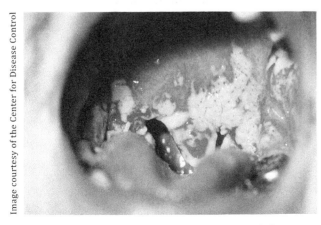

FIGURE 24.3   *Oral thrush due to Candida albicans*

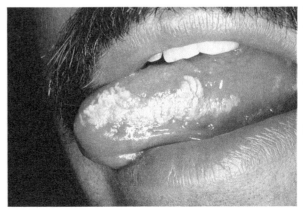

FIGURE 24.4   *Oral hairy leukoplakia due to Epstein–Barr virus*

Cutaneous Manifestations

-Viral infections of the skin and mucous membranes

-Exanthem of acute HIV is an erythematous morbilliform eruption of trunk and upper arms

-HSV-1 and HSV-2, VZV, CMV, HPV

Bacillary Angiomatosis

-Lesions characterized by vascular proliferation, hemorrhage, and necrosis

-Can be subcutaneous nodules

-Caused by *Bartonella henselae* (cat-scratch disease agent) and *Bartonella quintana*

Kaposi's Sarcoma

-Vascular neoplastic disorder

-Associated with presence of HHV-8; treated by radiotherapy

-Appear as cutaneous red–purple nodules or plaques

-Sites usually affected: legs, feet, mucous membranes, hard palate, nose, trunk, and scalp

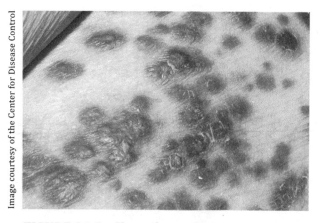

FIGURE 24.5   Kaposi's sarcoma

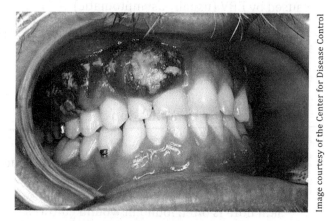

FIGURE 24.6   Oral Kaposi's sarcoma

Image courtesy of the Center for Disease Control

Scabies

-Common in AIDS patients

-*Sarcoptes scabei* mite: usually on palms, soles, trunk, or extremities instead of between fingers and on wrists (pattern in immunocompetent)

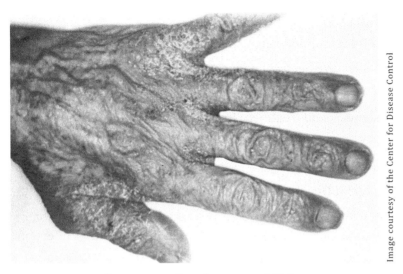

FIGURE 24.7 *"Norwegian" scabies in an AIDS patient*

Renal Disease and HIV

-HIV-associated nephropathy

-Occurs in 2% to 10% of cases

Ocular Infection and HIV

-Very common; ranges from benign HIV retinopathy to sight-threatening viral infections

-Most common viral cause is CMV—very serious!

-VZV retinitis: severe necrotizing retinitis

-Ocular toxoplasmosis

-*Pneumocystis jiroveci* choroiditis

Cardiac Manifestations of HIV Disease

-Common in HIV/AIDS

-Cardiac abnormalities include opportunistic infections or diseases of the myocardium (*T. gondii*, *T. cruzi*) or pericardium (TB, KS)

-Infectious endocarditis (especially in IDU)

-Accelerated atherosclerosis

-Pulmonary hypertension, dilated cardiomyopathy, left ventricular dysfunction

Pulmonary Disease and AIDS

-Leading cause of mortality and morbidity in HIV-infected patients

-Common causes of pneumonia in AIDS: *Pneumocystis jiroveci* pneumonia (PVP), bacterial pneumonia, *M. tuberculosis*, *M. kansasii*, *M. avium* complex, viral pneumonia, fungal pneumonia

Pneumocystis Pneumonia (PJP)

-Insidious onset, opportunistic infection

-Most people have been colonized with this as children

-Intact cell-mediated immunity important

-Early diagnosis and treatment important

-Treatment trimethoprim-sulfa

-No purulent sputum

Mycobacterial Disease

-Those infected with HIV have an increased risk for reactivation of latent infections and increased risk of symptomatic disease after infection

-Usually occurs as the first infectious complication of HIV

-Increased incidence of disseminated TB and MDR-TB, XDR-TB

-Opportunistic infections with *M. avium*-complex common (systemic infection with bacteremia, sepsis)

Protozoan Disease

-*Toxoplasma gondii*: fever, cough, dyspnea, septic shock

Gastrointestinal and Hepatobiliary Disease with HIV

-Esophageal disease: due to inflammation or ulceration caused by infectious agents and noninfectious processes

> *C. albicans*, CMV, HSV, VZV, *M. tuberculosis*, *H. capsulatum*, *P. jiroveci*, and primary HIV

-Stomach disease: CMV gastritis and Kaposi's sarcoma

-Gallbladder: CMV, cryptosporidium, microsporidium

-Liver: very common complication with HIV

> - Often CMV, EBV, HAV, HBV, HCV, adenovirus

> - Also Mycobacterium, esp. *M. avium*-complex, fungi

-Pancreas: disease often due to lifestyle choices (e.g., alcohol abuse) but also to CMV, Cryptosporidium, Candida, Toxoplasma, *P. jiroveci*

-Small and large intestine: diarrhea is a common problem in HIV

> -Small bowel diseases and colitis

> -Common with *Salmonella, Shigella, Campylobacter, E. coli, Listeria, C. difficile* in hospitalized patients, parasites such as cryptosporidium, *E. histolytica, G. lamblia*, also viruses such as CMV

> - CMV most significant cause of enterocolitis—can lead to intestinal perforation

> - Proctitis in HIV is usually associated with STI

Neurologic Manifestations of HIV

-Neurologic complications in 39% to 70% of patients

-Dementia, neuropathy, myelopathy

-(HIV)-1 enters the CNS soon after infection

-Cognitive impairment usually in later stages of AIDS

-Some neurologic complications are due to the toxicity of the drugs

-Headaches, seizures, strokes are common

-Brain abscesses with bacteria, fungi, and protozoa common

HIV AND PREGNANCY

Perinatal Transmission

-From 14% to 33% of babies are infected if mother has untreated HIV

-Less than 1% if mother has adequately treated HIV

-HIV can be transmitted to fetus during gestation (late pregnancy), at delivery, or by breast-feeding

-Maternal viral load most important factor in determining risk for fetus

-Vitamin A deficiency in pregnancy—adds increased risk of transmission

-Elective Caesarian reduce the risk of transmission

Impact of HIV on Pregnancy Outcome

-Maternal HIV is not associated with fetal anomalies, premature delivery, or low birth weight

-Infection of the embryo seems to occur more often in the last two months

-HIV **not** a cause of spontaneous abortion

-Mother's CD4+ count should be closely monitored and the appropriate anti retroviral therapy given

Pediatric HIV Infection

-Infection with HIV is usually asymptomatic during the first few months of life

-Mean age at onset of symptoms is 1 year

-Generalized lymphadenopathy, hepatomegaly, splenomegaly, failure to thrive, oral candidiasis, recurrent diarrhea, parotitis, cardiomyopathy, hepatitis, nephropathy, CNS disease, lymphoid interstitial pneumonia, recurrent invasive bacterial infections, opportunistic infections, and some malignancies

-*Pneumocystis jiroveci* pneumonia (PVP) is the most common serious opportunistic infection in children with HIV (three to six months of age)

Diagnosis of HIV

-Serology for demonstration of HIV antibodies

- ELISA tests, positives are confirmed by Western Blotting

-rtPCR for quantitative measurement of numbers of viral particles in blood

-Clinical assessment of the "indicator infections" and CD4+ levels

Transmission of HIV

-Transfer or direct contact with infected body fluids

-Blood most important, highest viral load (up to 100,000 viruses per ml)

-Semen also important (up to 50 viruses/ml)

-HIV does not survive long if in the environment

-Intimate sexual contact, breast milk, vertical transmission to the fetus, blood contamination from needles, organ transplants, artificial insemination, blood transfusion

-Vaginal intercourse more effective than other modes for transmitting virus from male to female

-Transmission is more efficient if there are lesions present in the area (e.g., soft and hard chancres)

Treatment and Prevention of HIV

Prevention: most important because there are no vaccines available yet

examples: condoms very important, reduction in IDU (intravenous drug users) numbers, changes in attitudes and behaviors

Vaccines:

-Rapid mutation of HIV causes extreme problems in production of an effective vaccine

- Vaccine projects are ongoing: for example, AIDSVAX in Thailand
- Most vaccines are made against the gp120 and the other glycolipid proteins in the envelope

Chemotherapy:
1. First target was the reverse transcriptase (AZT)
2. Nucleoside analogues block production of viral DNA
3. Protease inhibitors cut proteins that are inserted into the envelope of new viral particles
4. Integrase, which inserts the viral DNA into the host DNA
5. Chemokine receptor inhibitors next drugs coming

PROBLEM: rapid development of resistance to every drug yet introduced

Immunotherapy: has been started on a trial basis, using IL-2 (interleukin causing the production of antiviral proteins by other cells

-So far it has been found that the IL-2 may cause increases in CD4+ cells

Gene therapy: collect patient's own T cells and engineer them to recognize and destroy HIV-infected T cells (trials are ongoing)

Microbial agents as "biotherapy": genetically engineered cow virus that attaches to the gp120, enters the cells, and kills the cells infected with HIV

HAARTS = highly active antiretroviral therapy

-Not a magic bullet

-Potent cocktail of anti-HIV drugs

-Many unpleasant side effects including nausea; similar to cancer chemotherapy treatments

Deleterious side effects of HAARTS

-Nucleoside-related toxic effects: neuropathy, pancreatitis, hepatic stenosis, lactic acidosis, lipoatrophy

-Metabolic complications: fat redistribution, insulin resistance, hyperlipidemia

-Bone disease: osteopenia and/or osteoporosis

RISK FOR TRANSMISSION OF HIV TO HEALTHCARE WORKERS

-Total of 23 studies of needle sticks among HCW showed transmission in 20/6135 (0.33%) with HIV

HBV is 37% to 62%, HCV is 23% to 37%

-With mucosal membrane exposure (eye, mouth), risk is 0.09%

-As of June 2000, there were 56 HCW in the United States who had seroconverted and were diagnosed with HIV. Major occupations of these:

>Nurses (23)

>Lab techs (20)

>Physicians (6)

Note: all transmissions involved blood or body fluid.

Risks for Seroconversion

1. Deep injury
2. Visible blood on the device
3. Needle placement in an artery or vein
4. Source with late-stage HIV infection and high viral load

-Risk assessment will dictate what postexposure prophylaxis is used on the HCW

> examples: low risk with low viral load: two-drug combination
> high risk (major blood splash) from a patient with a high viral load: three-drug combination

-Greatest risk to seroconvert in the first six months

-PEP (postexposure prophylaxis) should be started early, preferably within 1 to 2 hours of exposure and up to 36 hours

-Four-week course of drugs, monitoring of antibody levels for at least one year

Common side effects of PEP (postexposure prophylaxis):

> Two drugs: 63% get side effects
>
> > nausea, vomiting, diarrhea, fatigue, headache
>
> Three drugs: 83% get side effects
>
> > same

Common Causes of Immunosuppression Other than HIV

Congenital Immune Deficiencies

> examples: CGD, agammaglobulinemia

Acquired Immune Deficiencies

- Caused by drugs, chronic disease (e.g., diabetes), cancers (e.g., Hodgkin's disease lowers the CMI), infectious agents (e.g., HIV), removal of spleen, transplants, and antirejection drugs taken (e.g., bone marrow, organs)

-Most common is the acquired immune defect

-Regardless of whether the patient has a congenital or acquired immune defect, he/she will have an increased risk for infection with both opportunistic and pathogenic organisms

-Antibiotic treatment is often not as effective in these patients as in patients with normal immune systems

-The normal immune system usually works in conjunction with antibiotics to eliminate or inactivate the infecting microorganism.

General Precautions for Preventing Infection in Immunocompromised Patients

-Includes all causes of immunosuppression, genetic or acquired

-Routine microbiological surveillance of rooms to detect fungi, Pseudomonas, etc.

-Laminar airflow or HEPA-filtered rooms for bone marrow transplants and oncology patients in areas with high incidences of mold infections

-Adequate hand washing still the best precaution

-Discourage any visitors with coughs or other infections

Chemoprophylaxis for Immunocompromised Patients

-Intravenous immunoglobulin administration in patients with recurrent bacterial infections or exposure to VZV

-Vaccination of patients if possible before splenectomy with *S. pneumoniae, H. influenzae, Neisseria meningitidis,* and hepatitis B

-Certain immunosuppressed may need prophylactic antibiotics

-Bone marrow transplants; usually use antifungals and antivirals

-Antivirals in all transplants (e.g., ganciclovir to prevent CMV)

-Prophylactic trimethoprim-sulfa against *P. jiroveci*

Interested? Want to learn more?

For more reading, several texts online at the U of A library are recommended:

1. Brooks, GF, Carroll KC, Butel JS, Morse SA, editors. Jawetz, Melnick, and Adelberg's Medical Microbiology, 24th ed. Blacklick OH-McGraw Hill; 2007.

2. Ryan KJ, Ray CG, editors. Sherris Medical Microbiology, 5th ed. New York – McGraw-Hill, 2010.

3. Mandell GL, Bennett JE,Dolin R, editors. Mandell, Douglas and Bennett's Principles and Practices of Infectious Diseases, 7th ed. Churchill Livingstone Elsevier, Philadelphia, 2010.

Chapter 25

Laboratory Techniques for Diagnosis of Infection

Learning Objectives:

1. Describe the most commonly used routine culture media for human pathogens.
2. Differentiate between aerobic and anaerobic cultures.
3. List the methods used routinely to identify bacteria.
4. Explain how hemolytic reactions, the coagulase test, and the catalase test can help to differentiate Gram-positive organisms from one another.
5. Familiarize yourself with the techniques that can be used for identification.

Culture and Identification of Bacteria

Although the trend in modern clinical microbiology laboratories is going toward the increased use of molecular biology for identifying and typing isolates of human pathogens, culture remains a mainstay in the diagnosis of infection. If we can isolate a pathogen from a clinical specimen, then we can perform antibiotic susceptibility tests on the isolate to provide good information for the treatment of the infection, and we can also type and subtype the organisms for epidemiological tracking.

Culture of specimens is normally done using a standard battery of culture media, unless there are specific concerns about the identity of the infecting organism (e.g., *Francisella tularensis*, *Legionella pneumophila*, *Mycobacterium tuberculosis*—all of which require special additives to the routine culture media to ensure growth and proper identification of the organism).

STANDARD CULTURE MEDIA FOR ISOLATION OF BACTERIA FROM CLINICAL SPECIMENS

Aerobic Cultures

Blood agar plate (incubated in 5% CO_2)

Chocolate agar place (incubated in 5% CO_2)—chocolate agar is blood agar that has been heated at 56 °C to lyse the red blood cells. Certain bacteria, for example, *Haemophilus influenzae* will not grow on blood agar but will grow on chocolate agar

MacConkey plate (for isolation of Gram negatives) incubated aerobically

Anaerobic Cultures

Blood containing prereduced agar incubated anaerobically

Selective culture plate usually containing laked blood (blood cells are hemolyzed)

Broth medium, usually thioglycollate

Specimens arriving at the lab are registered and sent for processing according to the origin of the specimen and any special clinical considerations. Gram's stains are done on the swabs, approximate numbers of the different types of bacteria seen and the presence/absence of neutrophils is noted, culture plates are streaked, and a portion of the specimen (sometimes the swab) is inoculated to an anaerobic broth medium. All plates are incubated at 37 °C for 24 hours before they are inspected for growth; then after suspected bacterial colonies have been subcultured, plates are returned to the incubators for further incubation. Some bacteria grow quickly and will appear as small colonies or "heaps" of bacteria on the surface of the agar plates after only 18 to 24 hours, and others need more time to become visible.

Once it has been ascertained that there is growth of bacteria, further identification is done to give the bacteria a name and/or serotype, which may be very important for epidemiological tracking purposes.

Laboratory Methods for Identification of Bacteria

1. **Morphology**: the appearance of "colonies" on agar plates gives a clue as to the identity of the bacterium, and the ability of the bacteria to grow on the different media types is also part of the identification process.

    *examples: appearance and color of colonies, presence of hemolysis on blood agar, and smell

2. **Gram's stain**: Gram-positive or Gram-negative cocci, bacilli, or spiral and any characteristic arrangements of the organism

3. **Growth characteristics**: that is, anaerobe, aerobe, facultative

    Requirement for 5% CO_2

    Odor: can distinguish certain bacteria based on the smell of the breakdown products they produce (sometimes this is a pleasant smell and sometimes not!)

4. **Further identification** of genus and species by testing for bacterial enzymes and by-products of metabolic processes. A few examples:

Staphylococcus aureus produces a DNase that breaks down DNA. This can differentiate it from other staphylococcal species that do not produce the enzyme. An agar plate is made containing DNA, and the staphylococcus strain bacterial strain is streaked on it and incubated overnight for growth. The next day the plate is flooded with HCl, which precipitates DNA in the plate and causes the agar to go cloudy. A clear zone around the growing staphylococcus strain indicates that this is an *S. aureus*.

Staphylococcus aureus also produces an enzyme called "coagulase," which converts soluble fibrinogen to insoluble fibrin. This is a test that differentiates *S. aureus* from other *staphylococci*. A positive coagulase test will result in the reporting of *S. aureus;* if the strain is coagulase negative, then "CNS" or coagulase-negative *staphylococci* will be reported. CNS will be typed and speciated if the specimen is from a normally sterile site but will not likely be worked up if the isolate is from a sore.

Coagulase Test

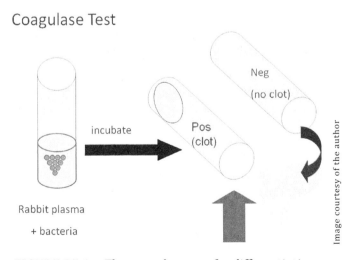

FIGURE 25.1   *The coagulase test for differentiating* S. aureus *from other* staphylococci

Hemolysis on blood agar plates in conjunction with specific colony morphologies is enough to allow the experienced bacteriologist to differentiate between most strains of beta-hemolytic staphylococcus and streptococcus, but if in doubt, a catalase test can be done.

Catalase Test

-Catalase breaks down hydrogen peroxide to CO_2 and H_2O; mixing the bacterial strain in a drop of hydrogen peroxide and then observing for bubbles of gas will give a positive test, indicative of the presence of the catalase enzyme indicating a staphylococcus strain.

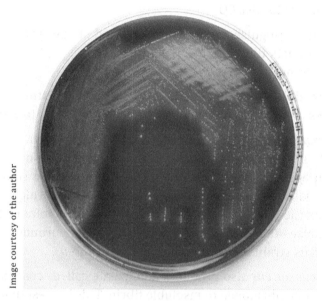

Image courtesy of the author

FIGURE 25.2   *Beta-hemolysis on blood agar*

Proteus species produce urease, which can be tested for by inoculating the bacterial isolate in a medium containing urea and a pH indicator. If the bacteria produce urease, urea will be broken down to ammonia, raising the pH of the medium and changing the color of the medium due to the pH indicator.

Bacteria can be tested for their ability to use certain carbohydrates for an energy source, and the breakdown product (often acid) will cause a change in pH of the medium, which can be seen if there is a pH indicator present. Enteric bacteria (Enterobacteriaceae—Gram-negative rods that grow on MacConkey medium) are often subtyped to the genus and species level using fermentation panels.

MacConkey culture media contains, in addition to nutrients for growth, crystal violet, which inhibits the growth of Gram-positive bacteria; bile salts, which inhibit the swarming activity of Proteus (necessary; otherwise any Proteus bacteria present can swarm all over the surface of the plate and hide other species that might be important); and neutral red, a pH indicator that is colorless at neutral pH and red at acidic pH. *Escherichia coli* can ferment lactose; *Shigella* species do not, so in this case, an *E. coli* would break down the lactose to acids and cause a change in the pH of the medium, shifting the color of the pH indicator from colorless to red. *E. coli* would then appear as red-colored colonies, and the *Shigella* remain as white colonies.

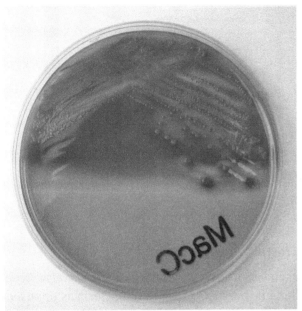 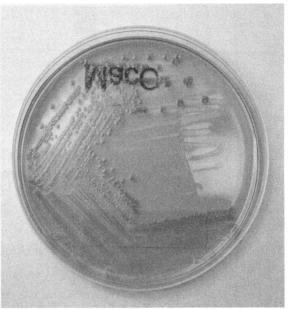

a *Lactose fermenter*   **b** *Lactose nonfermenter*

FIGURE 25.3 a and b   MacConkey agar: selective and differential for Gram negatives

There is a multitude of tests that can be done after the Gram's staining of the isolate in order to identify bacteria into families, genera, and species. Many diagnostic companies now make this easier by offering panels of media and tests for enzymes in an easy-to-perform test. Choice of identification tests depends on the characteristics of the bacterium isolated (e.g., fermenter, nonfermenter of lactose if a Gram negative, etc.).

Common Rapid Identification Systems for ID of Bacteria

1. **Multisystem tests** (i.e., Enterotube, API, Minitek): each of these are available for different types of bacteria (e.g., API Staph, API enteric, API anaerobic)

-Systems consisting of a plastic holder with many different types of media, the bacteria are inoculated to the system then incubated, and the reactions are read from all the different "test compartments" in the system. The probable bacterial ID can be determined for most bacteria that are medically important. A score is derived from the pattern of positive/negative reactions in the different tests, and this is compared to computer derived-lists, and a probable bacterial genus and species is arrived at.

2. **Slide agglutination**

-Bacteria are mixed with a reagent antibody; if the antigen and antibody bind, there will be visible agglutination

-Used often for identification of bacteria in CSF and for the subtyping, or grouping, of bacteria (i.e., hemolytic streptococci—groups A, B, C, G)

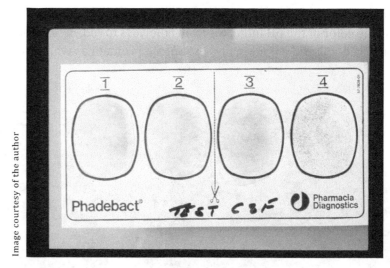

FIGURE 25.4   *Slide agglutination test*

3. Fluorescent antibody tests

-These tests are generally used when searching for a specific bacterial type in a specimen and can be done if there is a mixture of bacteria as opposed to the other typing procedures, which rely on a "pure culture"

-Reagent antibody labeled with a fluorochrome (e.g., fluorescein isothiocyanate or FITC) is allowed to react with the bacterial isolate or specimen, and after washing excess reagent away, slides containing specimens and antibodies are read in a microscope with an ultraviolet light source. Bacteria that match the specificity of the reagent antibody will glow bright apple green when UV light is shone upon them

-Typically used for *Bordetella pertussis*, cause of whooping cough, respiratory syncytial virus, among others

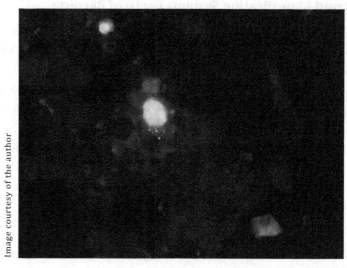

FIGURE 25.5   *Direct fluorescent antibody test (DFA)*

4. DNA composition and molecular biology techniques

-The DNA sequence of most bacteria have a set ratio of cytosine and guanine; the closer the match, the more related the bacteria

-Sequencing of RNA and DNA

-PCR: polymerase chain reaction (detection of specific sequences of nucleotides in a specimen)

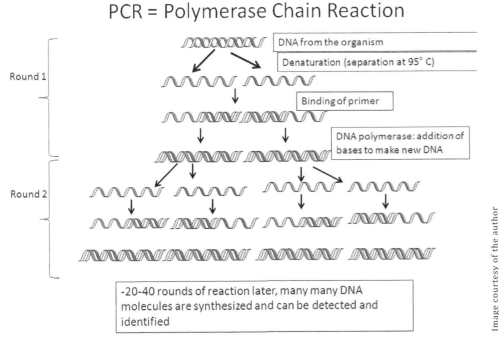

PCR = Polymerase Chain Reaction

DNA from the organism

Denaturation (separation at 95° C)

Round 1

Binding of primer

DNA polymerase: addition of bases to make new DNA

Round 2

-20-40 rounds of reaction later, many many DNA molecules are synthesized and can be detected and identified

Image courtesy of the author

FIGURE 25.6   *PCR reaction*

ANTIMICROBIAL SENSITIVITY TESTING

MIC = minimum inhibitory concentration

MBC = minimal bactericidal concentration

MIC: the lowest antibiotic concentration that prevents visible growth of bacteria

- Important to know so that antimicrobials are not overprescribed in unnecessarily high doses

- Important for choice of an antimicrobial to treat an infection caused by a specific organism

- Also important to know as there is some toxicity associated with some drugs, and if we know the MIC, we can dose under the level where the toxic effects begin

Methodology for Testing Antimicrobial susceptibilities

1. **Broth dilution**: bacteria are grown to a standardized concentration in broth, and different dilutions or amounts of an antibiotic are added. Broths are then incubated at 37 °C, and the tubes are observed for evidence of cloudiness signaling growth of bacteria.

    MBC occurs at the point where the antibiotic concentration was high enough to kill the bacteria.

2. **E-test**: bacteria are spread over the surface of an ordinary agar plate, and a plastic strip containing a gradient of antibiotic is placed on the plate. After overnight incubation, the zone of inhibition can be read off the plastic stick as the MIC.

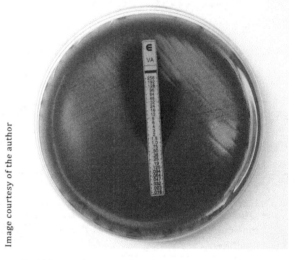

Image courtesy of the author

FIGURE 25.7   E-test for antimicrobial susceptibility testing

3. Disk diffusion test or Kirby-Bauer test

-Three categories of susceptibility

>   S = susceptible
>
>   I = intermediate
>
>   R = resistant

-Used for rapidly growing bacteria

-Bacteria are inoculated into a broth from a pure culture. When the organisms are growing at log phase (fastest growth phase), they are plated onto an agar plate in a standardized concentration. Small round disks impregnated with antibiotic are placed on the agar surface seeded with bacteria, and the plates incubated for growth

-Result: zones of inhibited growth around the antibiotic disks

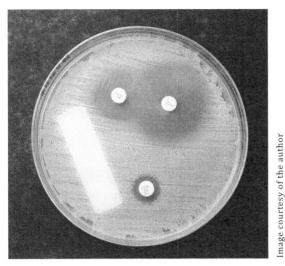

Image courtesy of the author

FIGURE 25.8 *Kirby-Bauer test for antimicrobial susceptibility*

-Interpretation is done by measuring the zones—the sizes of the zones have been tested and are already categorized as to group (S, I, R) for each bacterial genus

-Drugs giving intermediate values for a bacterium should not usually be used unless the infection is, for example, a urinary tract infection. In this case, a drug may act effectively even though it is officially "I" as the kidney works to concentrate antibiotics, and the level in the urine may be 100X greater than in the blood.

4. Testing for beta-lactamase production

Testing for this enzyme is always done for staphylococci, but also for some other bacteria like *Neisseria gonorrhoeae* and *Haemophilus influenzae*

-If a bacterium produces beta-lactamase, then all penicillin and cephalosporin antibiotics will automatically be classified as "R," resistant

-Can be done by placing a disk impregnated with nitrocefin on an agar plate seeded with bacteria (nitrocefin is a cephalosporin that will turn red when the beta-lactam ring is cleaved off)

5. Screening for vancomycin resistance

-Usually done by putting a disk impregnated with vancomycin on the agar plate (preseeded with the bacterium in question) and measuring the zone of inhibition after incubation

-All *enterococci* and some *staphylococci* are screened for this type of resistance

6. Screening for ESBL (extended spectrum) beta-lactamase in Gram-negative enteric bacteria

-Bacteria are plated on an agar plate containing cefpodoxime (a third-generation cephalosporin), and if they grow, then more tests must be carried out to determine if they are really ESBL

Diagnostic Immunology

-Antibodies to infectious agents present in patient serum can be used to diagnose disease.

-Presence of specific antibodies in a serum specimen is an indication that the individual has been exposed to the antigen (microorganism, in this case) and produced antibodies to the agent.

-For **diagnosis** of disease, it is not enough to show that the patient has long-lived IgG antibodies because this may be an old infection that is not relevant to the disease. IgG antibodies may either be a result of an ongoing infection or may be present as a result of earlier immune stimulation.

-IgM antibodies are usually considered an indicator of either a fresh, ongoing primary infection or a recent infection.

-Necessary to have two separate blood specimens with a time interval in-between (usually two weeks for a viral infection) to show that the level of antibodies has changed significantly from the first testing occasion to the second. A fourfold increase in antibody levels is usually the criterion used to designate a new versus an old infection.

4- fold rise in antibody?

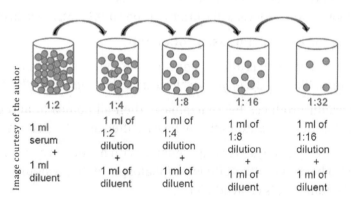

FIGURE 25.9   Fourfold increase in antibody titer

-IgE and IgD are not usually used for diagnosis of infections because the concentrations are too low in sera to be useful.

-IgA is a useful tool for some types of infections and is beginning to be used more and more for diagnosis because the half-life of IgA in serum is only five to six days compared to IgG, where the half-life is much longer.

METHODS USED IN THE LABORATORY TO DETECT ANTIBODIES

a.   Precipitation

b.   Agglutination

c. Neutralization

d. Complement-fixation

e. Fluorescent antibody techniques

f. ELISA (enzyme-linked immunosorbent assay) also called EIA (enzyme immunoassay)

a. Precipitation reactions

-Reaction of soluble antigens with IgG or IgM antibodies to form large complexes, which will precipitate or fall out of solution when the concentrations are optimal

-Individual antigen–antibody complexes join together to form lattices

-Prozone effect: no precipitation occurs because the antibody or the antigen is in excess. This is a cause of false-negative tests for antibodies

-Immunodiffusion tests are tests based on the precipitin reaction, but they are done in an agar gel medium, and the precipitate develops between the reactants, which are usually placed in small wells dug out in the agar

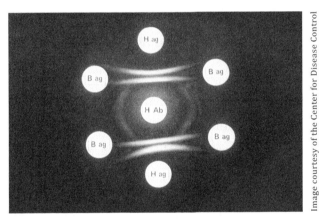

Image courtesy of the Center for Disease Control

FIGURE 25.10   Immunodiffusion

-Immunoelectrophoresis combines immunodiffusion and electrophoresis and is often used to separate proteins

*example: the Western Blot is a method used for the definitive diagnosis of HIV—the proteins extracted from the virus are separated by running them in an electrical field, where they migrate according to their charge. When the proteins are separated, the patient serum can be added, and the antibody–antigen reactions take place if there are antibodies present in the serum.

b. Agglutination reactions (can use to detect antigen or antibody)

-Agglutination involves insoluble antigens (or particulate antigens)

-Antigens may be cells or may be soluble antigen that is linked to a particle, (e.g., a latex particle)

-The antigen–antibody reaction results in a visible "agglutination" or clumping of the cells or particulate matter used in the test

-Two types of reaction

Direct agglutination

- Detects antibodies against large antigens (i.e., RBC, bacteria or fungi)

- Usually done in test tubes or in microtiter plates

- Serum is "diluted" in a serial manner, so the first tube contains, for example, half buffer and half antibody. The second tube could then contain 1/2 of the original antibody concentration, the third tube 1/4, and so on.

- Antibody titers are reported as, for example: "1/8". This is the last tube to show evidence of antibody activity, in this case, agglutination.

*Remember, an antibody titer of 1/128 is larger than a titer of 1/64. They are not ratios; they instead mean that you can dilute the serum 64 or 128 times and still get a positive test.

Indirect agglutination

- Antigens are coated on a particle-like latex or red blood cells, and the binding of antigen and antibody causes the particles to agglutinate together

- Often used for the rapid detection of organisms, for example, the rapid tests for *S. pyogenes* (strep Group A) in clinics

c. Neutralization reactions

Antigen + antibody block toxins or other harmful effects of a microorganism.

-Not used much in diagnostics today but was earlier used to identify, for example, a virus by observing the lack of infectivity after a virus had been treated with a specific neutralizing antibody

d. Complement-fixation reactions

-Used earlier for detection of syphilis, gonorrhea, and Mycoplasma antibodies

-Complement is "fixed" or activated during an antigen–antibody reaction and will lyse the red blood cells used as indicator system

-Very hard to standardize; poor sensitivity and specificity

e. Fluorescent antibody tests

-Two types: direct and indirect

-Antibodies are "conjugated" with a molecule called FITC (fluorescein isothiocyanate) that will emit a green color of light when excited by UV rays

-**Direct FA:** used to detect the organism directly in a specimen (see previous section)

-Indirect FA: used to detect the antibody in serum

-Uses "sandwich technique," where the organism is attached or fixed to a glass slide, and patient serum is added; if antibody is present, it will bind to the antigen. A second antibody is added—this is a reagent antibody with a conjugated FITC (e.g., antihuman IgG) molecule, and if patient IgG has attached, the complex will fluoresce in a UV microscope

-By using different dilutions of patient serum, an end point and "antibody titer" can be determined

f.   ELISA or EIA

-Enzyme-linked immunoassay

-Often uses horseradish peroxidase or alkaline phosphatase as the enzyme in the system

-Two types: direct and indirect

-Use "sandwich technique"

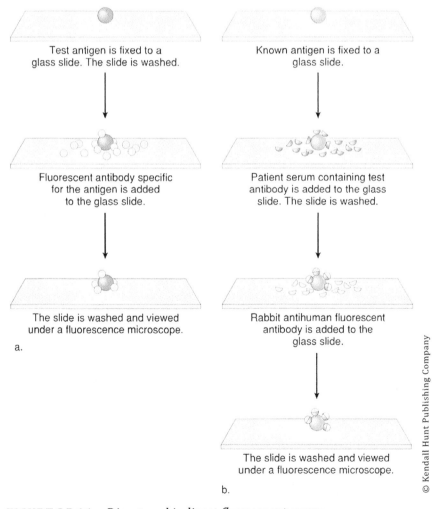

FIGURE 25.11   Direct and indirect fluorescent assay

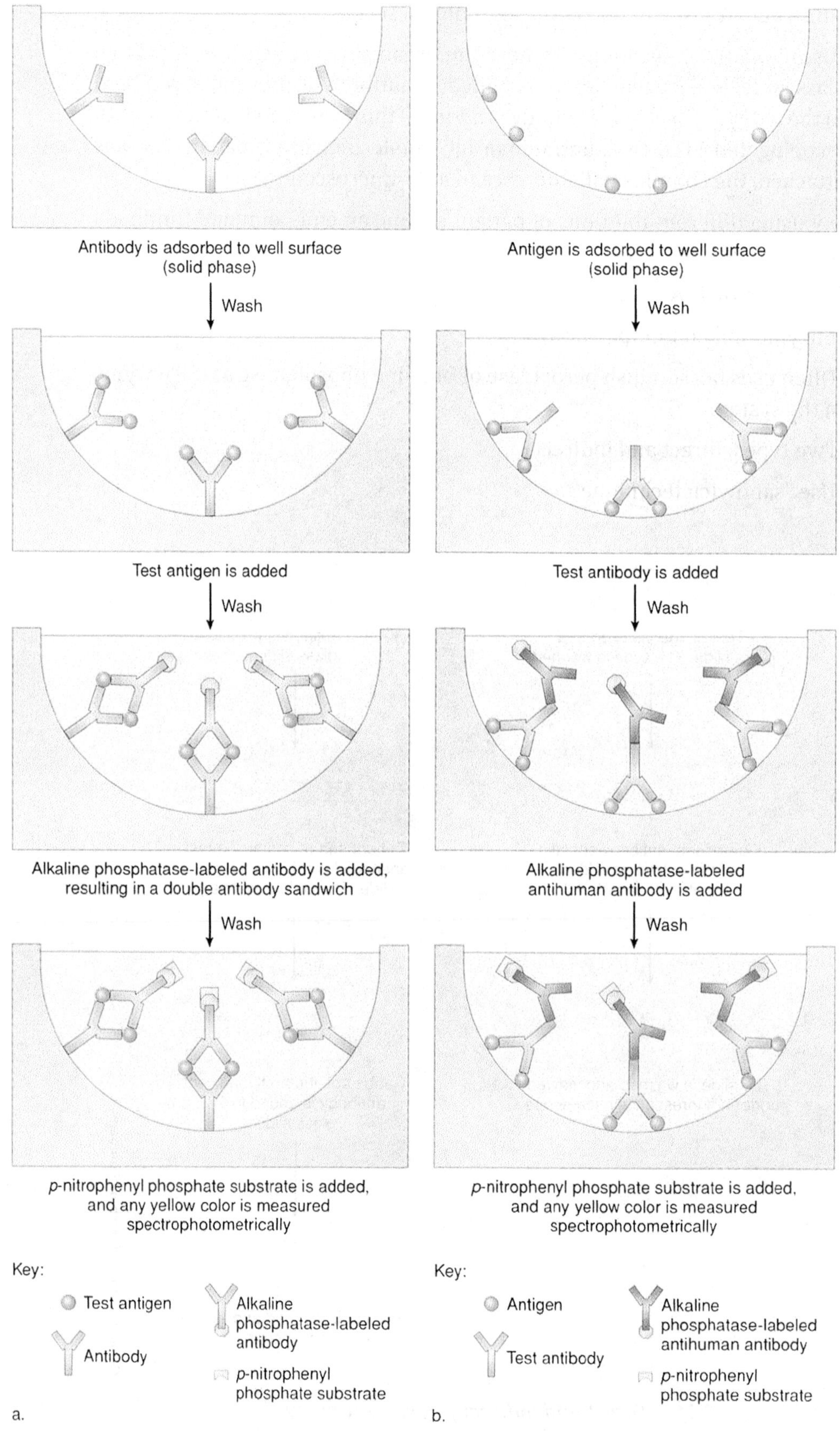

Antibody is adsorbed to well surface
(solid phase)

↓ Wash

Test antigen is added

↓ Wash

Alkaline phosphatase-labeled antibody is added,
resulting in a double antibody sandwich

↓ Wash

p-nitrophenyl phosphate substrate is added,
and any yellow color is measured
spectrophotometrically

Key:

● Test antigen

Y Antibody

Y Alkaline phosphatase-labeled antibody

▱ p-nitrophenyl phosphate substrate

a.

Antigen is adsorbed to well surface
(solid phase)

↓ Wash

Test antibody is added

↓ Wash

Alkaline phosphatase-labeled
antihuman antibody is added

↓ Wash

p-nitrophenyl phosphate substrate is added,
and any yellow color is measured
spectrophotometrically

Key:

● Antigen

Y Test antibody

Y Alkaline phosphatase-labeled antihuman antibody

▱ p-nitrophenyl phosphate substrate

b.

FIGURE 25.12   EIA technique

-Direct ELISA detects antigens, drugs, or toxins

- Specific antibodies (usually monoclonal antibodies) are fixed to plastic plates, and specimen is added; if the antigen is present, it binds; then another antibody which is specific for the desired antigen, is added; this will bind to the patient's antigen. This second antibody has an enzyme attached, and on the addition of the enzyme's specific substrate, the enzyme will cleave the substrate and produce a colored compound that can be measured quantitatively.

-Indirect ELISA detects antibodies

- Much the same technique as the direct, except that a known antigen is bound to the plastic, and patient's antibodies in the sample bind to it. An antihuman antibody that is bound to an enzyme is added, and if the complex is there, the enzyme will remain and be able to cleave the substrate, producing a colored product.

 *example: home pregnancy tests are based on this reaction

SPECIMEN COLLECTION

Types and amounts of specimen to be collected may differ from laboratory to laboratory, so find out what your local laboratory expects. Ask for a written description of their recommendations for specimen collection.

This will prevent you from wasting your time, the patient from getting mad and becoming uncooperative if he has to be sampled several times, and the lab from throwing specimens away and/or culturing unsuitable, poorly handled specimens that will not give a good, reliable result that can be used for patient treatment.

Always use Universal Precautions.

Considerations concerning the collection of samples for microbial analysis:

1. Specimen containers should be sterile and of a specified size and should also have properly fitting lids to prevent leakage. Special transport packages are provided (padded envelopes, reinforced boxes, etc.). Canada Post gets upset if a specimen spills and causes a dangerous mess.

2. The time for transport to the laboratory should be considered when determining how to store specimens in the clinic or ward before transport.

   examples: a urine specimen should be kept in the refrigerator until sent to the lab, and if it has to be sent a long distance, it should be sent refrigerated—this prevents the overgrowth of contaminants.

   Blood and sterile fluids (i.e., CSF) cultures should always be sent directly to the laboratory and kept, if possible, at 37 °C.

3. If specimens consist of pus from a deep abscess or any other type of infection that could likely be caused by an anaerobe, make sure that

the specimen is transported to the lab as quickly as possible, and use the special anaerobe media provided where possible.

4. Mark all specimen requisitions and specimen containers well—patient name, HC number, patient location, date of collection. You usually have computer-generated labels—use them, and add the date of collection and sometimes the time of collection.

5. Think about what kind of specimen you are taking, and try to avoid some common pitfalls that could destroy the accuracy of the results. A good example is the collection of blood cultures. These are often taken before the antibiotic therapy is initiated because the antibiotic may kill the bacteria or inhibit bacterial growth. Always indicate on the requisition if the patient is on antibiotics and, if so, which antibiotic.

6. Urine samples: try to ensure that the samples are midstream and that the patient has complied with the directions for cleansing. Normal flora in the GU tract can quickly overgrow and obscure the results.

7. Special instructions may apply for collection of samples for different diagnostic procedures.

   examples: Specimens for PCR: these are not going to be cultured, and there are special instructions for the collection of these swabs or fluids.

   Culture of open sore: Clean off debris first, and take swab sample from bottom of the sore

Top Organisms to Know

Top Fungi to Know

YEAST = ONE CELLED FUNGI

Candida albicans

Cryptococcus neoformans/gatti

Pneumocystis jiroveci

Malessezia furfur

Saccharomyces sp.

MOLDS = MANY CELLED FUNGI

Aspergillus species

Mucor species

DIMORPHIC FUNGI

Sporothrix schenkii

Histoplasma capsulatum

Coccidioides immitis

Blastomyces dermatitidis

Important Bacterial Pathogens —
Top Bugs To Know

a) **Staphylococcus**

S. aureus (coagulase +)

S. epidermidis (coagulase −)

S. saphrophyticus (coagulase −)

b) **Streptococcus**

α-hemolytic: S. pneumoniae (note this is diplococci not long chains)

β-hemolytic: S. pyogenes (Group A strep)

S. agalactiae (Group B strep)

γ-hemolytic: Enterococcus (Streptococcus faecalis/ faecium)

a) Without spores: Listeria monocytogenes

Corynebacterium diphtheriae

b) With spores: Bacillus species **(aerobic)**

e.g. B. anthracis

B. cereus

Clostridium species ***(anaerobic)***

e.g. C. difficile

C. perfringens

C. botulinum

C. tetani

Neisseria gonorrhoeae (diplococci)

Neisseria meningitidis (diplococci)

D. GRAM NEGATIVE BACILLI (PINK-RED RODS)-SHORT, LONG, FAT, THIN, CURVED, STRAIGHT

a) Aerobic and facultative Gram negative bacilli:

Escherichia coli (including O157:H7)

Pseudomonas aeruginosa

Salmonella

Shigella

Campylobacter

Yersinia

Francisella

Bartonella

Helicobacter pylori

Haemophilus influenzae

Bordetella pertussis

Pasteurella multocida

Vibrio cholerae

b) Anaerobic Gram negative bacteria:

Bacteroides

Fusobacterium

c) Anaerobic Gram positive pleomorphic bacilli:

Actinomyces (aerotolerant)

E. OTHER MEDICALLY IMPORTANT HUMAN BACTERIAL PATHOGENS THAT ARE NOT IDENTIFIED BY GRAM'S STAIN:

Mycobacterium tuberculosis and *Mycobacterium leprae* (cell wall not stainable using the Gram stain)

Mycoplasma pneumoniae (no cell wall)

Treponema pallidum (too small to see in Gram's stain)

Chlamydia trachomatis (intracellular, too small to see)

Top Parasites To Know

PROTOZOA = ONE CELLED PARASITES

Entamoeba histolytica

Giardia lamblia

Trichomonas vaginalis

Acanthamoeba species

Cryptosporidium parvum

Toxoplasma gondii

Trypanosoma cruzi and brucei

Leishmania species

Plasmodium species: *P. falciparum, P. malariae, P. vivax, P. ovale, P. knowlesii*

METAZOA = MANY CELLED PARASITES = HELMINTHS

A. Nematodes

Enterobius vermicularis (pinworm)

Ascaris lumbricoides

Trichuris trichuria

Hookworm

Anisakis

Trichinella

Filaria = blood roundworms (general)

B. Trematodes

Schistosoma: *S. hematobium, S. japonicum, S. mansoni*

C. Cestodes

Taenia saginata (beef tapeworm)

Taenia solium (pork tapeworm)

Echinococcus species (dog tapeworm)

D. Ectoparasites

Sarcoptes scabei

Pediculus humanus

Phthirus pubis

Appendix B

Case Questions

Central Nervous System (CNS) Infections Case 1: Sharing Saliva at New Years

- Nora, 18 years old, felt nauseated and weak one afternoon, three days after attending an all-night New Year's Eve party. Within 4 hours, her condition had deteriorated and she was severely ill with fever, nausea, confusion, stiff neck, and the beginning of a rash on her extremities.

- Alarmed, her parents took her to the ER. By this time she was floating in and out of consciousness, and the rash appeared as large, red–purple blotches on her arms, legs, and body.

- At the ER, CSF and blood cultures were drawn and antibiotic administered directly after.

- Within 15 minutes her condition had worsened and she was transferred to the ICU and put on a respirator. Within 30 minutes the results came from the lab. The cell count in the CSF was increased (predominantly neutrophils), protein levels were increased, and glucose levels were decreased. Gram-negative diplococci had been seen by the bacteriology lab.

- During this crisis, a 20-year-old male, Kevin, was admitted to hospital with a stiff neck and fever. A CSF was drawn on suspicion of meningitis, and antibiotics were initiated. It was later found that Kevin had attended the same party. After four days, his blood culture grew *N. meningitidis*. All partygoers were offered prophylactic antibiotics (ciprofloxacin).

1. **How is *N. meningitidis* spread?**

2. **What other organisms are Gram-negative diplococci?**

3. **What significance does an increased cell count, increased total protein, and decreased glucose level have in CSF?**

4. **What is the papular rash called?**

5. **Why did Nora suffer respiratory failure, and what other organs were likely affected?**

6. **What antibiotics are normally used in cases of meningococcal meningitis?**

7. **What are her chances for a total recovery?**

8. **What are Kevin's chances for a total recovery?**

9. **How could this have been prevented?**

Central Nervous System (CNS) Infections Case 2: Don't Eat That!

On October 15, 2001, a 40-year-old man was admitted to the hospital. He had a "splitting headache," his legs were unsteady, and his vision was blurred. During examination, it was apparent that there was something wrong with his throat. It wasn't sore, but it felt stiff and tight and he could not speak.

Over the next seven days, 28 people with similar symptoms were admitted to the hospital. Twelve of these required assistance with breathing (ventilation); none of them died. An investigation was undertaken to find out whether there were any common denominators for these 29 patients. The only finding was that all victims had been to a party at the local community hall on October 14.

Detailed histories were taken from the patients about what food they had eaten at the party, which was a potluck affair. There had been about 100 people at this party. It was found that all patients had eaten a venison stew with onions, carrots, and potatoes. Backtracking, it was found that the person responsible for making the stew had made it in small batches, then kept it in large clay pots in a root cellar for at least 24 hours before the party.

1. **What would the most likely causative organism be, given the fact that the dish was a stew containing meat and that the patients had neurological symptoms?**

2. **Does this scenario fit the descriptions we have learned about food poisoning?**

3. **Was this food infection or intoxication?**

4. **How could this food have become contaminated?**

5. **How could this have been prevented?**

Central Nervous System (CNS) Infections Case 3: Watch Your Feet

- A 63-year-old male alcoholic was taken to the emergency department with obvious gangrene of both feet. He was stuporous and during the evening had a seizure.

- Later the same evening he was noted to have opisthotonic posturing and to have developed increasing rigor, respiratory distress, and unresponsiveness.

- Necrotic blackened areas were present over both feet, and several draining ulcers were noted on heels and toes.

- Neurologically the patient responded to deep pain with a grimace. On the basis of these findings, the patient was treated with supportive therapy and ultimately recovered.

1. What organism caused his infection?
2. What virulence factor produced by this bacterium was responsible for his rigor and posturing?
3. How did this patient become infected with the organism?
4. What specific therapy is indicated?
5. How could this have been prevented?

Central Nervous System (CNS) Infections Case 4: Preventable Paralysis

- A 12-year-old male, who had been in apparent good health, complained of headache four days prior to admission at the emergency department of a major city hospital.

- Three days prior to being transported to the city, he complained of weakness in his legs, a stiff neck, upper stomach pain, and some growing weakness in his left arm. At this time he was hospitalized at a small country hospital, and a lumbar puncture was done.

- By the time he reached the city, he was in respiratory distress and could not talk. He was found to have no sensory or vibratory sensation. The CSF showed a pleocytosis with a WBC count of 58/mm^3 (2% neutrophils and 98% lymphocytes). CSF glucose and protein levels were normal.

- The immunization history was questionable because his parents did not believe in vaccination.

- Blood, CSF, and stool specimens were taken and sent to the lab. A virus culture of the stool revealed the diagnosis.

1. **Which virus was isolated from the patient's stools?**

2. **What is the epidemiology of this infection?**

3. **For which cell types does this virus show tropism?**

4. **What are the revealing symptoms?**

5. **Can this infection be treated with antivirals?**

6. **Is there a vaccine?**

Central Nervous System (CNS) Infections Case 5: What ..sackie

- The patient is a 3½-month-old male who presented in August with a two-week history of diarrhea, which abated with oral rehydration.

- One week later he developed a fever of 39.2 °C and respiratory symptoms. He was found to have some wheezing and otitis media.

- He was treated with a beta-lactam antibiotic for presumed respiratory infection. He continued to have a fever and developed irritability and vomiting. He returned to the clinic and was admitted.

- On admission he was irritable and had a temperature of 36.6 °C. He had tachycardia with a pulse of 180 beats/min. He was found to have anemia, and his WBC was 9300/mm³ (normal is 5,000–10,000) with 60% lymphocytes.

- A lumbar puncture was done, and he had a WBC of 75/mm³ with 72% neutrophils, 8% lymphocytes, and 20% monocytes; glucose and protein were normal. Antibiotics (ceftriaxone) were initiated on suspicion of bacteria. Gram's stain was negative for bacteria. His CSF was sent for viral culture.

1. **Does this patient have meningitis?**

2. **Which type of virus is likely responsible?**

3. **What is the transmission and pathogenesis of infection with viruses of this group?**

4. **What is the treatment, and how can the infections be prevented?**

Cardiovascular and Lymphatic Infections Case 1: Bull's-Eye

In early 1975 some mothers observed that a high number of children in a small rural area of the United States were diagnosed as having juvenile rheumatoid arthritis. This is usually a rare disease. An investigation was instigated, and the records of 51 cases of RA cases were studied in early 1976. On four different country roads, there was an incidence of 1:10 for the disease, and six families had several cases.

Suspicion was directed to arthropod bites, and an investigation of ticks and Lyme disease done. The months of June and July were responsible for 60% of the cases. It was found that there were 35 cases on the east side of the river and only 8 on the west side. This contributed to the suspicion of an arthropod vector.

In a simultaneous study, the number of ticks of species *Ixodes scapularis* from wild animals were measured and found to be more dense on the east side of the river. *Borrelia burgdorferi* was later isolated from the ticks and antibodies found in the children.

1. **What is *Borrelia burgdorferi?* How long does the tick have to be attached before the bacterium is transferred from tick to person?**

2. **What type of terrain is usually associated with ticks?**

3. **Can other organisms be transmitted by the same tick at the same time?**

4. **What is the normal reservoir for the ticks?**

5. **Arthritis and chronic neurological disorders are symptoms that develop from an untreated *Borrelia* infection. How do you diagnose this infection, given that the bacteria are very hard to grow in culture and are hard to locate in the tissues?**

6. **What treatment is given for Lyme disease?**

7. **Is there a vaccine?**

Cardiovascular and Lymphatic Infections Case 2: That Darn Cat!

- Two brothers, John and Peter, became ill after having been scratched by a new kitten an aunt had given to them.

- John is 5 years old and has been healthy all his life. He developed a 6-mm cutaneous papule on his right hand at the site of the cat scratch after one week. After another week the lymph glands in his right armpit were swollen. He recovered without antibiotic therapy.

- Peter, 3 years old, has an HIV infection acquired from a contaminated blood transfusion when the family was living in Africa. He developed three large, painless red skin lesions resembling tumors. Biopsy of the largest one showed proliferation of blood vessels and many bacteria. He was diagnosed with bacillary angiomatosis and treated for one month with erythromycin. He relapsed three weeks later and was treated again.

1. **Why did the two brothers have such different responses to the same organism?**

2. **What kind of organism is this?**

3. **Why did Peter relapse even after one month of antibiotics?**

4. **How could you diagnose this disease?**

5. **Do you think that the cat showed symptoms of infection?**

Cardiovascular and Lymphatic Infections Case 3: "Bad Air"

- This 35-year-old male seaman was admitted to the hospital after he returned home for leave. He had been travelling the world and had disembarked in several African countries including Kenya.

- Bob had been sick on ship with fever, malaise, and headaches and was treated empirically with chloroquine. Bob had initially felt better but became ill again on the way home.

- Laboratory studies done on the ship were consistent with the diagnosis of malaria. New blood tests were done, and the laboratory reported the finding of malarial parasites (*Plasmodium falciparum*, 5% infection) in the blood.

1. **What is the most likely explanation why the chloroquine did not cure this patient's malaria?**

2. **Which laboratory test would be used to confirm the diagnosis of malaria?**

3. **Which *Plasmodium* sp. causes the most severe disease and why? What are serious complications of infection with this parasite?**

4. **How is malaria transmitted?**

5. **How can this disease be controlled?**

Cardiovascular and Lymphatic Infections Case 4: The Rabbit Skinner

- This 40-year-old female noted an ulcer on the distal aspect of her right third finger approximately 12 days prior to admission. She developed chills and fever and was treated with oral antibiotics without success; she was then referred to a larger hospital.

- On physical examination, the patient was an obese female in moderate distress. Her temperature was 40 °C, her blood pressure was 146/82 mm Hg, her pulse was 120 beats/min, and her respiration was 18 breaths/min.

- Significant physical findings included an ulcerated lesion of the right third finger and associated enlarged axillary lymph nodes. Cultures (including blood and wound surface) were negative.

- Retrospective questioning revealed that the patient had butchered a rabbit one week prior to the onset of her illness.

1. **Which pathogen is the most likely agent of infection on the basis of the rabbit exposure?**

2. **Why should the laboratory be notified before sending cultures for this organism?**

3. **How can this disease be diagnosed?**

4. **Is this the most common manifestation of disease?**

5. **Can this disease be treated?**

6. **Is there a vaccine?**

Cardiovascular and Lymphatic Infections Case 5: Houdini's Scourge

- A 21-year-old man presented to the emergency room with three days of abdominal pain, which began as a diffuse, dull, continuous pain.

- The pain became crampy in the midgastric and lower abdomen. He noted a decrease in appetite but no nausea, vomiting, or diarrhea.

- On examination, the patient was febrile to 39.2 °C, tachycardic with a heart rate of 150 beats/min, and tachypneic with a respiratory rate of 52 breaths/min and had a blood pressure of 108/60 mm Hg. His physical examination was notable for midgastric and right lower quadrant abdominal tenderness.

- The white blood cell count was normal. Blood cultures were obtained on admission and were subsequently positive for an anaerobic, Gram-negative rod, at which time the patient was taken to the operating room for an exploratory laparotomy.

1. To which genus do you think that this bacterium belongs?

2. Upon learning of the positive blood culture, the surgical team opted for abdominal surgery. What type of lesion do you suspect they would find in the abdomen?

3. How would this intraabdominal infection be treated?

4. A culture specimen was taken from the abscess. What grew?

5. What other types of infection does this bacteria cause?

6. Which antibiotics would be used to treat the patient?

Cardiovascular and Lymphatic Infections Case 6: The Heart of the Matter

- The patient was a 43-year-old female with a history of mitral valve prolapse. She was admitted with a chief complaint of intermittent fevers for one month and headaches for three weeks.

- Two weeks prior to developing symptoms, she had undergone a dental surgery.

- She had a few small, red skin lesions and hemorrhages in her nail beds. All four blood cultures performed on admission were positive for Gram positive cocci in chains. These bacteria grew on blood agar plates with alpha-hemolysis.

1. **What is your diagnosis?**

2. **What is the likely source of this organism?**

3. **Why did she receive prophylactic antimicrobial agents before dental procedures?**

4. **What are the common complications of endocarditis?**

Immunology Topic 1: AIDS

Why do people with AIDS have so many problems with infections caused by organisms called "opportunistic pathogens"?

HIV virus seeks out and enters CD4+ (helper) T lymphocytes by latching on to the CD4+ receptor and a chemokine receptor. These cells are the lymphocytes that interact with "antigen-presenting cells," like macrophages, and send the signal that there is an invader to the CD8+ T lymphocytes (the killers). CD4+ cells also stimulate B lymphocytes to start maturing into antibody factories. When the HIV virus enters the CD4+ cells, it takes over the cell and uses all the nucleotides, etc., for replication of new HIV virus particles. The CD4+ cell then dies because none of its own DNA or proteins are being produced. This leads to a reduced number of CD4+ cells, which in turn leads to a reduced number of CD8+ killer cells and an impaired ability to deal with infections. When HIV infections have progressed to the point where the patient is said to have AIDS, the numbers of CD4+ cells are far below normal (normal is 800 to 1000 cells/mm^3). When the level of CD4+ gets below 200 to 400, the problems with opportunistic infections usually start.

We who have normal immunity and normal amounts of functioning CD4+ cells can react to invasion by organisms and get rid of them quickly. These organisms may be either "primary pathogens" or "opportunistic pathogens." AIDS patients cannot destroy these organisms and so get overwhelming infections that eventually lead to death (often by pulmonary infections).

Immunology Topic 2: Antiinflammatories Like Cortisone and NSAIDs: How Do They Work?

We have all heard about people with inflammatory disorders like rheumatoid arthritis, lupus, etc., being treated with cortisone. So what does cortisone do?

Cortisone, or corticosteroids, is a cholesterol derivative. There are a number of different drug derivations; some include prednisone, prednisolone, and methylprednisolone. Treatment with these substances results in a number of effects on immune functioning, including reduced numbers of white blood cells like lymphocytes and reduced amounts of cytokines. Because cortisone derivatives are very lipophilic, they can easily pass through the cell membranes and reach the nucleus of the cells where they a stimulate production of an inhibitor of NF-κB. Reduced activity of NF-κB will prevent activation of cells such as T cells and the production of cytokines. Cortisone also causes reduced phagocytic cell activity of macrophages and neutrophils.

NSAIDs

This abbreviation is one that you'll see often. It stands for nonsteroidal anti-inflammatory drugs. These drugs are the most frequently used drugs for treating inflammation and pain. Salicylate, found in aspirin, is one such drug.

The mechanism by which these drugs work is by inhibition of the cyclooxygenase pathway that produces prostaglandins and thromboxanes from arachidonic acid. A reduced prostaglandin production results in a decrease of vascular permeability and in neutrophil chemotaxis, so the inflammatory response will be limited. The pathway involved in prostaglandin synthesis is regulated by two enzymes, Cox-1 and Cox-2 (cyclooxygenase-1 and cyclooxygenase-2). The inhibition of Cox-2 seems to be the most important effect of the NSAIDs.

Immunology Topic 3: DiGeorge's Syndrome

This is also called congenital thymic aplasia. The most severe form is a total absence of a thymus, which is the source of all T cells. B cells are present in normal numbers, but because there are no T cells, the B cells do not get activated. As a result of this disease, patients suffer from chronic diarrhea, viral and fungal infections, and a general failure to thrive. Transplantation of the thymus can be done.

Immunology Topic 4: Leukocyte Adhesion Deficiency

What happens if our neutrophils are defective in their capacity to adhere to the blood vessel lining (endothelium)?

In the normal course of events, neutrophils circulate around in the blood. If they get the "scent" of an invader, they stop, move to the side of the blood vessel, and stick to it by adhesive molecules like the "selectins" or "integrins." From here they can bore their way through the blood vessel wall between the different cells and get out into the tissues where they can track down the invader, phagocytose it, and kill it.

In the case where the neutrophil is lacking in these adhesive molecules, the patient will suffer from recurrent severe bacterial infections that are eventually fatal. There is a disease, leukocyte adhesion deficiency, where this happens—the neutrophils are not handicapped in killing functions, but they never get to the site of infection, so the infection gets out of control early, like a wildfire.

Bone marrow transplantation can be done in infants with this syndrome—they get functional neutrophils this way that have these "adhesins" on their surfaces.

A bit of trivia: cattle have the same type of disease, but it is called BLAD (bovine leukocyte adhesion deficiency). Because of selective breeding of cattle, this disease was once common (10% of cattle in dairy herds had the gene). Sires are now routinely screened and eliminated from the breeding pool.

Immunology Topic 5: MHC Class II Deficiency

What happens if there is no MHC II on the membranes of our macrophages and B-lymphocytes?

Lack of MHC II is an inherited X-linked disease. The health problems show up early in infancy. These babies look at first as if they have severe combined immunodeficiency (SCID) but do have T lymphocytes, unlike the people with SCID (e.g., bubble boy). With an MHC II deficiency, the patient will have a lot of trouble with pyogenic and opportunistic infections. These patients do not have helper T lymphocytes (CD4+). This means that they don't produce many antibodies either because the CD4+ cells are the type of cell that tells the B lymphocytes to turn on and make antibodies to a certain pathogen. Many of these patients succumb to infection.

This disease is also called "bare lymphocyte" syndrome.

Immunology Topic 6: Multiple Myeloma

This is a disease of the bone, as the tumor cells arise in the bone marrow. Multiple myeloma is caused by B cells becoming cancerous and multiplying without being stopped from doing so by the normal cellular inhibitory mechanisms. This results in tumors of plasma cells that produce a single type of antibody in very high amounts. These malignant plasma cells produce more light chains than heavy chains, so there will be a lot of light chains excreted in urine. These protein antibodies can be detected in the urine and are called "Bence-Jones" protein.

The tumors grow in the bone marrow and cause a disintegration of the bone. These patients also usually become anemic (too few red blood cells or erythrocytes), have low platelet counts (platelets come from megakaryocytes in the bone marrow), and have low numbers of other white blood cells like neutrophils because the plasma cell tumors crowd out the other blood cells in the bone marrow.

Immunology Topic 7: Neutropenia

What happens if we have too few neutrophils?

Usually we are very susceptible to "pyogenic infections." These are infections where there is a lot of pus. They may be caused by a variety of bacteria, like *Staphylococcus aureus.* In this case, the neutrophils, which are the phagocytes (means eater and killer cells), do not have a chance to contain the infection because there is too few of them. An example of this is a disease called "Felty's syndrome"—in this disease, which is a complication of rheumatoid arthritis, the patient has a decreased number of neutrophils and is very susceptible to infections. Remember that the neutrophil, dumb and unspecific as it is, is the cell that first responds to an infection and attacks the bacteria immediately.

What happens if the neutrophils are normal in number but do not function as they should?

In this case, there are a lot of pyogenic infections as well. Usually the lack of functioning is due to a defect in the killing of phagocytosed bacteria. The bacteria are phagocytosed normally, but when the phagosome and the lysosome fuse, the enzymes are just not there to chew up the bacteria. The bacteria survive and perpetuate the infection, and there are many abscesses. Examples of this are Chediak-Higashi syndrome and chronic granulomatous disease.

In CGD (chronic granulomatous disease). Here, the level of hydrogen peroxide and other substances that could kill bacteria may be totally zero or almost zero. In this disease, the mononuclear phagocytes finally get wind of the fact that there has been an invasion as it becomes a "chronic infection," and they rush to the site, phagocytose, and end up usually being able to chew up some bacteria. Some of these pieces of bacteria are moved out to the cell membrane where they are glommed on to by the MHC II complex. This sets the adaptive (also called acquired) immune system going, and you get more mononuclear phagocytes being recruited to help. Eventually this results in a "granuloma," which is a big collection of mononuclear phagocytes.

In some acute leukemias there is a lack of neutrophils as well—and the same problems with infections by pyogenic bacteria.

Immunology Topic 8: Peanut Allergies

These are examples of acute systemic anaphylaxis. This is a Type 1 IgE-mediated hypersensitivity reaction to antigens (peanuts) that is so dramatic and overwhelming that the patient can die. This will not happen on the first exposure to an antigen because the IgE antibodies have to be formed first. So, it may happen on the second and subsequent exposures. These IgE-peanut antibodies will bind to the surface of mast cells. If there is another exposure to peanuts, there is cross-linking of the IgE on mast cells, and this stimulates the mast cells to start pumping out histamine and leukotrienes. Histamine increases the permeability of the blood vessels (so they leak and the blood pressure drops), and leukotrienes affect smooth muscle, causing bronchospasm and swelling of the throat.

Acute anaphylaxis is a medical emergency and requires immediate therapy. People known to have such reactions should have medical alert bracelets and always carry an EpiPen™ with them. Epinephrine acts to inhibit the contraction of smooth muscle so the airways would not close and spasm and contracts the blood vessels, stopping any leakage and preventing a drop in blood pressure.

Immunology Topic 9: Severe Combined Immunodeficiency Syndrome (SCID)

This is the disease made famous by the bubble boy. It is often (55% of the time) an X-linked hereditary disease in which the individual lacks T cells. There are other underlying genetic defects that also result in this syndrome. Because there are no T cells, any B cells that are there will not be stimulated and will not mature to plasma cells, so the patient will not have any chance of defeating an infection.

There are many genetic variants of SCID, but they all boil down to the same thing: no T cells. As a result, there are no immune responses mounted to infection. These patients usually have neutrophils that function, but this is not enough for survival, and most infants die in the first few years of life of overwhelming infections. Infants diagnosed with SCID can be saved by bone marrow transplantation.

Immunology Topic 10: Selective Deficiencies of Immunoglobulin Classes

There are a number of immunodeficiency states characterized by significantly lowered amounts of specific immunoglobulin types. The most common is IgA deficiency, which affects 1 out of 300 individuals. Many of these are asymptomatic, but other patients may have severe problems. Recurrent respiratory and genitourinary infections are common. If treatment is necessary, immunoglobulin can be administered.

Immunology Topic 11: T-Cell Lymphoma

This is a tumor that occurs when mature T cells or their precursors in the thymus become "transformed" or cancerous and grow uninhibitedly. There are different types of T-cell lymphomas depending on the stage of the cells when they are transformed into cancer cells.

Some viruses can transform cells into cancer cells—these are the oncogenic viruses. An example is HTLV 1, which is a retrovirus closely related to the HIV virus. HTLV 1 infects mature CD4+ cells and transforms them into cancer cells—resulting in adult T-cell leukemia.

Immunology Topic 12: What Happens if You Do Not Have Any B-Lymphocytes?

One of the most important functions of the adaptive or acquired system is the ability to make antibodies. Normally 30 billion B lymphocytes are released into the bloodstream daily. The reason for not having B cells is usually an X-linked genetic disease, X-linked agammaglobulinemia.

These patients can be administered gamma globulin and in this way gain some antibody. They are susceptible to recurrent infections. Gamma globulin is prepared from human plasma at the blood bank. Plasma is pooled from >1000 donors and fractionated at very low temperatures ($-5\ °C$) to remove the gamma portion of the serum proteins because this is the part that contains the antibodies.

Immunology Topic 13: X-Linked Agammaglobulinemia (A B-Cell Defect!)

This disease is also called Bruton's hypogammaglobulinemia and is characterized by very low levels of IgG and the total absence of other antibody classes. These patients have **NO** circulating B cells. Because they cannot make enough antibody, they suffer from recurrent infections starting at about nine months of age when the maternal antibody disappears from their systems. A treatment often used is the administration of immunoglobulin (pooled antibody), but the patients usually do not survive into their teens.

Immunology Topic 14: X-Linked Hyper-IgM Syndrome

This is a disease that results from a defect in T-cell surface molecules. The syndrome is characterized by a lack of IgG, IgA, and IgE, together with an overproduction of IgM. There are a normal number of B cells, but they don't produce all kinds of antibody. Patients usually suffer recurrent infections, especially severe respiratory infections.

Lower Alimentary Tract Infections (LATI) Case 1: What? A Worm?

- A distraught mother phoned her local district nurse and hysterically told the nurse that she had found large worms in her baby's diaper. She was told to calm down and bring the child into the clinic for an examination and to also bring the worms. The mother had been so upset by the worms that she had thrown the diaper away immediately and did not have the "evidence."

- Mother and child went to the clinic, and during the hour-long wait to see the nurse, the child, who was an obviously healthy 8-month-old, spent the time playing with the Legos from the toy box of the waiting room.

- All of a sudden the mother noticed a long white object sticking out of the child's nose and on closer inspection found this to be the same type of worm that she had found in the diaper.

- The worm was sent to the laboratory, and in addition, fecal samples were taken. The parasitology lab identified the worm. Typical fertilized eggs were found in the feces.

- The patient was treated and the infestation cured.

1. **What is the causative organism?**

2. **What is the most likely source of infection for this parasite in a small child?**

3. **What symptoms are usual in this type of infection?**

4. **Is the child infectious?**

5. **Why were worms crawling from the nose if this is an intestinal parasite?**

6. **What is the significance of the finding of fertilized eggs as opposed to unfertilized eggs?**

Lower Alimentary Tract Infections (LATI) Case 2: Passing the Gas

- A 22-year-old man became ill with stomach cramps and diarrhea, which he thought was a stomach virus, so he expected to be healthy in a day or so.

- After a week, his symptoms were, if anything, worse, and in addition to cramps and diarrhea he experienced a great amount of gas. He finally went to his doctor, who found out that the man had recently been on a hiking trip in the mountains and had been drinking clean "fresh" cold water from mountain streams.

- The doctor ordered a stool sample, which was sent to the laboratory for bacteriology and parasitology.

- The bacteriological results were negative for *Salmonella, Shigella, Yersinia,* and *Campylobacter.* The results from the parasitology lab were, however, positive for a flagellate.

1. **What organism is the most probable cause of his symptoms?**

2. **The man claimed that he had only been drinking from clear, running streams. What could the source of the organism be?**

3. **How could he have prevented this event?**

4. **The patient is an otherwise totally healthy individual. What would the likely treatment be?**

5. **Is he likely to infect the other members of his household?**

Lower Alimentary Tract Infections (LATI) Case 3: A Spore-ific Experience

- The patient is a 37-year-old male from Ontario with hemophilia. He contracted HIV from the blood products that he received in the early 1980s and recently has been diagnosed with AIDS.

- Three months ago he was hospitalized with *Pneumocystis jiroveci* pneumonia, for which he was treated. His current treatment regimen includes factor VIII, suppressive trimethoprim-sulfamethoxazole, and a cocktail of anti-HIV drugs. He presents with a three-day history of voluminous diarrhea, 5-kg weight loss, and profound dehydration.

- Stool samples were examined, and no white blood cells were seen. Tests for *Salmonella, Shigella, Campylobacter,* and *Yersinia* were negative. Parasitology was negative. He had no recent travel history and had not recently consumed shellfish.

1. Which type of enteric pathogens are usually ruled out by a negative test for fecal leukocytes and occult blood?

2. Why was it important to get a travel history from this patient?

3. Considering that he has been treated with antibiotics for an extended period, what organism should be tested for?

4. Is this pathogen usually detected by culture or by a technique that detects the toxins produced by the bacteria?

5. Is this infection treatable in this patient?

Lower Alimentary Tract Infections (LATI) Case 4: Human-to-Human Bug

- A 30-year-old dairy farmer took a holiday in Turkey. On his arrival home to his farm outside of Grande Prairie, he experienced a sudden onset of fever, stomach pain, nausea, vomiting, and diarrhea. Thinking that he had the flu, he crawled into bed and decided to ride it out.

- Three days later, when he had not improved, he got his neighbor to drive him to town to the doctor. By this time he was very lethargic and was admitted to the hospital, where tests were done.

- A lumbar puncture was done because of his altered mental status and fever. The CSF was negative for microorganisms. He was treated with IV fluids and ampicillin. His condition improved. A stool specimen was taken, and the presence of fecal leukocytes and occult blood indicated that a stool culture should be done. The organism isolated was a lactose nonfermenter and was nonmotile.

1. Which organisms can cause bloody diarrhea with fecal leukocytes?

2. Considering that the organism was lactose negative and nonmotile, which of the above organisms are the most likely etiologic agent?

3. Would a travel history have been important?

4. Was it appropriate to treat this patient with antibiotics?

5. Was susceptibility testing necessary for the appropriate choice of antibiotic?

6. Is it important to type this isolate and why?

Lower Alimentary Tract Infections (LATI) Case 5: CMV–What Is That?

- The patient was a 59-year-old female who underwent a cardiac transplant six months earlier for an idiopathic cardiomyopathy. Since the transplant she has done reasonably well, with the exception of two acute episodes of rejection, which were treated with high doses of steroids.

- One week prior to this admission, she complained of malaise, fatigue, low-grade fever, and mild dyspnea on exertion. She was admitted to determine the etiology of her complaints. She was found to be anemic and had a low white blood cell count. She was transfused with 3 units of blood and underwent upper GI endoscopy, which revealed nodular gastric erosions.

- Biopsies and brushings were taken. A chest X ray revealed diffuse infiltrates. A bronchoscopy was done, and washings were sent for culture and acid-fast bacilli. Gram's stains were negative. The next day, H and E stains of the gastric lesion revealed the organism. Viral cultures were positive two weeks later.

1. **Which opportunistic infectious agents can cause pneumonitis and gastritis? What was the most likely etiology of her infection?**

2. **Which other two types of patient populations are subject to serious infection with CMV?**

3. **Which clinical manifestations are caused by this virus other than fever, leukopenia, gastritis, and pneumonitis?**

4. **This patient and her donor were seropositive for the virus. What are all of the likely sources of her infection?**

5. **Which other opportunistic infections may she develop?**

Lower Alimentary Tract Infections (LATI) Case 6: Infectious Hepatitis?

- The patient was a 32-year-old male who presented to the emergency ward with a three-day history of fever (max temperature 40 °C), malaise, and back pain. Lab data showed a WBC count of 4700/mm³ and abnormal liver function tests. Blood cultures were done but were negative for bacteria.

- He developed anorexia and jaundice in addition to fevers and malaise. He denied a history of intravenous drug use, sexual contact (for two months), and transfusions. Five weeks ago he was visiting friends in New York City, and they ate raw oysters. Recent telephone contact with one of the friends revealed that he had the same type of illness.

- On examination the patient was mildly icteric. There was no rash or lymphadenopathy, but there was a tender liver, which was enlarged. Blood was sent for diagnostic testing.

- Over the next month his symptoms resolved, and the liver function tests returned to normal limits.

1. **What is the differential diagnosis for this patient bearing in mind the abnormal liver enzyme tests?**

2. **What is the likely etiology of his infection? How did he contract it?**

3. **What is the usual disease outcome?**

4. **How is it diagnosed?**

Lower Alimentary Tract Infections (LATI) Case 7: Diarrhea Due to a Wheel-Shaped Virus

- The patient was a 1-year-old male, admitted to the hospital in December because of fever and dehydration.

- His parents reported that he had a one-day history of fever, diarrhea, emesis, and decreased urine output. On admission, his vital signs revealed a temperature of 39.5 °C, slight tachycardia with a pulse of 126 beats/min, and respirations of 32 breaths/min. He was very somnolent. His general physical exam was unremarkable except for hyperactive bowel sounds.

- Stool, blood, and urine samples were sent for culture. A stool sample was also checked for O&P (ova and parasites). There were no fecal leukocytes.

- The patient was given intravenous saline and had nothing by mouth. Over the next 48 hours his symptoms abated. Once he was rehydrated and was tolerating oral feedings, he was discharged home. All routine cultures gave negative results, but a rapid viral diagnostic test was positive.

1. **What is the differential diagnosis?**
2. **What is the most common agent of pediatric gastroenteritis?**
3. **What rapid diagnostic test was used for diagnosis?**
4. **Which treatment is effective?**
5. **What special infection control procedures are necessary in the hospital setting when caring for a patient with gastroenteritis?**

Lower Respiratory Tract Infection (LRTI) Case 1: A Child with Difficulty Breathing

- A 2-year-old child is brought to the emergency ward in January because of escalating breathing problems that began with a "cold."

- In the emergency department, a blood oxygen level is done, and it is found that the oxygen saturation is 85%.

- The child is admitted to the pediatric department, and laboratory tests are done.

1. **What would the first test to be done likely be?**

2. **What should be done to protect the other children in the ward if the DFA (Direct Fluorescent Antibody) is positive?**

3. **What are risk factors for acquiring this infection?**

4. **Should antibiotics be administered to this child?**

5. **Would antivirals be administered to this child?**

6. **Is there a vaccine for this infectious agent?**

Lower Respiratory Tract Infection (LRTI) Case 2: Are Grandchildren Dangerous?

- A 64-year-old grandfather of 10 grandchildren, aged 3 months to 10 years, was admitted to the hospital with a severe pneumonia on January 8.

- He had a preexisting heart problem and had already had three major heart attacks.

- Diagnostic tests were taken to determine the cause of his pneumonia.

- It was established early that the patient did not have a bacterial pneumonia because the CRP was normal and the white cell count was only slightly elevated with no increase in neutrophils.

- One of the residents had recently done a rotation in pediatrics, where an epidemic of RSV has just occurred. He decided to take a nasal aspiration and ordered a DFA RSV. The lab report was positive.

1. **What was the likely source of his infection?**

2. **What is the usual age group of patients who get symptomatic disease with this organism?**

3. **How is it spread?**

4. **How does the CRP reflect bacterial/viral diseases?**

5. **What does the white blood cell count tell us about infections?**

6. **What is the predominant type of leukocyte that increases in numbers during a bacterial infection? A viral infection? Are there any characteristic features of the cells?**

Lower Respiratory Tract Infection (LRTI) Case 3: The Spelunker

- A 14-year-old boy was hospitalized with suspected pneumonia. A chest X ray was done, and nothing remarkable was seen. His white blood count was normal, his CRP was only slightly high, and he had a fever of 40 °C.

- He was generally in very bad shape, had lost 30 lbs in the past two months, and had night sweats and fatigue. In addition, he had blood in his urine.

- He became worse while the testing was being done and was treated with azithromycin on the suspicion of *Mycoplasma pneumoniae*.

- Subsequent tests were negative for this bacterium, and the antibiotic was stopped after two days. TB was suspected and a new chest X ray was ordered, which showed a suspicious lesion looking like a granuloma. However, TB tests were negative as well.

- A travel history was done, and it was found that he had travelled extensively in the United States during the past four months, including Arizona and Nevada. While in Arizona, he visited caves.

1. **Is the travel history important for determining the cause of the infection?**

2. **What is a possible cause of this infection?**

3. **Would this infection be treated, and with what?**

4. **Is this organism found in Canada?**

Lower Respiratory Tract Infection (LRTI) Case 4: Old Man's Friend

- A 92-year-old previously healthy male was struck with the sudden onset of tightness in the chest, which rapidly progressed to the point where he had difficulty breathing.

- He had no upper respiratory tract symptoms and no fever initially.

- Within 3 hours of onset, he had a fever of 39.5 °C and felt very ill.

- He was transported to the emergency ward at the local hospital.

1. What tests were likely done at the emergency ward?

2. What was the likely causative organism?

3. Within 4 hours of being admitted to the hospital, the patient started to develop sputum and a cough. A sample was taken, and Gram-positive diplococci with many neutrophils were seen in the Gram's stain. What is the main virulence factor associated with this bacterium?

4. This patient had pneumonia, which had disseminated, causing bacteremia. What antibiotics would likely have been used to treat his condition?

5. Could this have been prevented? Is there a vaccine?

Lower Respiratory Tract Infection (LRTI) Case 5: Should Have Given Him a Dog, Not a Bird

- Gus, an 11-year-old boy, had nagged his parents for the better part of a year about getting a dog.

- His parents both worked and didn't think that it was appropriate to buy a dog at the present time; however, they promised that he could have a pet bird. The whole family went to the pet store to check out the birds available and bought a parrot, which they took home that day.

- Four days after bringing the bird home, Gus became very ill with the following symptoms: chills, fever (temp 41 °C), malaise, headache, anorexia, sore throat, and photophobia.

- One day later he developed a cough and mental confusion, and his 8-year-old twin sisters both developed fevers.

- His parents became alarmed and took all three children to the hospital. On admission, chest X rays and blood tests (including a blood culture) were done.

- Two days later it was found that four children in his school class sitting close to his desk fell ill with the same symptoms.

1. **What is the probable diagnosis?**

2. **Considering the history given, what could the causative organism be?**

3. **What is the source of this infectious agent, and how can it be diagnosed?**

4. **What would the results from the blood culture be?**

5. **The bird was totally healthy—could it have been the reservoir of infection?**

6. **Will penicillin effectively treat this infection?**

7. **What antibiotics could be used to treat this infection?**

8. **Could the twin sisters and the four children have been infected by direct transmission from the index case?**

9. **What other steps should be taken in this case to ensure that no one else becomes ill?**

Lower Respiratory Tract Infection (LRTI) Case 6: A Virus and a Bacteria?

- A 34-year-old man was healthy prior three days to admission when he had onset of fever, weakness, fatigue, headache, sore throat, and a cough productive of white sputum.

- He developed shortness of breath and was admitted after a chest X ray showed bilateral lung infiltrates consistent of pneumonia. A blood gas analysis was done, and he had hypoxia: the pO_2 was 48 mm Hg as compared with the normal of >93 mm Hg.

- His shortness of breath increased rapidly, and he became cyanotic and febrile (39.7 °C) with a respiratory rate of 44 breaths/min and labored respiration. His sputum became bloody with clumps of tissue. Gram's staining of sputum showed clumps of inflammatory cells and clusters of Gram-positive cocci.

- Despite appropriate antibiotic therapy and intensive care, he died. This occurred in the month of January.

1. The sputum Gram's stain was most consistent with which pathogen?

2. In addition to the bacterial infection, his symptoms were otherwise diffuse and suggest a viral infection. Which viral illness is most likely?

3. How is the presence of these two processes related?

4. Which other bacterial causes of pneumonia can complicate viral pneumonia?

Lower Respiratory Tract Infection (LTRI) Case 7: More Than Spots

- A 9-year-old girl was taken to her pediatrician in February because of fever and rash for two days. She also had a headache, sore throat, and mild cough. There were no gastrointestinal symptoms. No one in the household was ill, but she had a classmate with a similar illness.

- On examination she was alert and in mild distress. Her temperature was 38.3 °C, pulse rate was 110 beats/min, blood pressure was 90/60 mm Hg, and her respiratory rate was 40 breaths/min.

- She had a mild conjunctivitis. Her posterior pharynx was injected, and petechiae were present on her soft palate. The buccal mucosa had scattered raised papular lesions. She had a macular rash on her trunk, face, and arms.

- Her chest X ray was normal. A throat swab was sent for bacterial culture, and blood was drawn for viral serology.

- It was later found that the throat culture was negative for Group A streptococci. Acute and convalescent serum specimens revealed the diagnosis, and the school nurse was notified.

1. **What is the differential diagnosis in an individual who presents with the symptoms cited in this case, with specific emphasis on the skin rash? What is the agent of the patient's infection?**

2. **How is the diagnosis of this infection usually made?**

3. **Describe the clinical course of infection and the major complications.**

4. **How can infection with this virus be prevented? Why has there been a recent resurgence in cases?**

5. **How should her case be treated? Are there any specific treatments available?**

Lower Respiratory Tract Infection (LRTI) Case 8: Is That a Seal or a Child?

- The patient was a 1-year-old boy who was brought to the clinic in January because he developed fever, chest congestion, rhinorrhea, and a "barking" cough three days previously. His appetite was fair. There was no sputum production, nausea, or vomiting.

- His medical history was significant only for recurrent otitis media. On examination, his temperature was 38.4 °C. He was in no acute distress and had audible obstructive upper airway sounds. His throat was erythematous. The clinical impression was that he had croup.

- Specimens were sent for viral cultures. He was managed with therapies for symptomatic relief including the use of a humidifier in the home. Ten days later a virus was identified from a nasopharyngeal specimen.

1. **What are the various etiologies that can cause this clinical picture?**
2. **What is the epidemiology of this virus?**
3. **What is the spectrum of clinical illness that can result?**
4. **Will this child be immune to future infections with this virus?**
5. **What therapy is indicated?**

ObGyn and STI Case 1: Nongonococcal Urethritis

- A 20-year-old, second-year male student had a painful urethral discharge and was seen by Student Health. A smear of the discharge showed typical Gram-negative intracellular diplococci, and a culture was taken.

- He was given ampicillin in a dose sufficient to eradicate most penicillin-sensitive gonococci. The discharge diminished and became less purulent, but a week later it was still present, and he still had pain on urination. The initial culture was positive for penicillin-sensitive gonococci, but the subsequent culture was negative both in smear and culture.

1. **Was this a "treatment failure"?**

2. **What is a possible organism causing this persistent trouble?**

3. **Why was the initial treatment inappropriate?**

4. **Why did the ampicillin treatment not eradicate the *C. trachomatis*?**

5. **When it was seen that there were Gram-negative diplococci in pus cells on the direct smear, why did they bother with a culture?**

6. **What should the health service do to follow up this case?**

ObGyn and STD Case 2: B Is Bad for Babies

* A healthy 7 lbs, 4 oz baby boy was born to a 24-year-old mother.

* Within 8 hours, the baby's condition had changed dramatically: it was listless and irritable and cried weakly.

* Two hours later the baby started turning blue, and blood gases were done to check the oxygen saturation. It was found that the oxygen levels were extremely low, and the baby was put on oxygen.

* Blood cultures were drawn and sent to the lab, and antibiotics were started because of the suspicion of sepsis, despite the fact that the baby did not have a high fever.

1. **What was the reason for the baby's condition?**

2. **The clinical history of the mother is examined closely. She had been living in a northern community far from medical services and had not gone in for the normal prenatal routine checkups. No test had been done for GBS toward the end of her pregnancy. If she had been found to be positive, would she have been treated, and what type of antibiotic administered?**

3. **Could the baby have died from this infection?**

4. **Is the mother usually ill at the same time as the baby?**

5. **What type of culture(s) would have been taken from the mother?**

6. **What type of antibiotic treatment would the baby have been given?**

7. **Why the combination?**

8. **If the baby was treated with an aminoglycoside, what precautions should be taken to ensure the dosage is correct?**

ObGyn and STI Case 3: What Is That Crawling?

An 18-year-old girl visited her GP because of complaints of extreme itching in the groin area. She was sexually active and had recently taken up with a new boyfriend.

1. What is the first thing the doctor would probably do?

2. If either "crabs" or eggs are found, what would the likely course of action be here in terms of treatment?

3. Are the lice likely to spread a sexually transmitted disease?

4. When the girl tells her new boyfriend about this in order to get him to treat himself as well, she notices that his eyelids are reddish and swollen, then thinks that she sees some movement. What could this be?

ObGyn and STI Case 4: Infertile? Why?

- A couple makes an appointment at the gynecologist because they have trouble conceiving; nothing has happened for more than two years of trying.

- They are in their early thirties and have established jobs and a house, and they have attained a standard of life that they think is adequate for starting a family.

- Both partners have been sexually active for 15 years but have been together only 5 years.

- The gynecologist is a specialist in infertility and begins an investigation of their problem.

1. What is the gynecologist likely to do first?

2. The numbers and viability of the sperm (including motility) seems to be normal. What would the next step likely be?

3. On laparoscopy, it is found that the fallopian tubes are scarred and that there are abundant lesions in both fallopian tubes creating a blockage. What could be the cause of this type of scarring?

4. Can the tubes be cleared and the blockage removed to restore normal transport of egg from ovary to and through the fallopian tubes?

5. Will a cervical culture for *Chlamydia* likely be positive in this woman at this time? What about a biopsy from the fallopian tubes? What about antibiotic treatment?

6. What could be another consequence of scarring and blockage in the fallopian tubes?

7. Can other organisms cause this scenario?

8. What could be another consequence of scarring and blockage in the fallopian tubes?

9. Can other organisms cause this scenario?

ObGyn and STI Case 5 TSS: What's That?

- A 16-year-old female was well until two days prior to presenting to the ER, when she had a fever of 39.9 °C and vomiting.

- On the morning of admission, she had loose stools, continued fever, and vomiting. She was seen by a GP, who noted that she was hypotensive (bp 76/48 mm Hg) with a heart rate of 120 beats/min and a temperature of 38 °C. She had an erythematous rash.

- Blood, throat, and vaginal specimens were sent for culture; the patient was given intravenous fluids and intravenous antibiotics.

- Lab results showed abnormal liver function and abnormal renal function in addition to a WBC of 14,000/mm^3 (normal 5,000–10,000) with 78% neutrophils and 18% band forms. The patient began her menstrual period four days prior to admission and uses tampons.

1. The patient's symptoms are most representative of which syndrome?

2. The vaginal culture was positive for a heavy growth of catalase-positive, Gram-positive cocci. Which organism would you expect this to be?

3. Which virulence factor does this organism produce that is believed to be responsible for the signs and symptoms seen in this patient?

4. What is the significance of the tampon use in this patient?

5. Is TSS as a syndrome restricted to tampon-bearing women?

ObGyn and STI Case 6: B19–Is That a Vitamin?

- The patient was a 19-year-old pregnant female who presented at 22 weeks of gestation with signs and symptoms of preeclampsia.

- An ultrasonogram revealed intrauterine fetal demise. Hydrops (abnormal accumulation of fluid in tissues) was present.

- Induced labor and delivery were performed, and a stillborn female fetus was delivered. An autopsy was performed on the fetus, and severe autolysis was evident. This is consistent with intrauterine fetal death.

- On histopathological exam of the fetal tissues, characteristic intra-nuclear viral inclusions were seen in erythroid precursor cells in the bone marrow and liver. Serological evidence of acute infection due to maternal exposure to a virus supported the diagnosis.

1. **What is a possible viral etiology in this case?**
2. **Name three modes of transmission of this virus.**
3. **What laboratory test would be used to ascertain infection?**
4. **What other clinical syndromes does parvovirus B19 cause?**
5. **What other viruses can be congenitally acquired?**

ObGyn and STI Case 7: Herpes, a Friend for Life

- The patient was a 20-year-old previously healthy female who presented to the emergency ward with a four-day history of fever, chills, and myalgia. Two days prior to this, she had noticed painful genital lesions.

- On the day of admission she developed headache, photophobia, and a stiff neck. She admitted to being sexually active but had no history of sexually transmitted infections.

- A pelvic examination revealed extensive vesicular and ulcerative lesions on the left labia minora and majora with marked edema. Specimens were taken for culture of *N. gonorrhoeae*, *C. trachomatis*, and viruses.

- CSF was taken and showed a leukocyte count of $41/mm^3$ with 21% PMN and 79% mononuclear cells. The CSF was sent for bacterial and viral culture.

- By the time the results came back from the lab, she was improving and was released home with oral medication.

1. What organisms can cause ulcerative genital lesions?
2. What complication of her underlying illness developed?
3. What specific treatment did she get?
4. Is she at risk for recurrences?

Skin Case 1: The Wrestlers at Camp

- A wrestling camp was held July 1 through July 28 and attended by 175 male high school wrestlers from throughout Canada.

- On July 19, seven wrestlers developed painful vesicles on various parts of their bodies, including head and neck, extremities, trunk, and eye.

- Bacterial and fungal cultures taken were negative.

- A questionnaire was administered to wrestlers by telephone following the conclusion of the camp:

Results:

61 of 175 were found to have had cutaneous vesicles.

- All wrestlers had onset during the camp session or within one week after leaving camp.

- Those who reported wrestling with a participant with vesicles were more likely to have the infection themselves.

- 38 wrestlers reported past history with cold sores.

- The attack rate was 24% for wrestlers with a past history of cold sores and 38% for those with no history of cold sores.

1. **What disease(s) do you suspect?**

2. **How was this disease transmitted? Where did the organism come from?**

3. **How is this disease treated?**

4. **How do the drugs used for treatment inhibit the replication of the organism?**

5. **What is a possible explanation for the lower attack rate for wrestlers with past history of cold sores?**

6. **How can such outbreaks be prevented?**

Skin Case 2: The Terrible Burn

- A 9-year-old boy suffers third-degree burns over 60% of his body before being rescued from a fire in his mother's apartment.

- Despite precautions in the hospital, his wounds become infected and produce blue–green colored pus.

1. **What is the most likely cause of this infection?**

2. **What are the main virulence factors for this organism?**

3. **Where could this organism have come from?**

4. **Why did this infection occur in the first place?**

5. **The pus seen was blue–green in color rather than the normal green–gray of pus. Why? How would this patient likely be treated?**

Skin Case 3: Nasty Crusty sores

* A 4-year-old child attending day care develops lesions on his face, which spread to his extremities and torso. The lesions are very thin walled and yellow, and they break open easily, then crust over.

* His mother is upset and calls the day care center to ask if any of the other children have the same rash. She is told that two children did not come to day care that day because of a rash and that the personnel had already taken 10 calls from other concerned parents about the same type of rash. The first case had occurred three days ago, and the parents of that child had taken him to a MediCenter, where they had done bacterial and viral cultures.

The lab findings were negative for viruses but showed moderate growth of

Staphylococcus aureus

Staphylococcus epidermidis

Streptococcus pyogenes, group A

Streptococcus mitis

Propionibacterium sp.

Corynebacterium sp.

and sparse growth of *E. coli*

1. **How should the laboratory report be interpreted? What is important?**
2. **What is the Gram morphology of these suspected organisms?**
3. **How is this disease transmitted? Is the child infectious?**
4. **What is this disease called?**
5. **How should it be treated?**

Skin Case 4: Can't Be Too Careful!

- A 64-year-old farmer presented at a GP's office just before closing time after cutting the top of his thumb off with an axe. He had recently been treated for pharyngitis but had recovered fully.

- The artery in his thumb was severed; the thumb was pumping blood. After six stitches and a pressure dressing, he went home to bed.

- Six hours later he woke up and had a severe throbbing in his finger, with pain radiating up his arm. He turned the light on and saw bright red streaks originating from the bandage up the inside of his arm.

- Because it was 3 a.m., he took three extra-strength Tylenol plus a sleeping pill. He is successful at falling asleep but awoke in the morning with a high fever, delirium, and a very swollen arm that was turning bluish.

- His wife called an ambulance. At the ER, a blood culture was taken, and he was given a broad spectrum antibiotic IV. Within 30 minutes of arrival at the hospital, it is obvious amputation had to be done.

1. **What most likely grew in his blood culture?**

2. **Why did the patient get red streaks up his arm? What is this called?**

3. **What would have happened if the surgeons had not amputated his arm?**

4. **Couldn't intravenous antibiotics have saved the man's arm?**

5. **How could this have been prevented?**

6. **How did the microorganism get into the wound?**

Upper Respiratory Tract Infection (URTI) Case 1: Coughing, Sniffling, and Sneezing

* Ernie is in fourth grade and in good health. His classmates are all sniffling and sneezing, and it is obvious that there is an infection going around in the class.

* That evening, Ernie's eyes are "scratchy," and he feels a sore throat coming on. Mom gives him a Tylenol and sends him to bed

* The next morning, Ernie has a full-blown cold and stays home from school.

1. **People often bring up the "cure for the common cold" as a noble idea for basic research. Why is there no one cure or vaccine for the common cold, and why do we keep on getting sick?**

2. **What would be the basis of a "cure"?**

3. **What is the usual cause of the common cold? Name a few other viruses that can cause the same symptoms.**

4. **Why doesn't the usual cause of the common cold cause pneumonia?**

5. **What complications could arise from this infection?**

Upper Respiratory Tract Infection (URTI) Case 2: Ear Infection

- An 8-month-old boy becomes increasingly restless and irritable over a 24-hour period.

- He cries and cannot be consoled; he also tugs at his left ear.

- He develops a fever, and his parents become distraught and call a pediatrician.

1. **What organism(s) might be the cause of these symptoms, and how does it cause these symptoms?**

2. **What unusual feature might you see if you used an otoscope to look in the ear, and what is the reason for this?**

3. **How might the child be treated?**

4. **What difficulty might there be with using penicillin as a treatment?**

5. **What consequences may arise from this type of infection?**

Upper Respiratory Tract Infection (URTI) Case 3: A Bad Sore Throat

- A 21-year-old male appears at a MediCenter complaining of a "strep" throat and demanding antibiotics.

- He has had a very sore throat for three days and cannot eat or drink because he is so swollen and in pain.

1. **Should the doctor believe the man, and what should the doctor do?**

2. **What is the cause of "strep" throat?**

3. **Is antibiotic therapy always indicated for strep throat?**

4. **Why don't we have a vaccine for this common and potentially dangerous bacterium?**

5. **What would be the best choice of antibiotic for this infection?**

6. **What complications could arise from this infection?**

Upper Respiratory Tract Infection (URTI) Case 4: Diphtheria: Isn't That Eradicated?

- Lila and her husband live in a sparsely populated area in the far north of Canada where there is limited access to health care.

- They have always relied on the local "medicine woman" for help.

- Their daughter, Minnie, a 5-year-old girl, is noticed to have difficulty breathing.

- They worry because she is so ill and the medicine woman has not been able to help her, so they call the health clinic 400 km away and consult with the healthcare personnel there.

- When the nurse hears that the child has never been vaccinated for any diseases, she advises them to bring her to the clinic as soon as possible.

- Observing the back of the child's throat, the doctor notices a leathery gray–white membrane that bleeds when he tries to dislodge it.

1. **What is the likely causative organism?**

2. **Describe the process of lysogeny in bacteria.**

3. **What pathogenic process caused the formation of the leathery gray–white patch?**

4. **What should be done to treat the child and why?**

5. **What is the diphtheria toxoid often combined with in a vaccine preparation?**

Upper Respiratory Tract Infection (URTI) Case 5: Just Kissing?

- An 18-year-old female presented to the ear, nose, and throat clinic complaining of hoarseness and difficulty swallowing. She had a one-week history of fever, sore throat, fatigue, and muscle aches.

- She had enlarged tonsils and swollen cervical lymph glands in addition to splenomegaly. Her WBC was 7,000/mm^3 (normal 5,000–10,000) with 40% neutrophils, 28% lymphocytes, 12% atypical lymphocytes, and 20% monocytes.

- Liver function tests were elevated. Chest X ray was negative. A throat culture was negative for beta-hemolytic streptococci. A monospot and specific viral serology were ordered.

- When the results came, she was put on steroids and kept in the hospital for another four days until the tonsillar enlargement had reduced.

1. **What was the likely etiology of her infection?**

2. **How might she have contracted this infection?**

3. **What could this virus do to an immunosuppressed patient?**

4. **What is a complication of this infection caused by an antibiotic?**

5. **Why was this patient given steroids?**

6. **What are "atypical lymphocytes," and are they specific only for EBV infection?**

Wound Case 1: From the Mouths of Cats

- Alice, a 74-year-old woman from Beaumont, was admitted to the hospital because of a fever and a preexisting heart condition. She had a large leg ulcer. Blood cultures were drawn; the ulcer was cleaned and dressed. She was given IV cephalosporin for a suspected Gram-negative sepsis. Her fever disappeared, and she was discharged to her home before the lab findings were reported (Gram-negative coccobacillus).

- One week later she was again feverish, and her son took her back to the hospital, where a repeat blood culture was done. When the blood cultures grew a Gram-negative coccobacillus, she was treated with ampicillin and sent home again.

- Alice had another relapse three weeks later with the same symptoms, and blood cultures once again showed the growth of a Gram-negative coccobacillus.

- The laboratory typed all of the blood isolates from Alice to *Pasteurella multocida.*

Because this is an uncommon cause of sepsis for a patient like Alice, a nurse was sent home to investigate the home environment. It was found that Alice had three cats. Every time she removed the dressing from her leg ulcer, one of the cats would lick the wound, thereby inoculating it with more *P. multocida,* a common inhabitant of cat and dog mouths.

1. **What is the treatment of choice?**
2. **What is the usual mode of transmission for this agent?**
3. **Should all patients with animal bites receive prophylactic ampicillin?**

Wound Case 2: Gangrene

- The patient was an 85-year-old female with an advanced squamous cell carcinoma of the bladder who was admitted for treatment of a presumed cellulitis of her right lower leg.

- The patient appeared chronically ill. The right heel had a bluish hematoma and blister with 6 by 6 cm of reddened tissue.

- Lab studies on admission showed an elevated WBC of $43,200/mm^3$ with a left shift. She was treated with intravenous antibiotics for two days, but her condition did not improve. She underwent an X ray of the right ankle and foot, which demonstrated extensive gas in the soft tissues.

- She was surgically debrided and eventually had a below-the-knee amputation. A Gram's stain of the wound aspirate showed a few polymorphonuclear leukocytes and many boxcar-shaped, Gram-positive rods. No growth was seen on aerobic cultures.

- The patient's condition worsened, and she died.

1. **Which genus of bacteria can cause the type of infection described in this case?**

2. **What is the explanation for the finding of gas in the tissues?**

3. **Which virulence factors are produced by *Clostridia*?**

4. **What are characteristics typical of gas gangrene?**

5. **Why was it necessary to amputate her leg?**

6. **In what way could this woman have become infected?**

Wound Case 3: An Unfortunate Tub Experience

- A 42-year-old man with advanced MS is paralyzed and institutionalized. He is receiving physiotherapy involving bathing in warm water to improve the circulation in his legs. Because he is totally incontinent, he is not allowed in the larger pool with the other patients and instead has his own tub of water.

- The baths last for 45 minutes every day. He is returned to his room and put to bed. There is a shortage of nursing staff, and he is not turned as often as he should be to prevent formation of bedsores.

- As a result, he develops a bedsore on his left hip, which proves very difficult to treat.

- A bacterial culture is finally taken of his sore because it will not heal and smells terrible. The lab report reads:

Heavy growth of :	Moderate growth of:
Escherichia. coli	Streptococcus Group G
Klebsiella oxytoca	Bacteroides fragilis
Enterobacter cloacae	Prevotella melaninogenicus
Proteus mirabilis	Enterococcus faecalis
Pseudomonas aeruginosa	

1. **Is this a normal pressure sore?**
2. **What do the findings of the laboratory report indicate?**
3. **The attending resident gets upset when he sees the report and, because there are so many bacteria, doesn't know if he should start treating the patient or which antibiotic to use if he does treat. What should he do at this point?**
4. **Despite the nursing shortage, the resident finds that the hygienic care of the patient while on the ward is excellent and that he never has been left lying in fecal material. What would his next logical step be?**
5. **How do you think the sore was infected with a mixture of bacteria reminiscent of fecal flora?**
6. **How should the infected pressure sore be treated?**
7. **How could this have been avoided?**

Wound Case 4: What's That in Your Face?

- Ruth, 36 years old, lives at home with her mother in a small town in the prairies. Ruth is shy and unemployed and has no friends. She leaves the house only to go to the grocery store and buy baking supplies because she and her mother earn some income baking pastries and breads for the local bakery.

- Ruth begins to have problems with the skin on her face, developing large boil-like abscesses on her cheeks and neck. Her mother forces her to go to the doctor, a newly arrived bachelor in town. The doctor cannot find any apparent signs of disease except for the welts. He prescribes oxacillin and tells her to come back in two weeks.

- Ruth goes back in two weeks, and the doctor is surprised that the welts are now worse. Perplexed, he tries treating with cortisone. This also makes the lesions worse.

- While treating Ruth, the doctor notices that she is very attentive to him and unsettlingly difficult to get rid of. She has other abnormal personality traits, such as never making eye contact, so he decides to visit the home and speak with the mother. A pattern of antisocial behavior was established, but the mother could not shed any light on the cause. It becomes more and more evident that Ruth has a crush on the doctor, and he comes to believe that she is inflicting the wounds on herself.

- When he finally asks her, she admits that she has been injecting baker's yeast (*Saccharomyces* sp.) into her skin to get his attention. She was sent to a local psychiatric clinic and treated for her problems. The skin lesions disappeared, and Ruth was able to leave home and move into her own apartment.

1. **What causative organism did the doctor first suspect when he prescribed oxacillin?**
2. **Why did the antibiotic and the cortisone exacerbate the condition?**
3. **Is baker's yeast usually pathogenic?**
4. **What risks could Ruth run by injecting herself with an infectious agent?**

Wound Case 5: Complications of Health Care

- This 71-year-old woman was admitted with a recurrence of her poorly differentiated squamous cell carcinoma of the cervix. She underwent extensive gynecological surgery (excision of the organs of the anterior pelvis) and was maintained postoperatively on broad-spectrum intravenous antibiotics. The patient had a central venous catheter placed on the day of the surgery.

- Beginning three days postop, the patient had temperatures of 38.0 °C to 38.5 °C, which persisted without a clear source. On day eight postop, she had a temperature of 39.2 °C.

- Cultures of blood and of the tip of the central line both grew an agent that was ovoid and reproduced by budding.

1. What is the likely identity of this woman's infecting organism?

2. Is the organism part of the normal flora of humans?

3. How did treatment with broad-spectrum antibiotics predispose this patient to infection with this organism?

4. The same organism was present in a positive culture of blood and in a culture of the central venous catheter tip. What does this suggest in terms of the portal of entry of the organism causing the infection?

5. How likely is antifungal treatment to eradicate the infection? What should be done to do this?